Encyclopedia of Electromyography: Advanced Researches

Volume II

Encyclopedia of Electromyography: Advanced Researches

Volume II

Edited by **Michael Backman**

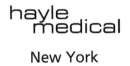

hayle
medical

New York

Published by Hayle Medical,
30 West, 37th Street, Suite 612,
New York, NY 10018, USA
www.haylemedical.com

Encyclopedia of Electromyography: Advanced Researches
Volume II
Edited by Michael Backman

International Standard Book Number: 978-1-63241-160-0 (Hardback)

Contents

Preface

This book on Electromyography (EMG) encompasses a broad range of subjects including Evoked Potentials, EMG in combination with other technologies and New Frontiers in Research and Technology. The authors have varied in their approach to their subjects, from reviews on different aspects of the field to experimental studies with exciting new findings. The experts have analyzed literature related to applied surface electromyography parameters for evaluating muscle function and fatigue to the constraints of different analysis and processing techniques. It also describes emerging applications where electromyography is employed as a means to regulate electromechanical systems, water surface electromyography, scanning electromyography, EMG measures in orthodontic appliances and in ophthalmological field. These original approaches to the usage of EMG measurement and new researches in the field will be of great interest to readers.

After months of intensive research and writing, this book is the end result of all who devoted their time and efforts in the initiation and progress of this book. It will surely be a source of reference in enhancing the required knowledge of the new developments in the area. During the course of developing this book, certain measures such as accuracy, authenticity and research focused analytical studies were given preference in order to produce a comprehensive book in the area of study.

This book would not have been possible without the efforts of the authors and the publisher. I extend my sincere thanks to them. Secondly, I express my gratitude to my family and well-wishers. And most importantly, I thank my students for constantly expressing their willingness and curiosity in enhancing their knowledge in the field, which encourages me to take up further research projects for the advancement of the area.

Editor

Part 1

Evoked Potential

Visual and Brainstem Auditory Evoked Potentials in Neurology

Ashraf Zaher

Department of Neurology, Faculty of Medicine, University of Mansoura, Mansoura, Egypt

1. Introduction

Historically, Richard Caton (1875) discovered evoked potentials and the electroencephalogram (EEG) at the same time. The evoked potentials provided a useful tool for neurophysiological research (Shagass, 1976).

Evoked potentials are the voltage changes generated in the brain, the sense organ and the pathway leading to the brain in response to an external stimulus. This stimulus has to be somewhat above its subjective detection threshold so as to be clearly discernible, as well as to be of abrupt onset and /or offset so, that discrete volley is set up in the afferent pathway, hence capable of eliciting distinct cortical potential changes (Kriss, 1980).

Chiappa et al., 1987 defined an evoked potential as the record of the electrical activity produced by groups of neurons within the spinal cord, brain stem, thalamus or cerebral hemispheres following stimulation of one or another specific system by means of visual, auditory, or somatosensory input.

EEG recording may be obtained in a relatively direct manner by amplifying and displaying the activity picked up by electrodes placed on the scalp (Shagass, 1976), but most evoked potential (EP) activity due to their low amplitude, 0.1-20 microvolts relative to the normal background activity of EEG, their activity can not be clearly displayed, however with the development of micro-computers in the seventies (special signal averaging process) helping the extraction of the evoked potential from the EEG activity which is of much greater amplitude leading to their widespread clinical use (Kimura, 1985).

2. Visual evoked potentials (VEPs)

2.1 Introduction

The visual evoked potentials (VEPs) result from change of brain activity following application of intermittent visual stimulus to the visual system. They provide a quantitative measure of the functional integrity of the visual pathways (Celesia, 1988). The function measured includes that of the optic nerve, through the optic chiasma and tract, to the lateral geniculate bodies and the geniculocalcarine projection to the visual cortex "area 17" (Yiannikas and Walsh, 1983).

Since the VEP measures the pathway from the retina to area 17, a normal P100 does not exclude lesions of the visual pathway beyond area 17. For this reason, the VEP may be normal in patients with the diagnosis of cortical blindness. The usefulness of VEP is limited in malingering and hysterical visual loss (Bodis-Wollner et al., 1977). It is useful when a normal VEP is recorded, but abnormal responses are of limited diagnostic value in such cases.

The most important fact to consider is that, although the axons from the nasal half of the retina decussate at the optic chiasm, the temporal axons do not. Therefore, retrochiasmatic lesions may not be detected by full-field checkerboard stimulation. VEPs are most useful in testing optic nerve function and less useful in postchiasmatic disorders. In retrochiasmatic lesions, the MRI is a more useful test. Partial-field studies may be useful in retrochiasmatic lesions; however, they are not performed routinely in clinical settings (Chiappa, 1990).

Recordings of this evoked potential are recognized as a reliable diagnostic procedure in the investigation of lesions of the anterior visual pathway (Halliday et al., 1976). However, it is not specific with regard to etiology. A tumor compressing the optic nerve, an ischemic disturbance, or a demyelinating disease may cause delay in the P100; only additional clinical history and, often, MRI are needed to uncover the etiology (Leslie et al., 2002).

2.2 Normal components of pattern reversal visual evoked potential (PRVEP) (Figure 1)

The cerebral pattern reversal evoked potential to full field stimulation consists of three peaks in normal subjects. The peak polarities are negative, positive and negative (NPN) and the mean peak latencies are 70, 100 and 145 milliseconds (msec) respectively. The first negative wave (N1 or N70) may be difficult to identify in some normal subjects and many patients likewise, the second negative peak (N2 or N145) is too inconsistent in latency and amplitude to be of clinical value. Thus, waveform identification in the pattern shift visual evoked potential consists of the large positive peak (P1 or P100). Depending on the stimulating device in use, and the presence or absence of abnormalities, it may be found any where from 90 to 250 msec (chiappa, 1982).

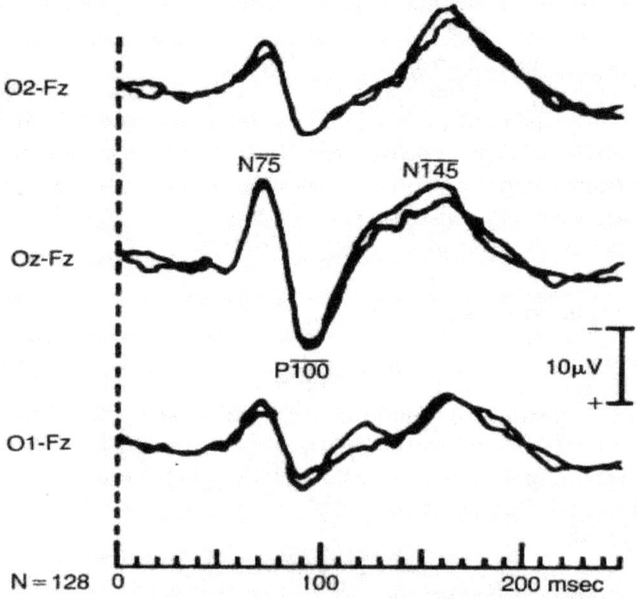

Fig. 1. Normal Visual Evoked Potential (VEP) (Poon's, 2003a).

	Latency (msec.)	R-L Difference	Amplitude (µV)	R-L Difference
N70	71.1 (<81.8)	9.4	3.8 (>0.1)	5.1
P100	95.8 (<112.0)	9.3	10.1 (>1.8)	7.0
Steady state P1	95.5 (<118.1)	21.0	8.3 (>6.1)	6.1

Table 1. Visual Evoked Potential Normative Data From Celesia (1985).

	Full field VEP			
	Mean	Range	SD	Mean + 3 SD
P100 latency	102.3 msec.	89-114	5.1	117.6
L-R difference	1.3 msec.	0-6	2.0	7.3
P100 amplitude	10.1 uV	3-21	4.2	22.7
P100 amp. Diff.	1.6 uV	0-5.5	1.4	5.8

Table 2. Visual Evoked Potential Normative Data From Chiappa (1990).

Check size	VEP Check Size Effects						
	Latency (msec.)				Amplitude (uV)		
	Latency Mean (SD) (Range)	Latency ULN	L-R Diff Mean (SD) (Range)	L-R Diff ULN	Amplitude Mean (SD) (Range)	L-R Diff Mean (SD) (Range)	L-R Diff ULN
17"	106.8 (6.4) (96.7-128.8)	126.0	2.73 (2.32) (0-8.80)	9.7	8.34 (3.71) (1.6-18.7)	1.48 (1.19) (0.2-5.2)	5.1
35"	102.9 (7.4) (88.6-121.4)	125.1	2.53 (2.91) (0-13.4)	11.3	7.13 (3.68) (1.0-19.8)	1.69 (2.00) (0-8.6)	7.7
70"	103.8 (6.9) (88.2-122.5)	124.5	2.18 (2.59) (0-12.7)	10.0	7.95 (3.64) (1.8-19.8)	1.29 (1.16) (0-4.8)	4.8
144"	107.3 (8.8) (91.1-130.6)	133.7	2.44 (2.55) (0-12)	10.1	7.72 (2.95) (1.5-16.1)	1.36 (1.22) (0-5.4)	5.0
288"	113.5 (11.8) (91.4 -142)	148.9	3.95 (4.03) (0 -15.2)	16.0	7.31 (2.74) (2.6 -14)	1.10 (1.05) (0 -3.9)	4.3

ULN = Upper Limit of Normal (Mean + 3 SD) (Chiappa, 1990).

Table 3. Check size 25.8" (Chiappa, 1990).

P100 is usually seen in all normal subjects and has a variability small enough to make it reliable in clinical practice, in addition to measuring the absolute latency of P100, determining the inter-ocular latency difference, amplitude, inter-ocular amplitude difference ratio and duration of P100 has increased the diagnostic yield of the test (chiappa, 1983).

The "W" morphology is most often an individual variation, although decreasing the stimulation frequency from 2 Hz to 1 Hz usually converts the W shape into a conventional P100 peak. Check size and alternation rate are factors in this; the responses can be manipulated to a "W" or a conventional P100 response by changing these parameters. Large checks tend to produce VEPs similar to those produced by flash stimulation (Leslie et al., 2002).

Blumhardt and Halliday, (1979) noted that the ipsilateral hemisphere evoked potential was actually a series of waves with negative components preceding and following P100 wave at latencies of approximately 75, 145 msec respectively. The contralateral hemisphere response consists of a triphasic complex occurring synchronously but of opposite polarity with a major negativity at about 100 msec and smaller positive deflections at 75 and 145 msec. Maximum value for P100 is 115 msec in patients younger than 60 years; it rises to 120 msec thereafter in females and 125 msec in males. Even though published norms are available in the medical literature, each individual laboratory should have its own norms to control for lab-to-lab variability in technique (Leslie et al., 2002).

2.3 Generator source of pattern reversal visual evoked potential (PRVEP)

In relation to the generator sources of PRVEP Chiappa,(1983) claimed that P100 is generated in the striate and pre-striate occipital cortex as a result of both primary activation and subsequent thalamocortical volleys. However, the exact sources of P100 are not well defined. Positron tomographic mapping of human cerebral metabolism during reversal checkerboard stimulation revealed strong activation of both primary and association visual cortical areas (Phelps et at., 1981).

Ikeda et al., 1998 studied generators of VEP by dipole tracing in the human occipital cortex. Current source generators (dipoles) of human VEP to pattern-onset stimuli were investigated. A visual stimulus, a checkerboard pattern, was presented for 250 ms in each of the 8 quadrants. Central and peripheral parts of each of the 4 quadrant fields were evaluated. The results from these analyses of VEP indicated topographic localization of the dipoles around the calcarine fissure.

2.4 Principles of recording of VEP
2.4.1 Technical details (Leslie et al., 2002)

Dark room; Patient seated 70-100 cm from the screen; Corrective lenses used if necessary (acuity check prior to commencement of VEP); Pupil size and any abnormality should be noted(The pupils should not be dilated by mydriatics to prevent interference with accommodation); Sedation should not be used, and note should be taken of medications that the patient is taking regularly; Checkerboard pattern is used as stimulation; Check size of approximately 30 seconds of visual angle; Contrast between 50-80 percent; Stimulus rates of 1-2 Hz are recommended (producing a reversal every 500 msec); Filter setting should be 1 to 200 Hz bandwidth (outside limit is 0.2-300 Hz); The recommended recording time window (i.e. sweep length) is 250 ms; 50-200 responses are to be averaged; A minimum of 2 trials should be given.

2.4.2 Stimulation procedures

There are two general types of visual stimuli that are most often used to elicit visual evoked potential. These are the un-patterned flashing lights and the patterned stimuli which in clinical laboratories are usually checkerboards (Sokol, 1980).

Unpatterned flashing stimuli can be produced with a photo stimulator similar to that used in EEG recordings for photic driving. The intensity, color and rate of stimulation of the flash light can be varied. But, the variability in amplitude and latency of the evoked potential is much greater than in patterned stimuli (Halliday, 1982).

Patterned stimuli can be presented in three ways. These are the flashing patterned stimulus, the pattern onset, offset and the pattern reversal. A flashing patterned stimulus is produced by placing a photo stimulator behind a large photographic transparency of black and white checks (Harter and White, 1968). In pattern onset, offset the checks appear for discrete amount of time (500 msec) and then disappear. While, in the pattern reversal stimulation, checks are visible all the time. In order to maintain a constant luminance level, one half of the checks increases in luminance, while the other half decreases. This can be accomplished electronically by using T.V. monitor to generate the checks (Arden et al., 1977b).

Checkerboard pattern reversal are the most frequently used stimuli in clinical investigations of the visual pathway as they evoke relatively large potentials (Halliday et al.,1987 and Chiappa, 1988) with variability in latency less than in flash stimuli and it is more sensitive to the presence of conduction defects in the visual pathway (Chiappa, 1982). The fovea is estimated to generate 65% of the pattern-reversal response; flash stimuli, in contrast, tend to generate response from the peripheral retina as well. The insensitivity of flash VEPs, particularly in retrochiasmatic lesions, has been based on diagnostic studies in which patient recordings must differ from normative population data by 2 standard deviations (SDs) to be considered abnormal (Berson, 1994).

Characteristics of pattern reversal stimulation

Erwin, 1980 outlined seven basic characteristics of pattern-reversal stimulation:
1-The rate of pattern-reversal is the number of times that the pattern changes within a second. The direction of pattern reversal is not considered since usually all the pattern reversal responses are averaged together. 2-The reversal time is the total time taken to change from one pattern to its opposite. 3-Stimulus luminance is an essential attribute for visual stimulus. 4-The type of the pattern is obviously important. The most commonly used stimulus is a checkerboard. 5-Vertical-horizontal orientation of the pattern evokes larger responses than oblique orientation. 6-The size of the pattern elements can be described in two ways. The visual angle subtended by each element can be measured. As well, the spatial frequency (the number of intensity cycles through light and dark per degree of visual field) can be used. Another aspect of the stimulus related to the spatial extent of the pattern elements is the spatial rate of luminance change. 7-Two of the most important aspects of the stimulus are its field size and relationship to fixation.

2.4.3 Electrode montage
Responses are collected over Oz, O1, and O2 and with hemifield studies at T5 and T6 electrodes using the standard EEG electrode placement. Scalp electrodes are positioned as follows:
a. Electrode number one: 5 cms above the inion posteriorly in the middle line (Oz).
b. Electrodes number two and three: 5 cms lateral on either side of electrode one (O1, O2).
c. Two additional electrodes: 10 cms away on each side from the middle electrode (T5, T6). Optional to be used in hemifield studies.
d. Reference electrode: is usually FZ. (e) Ground electrode: over the ear lobule (Halliday, 1982).

Both eyes are tested at first, then each eye is tested at a time, (while the other is covered with an eye patch) to avoid masking of a unilateral conduction abnormality. The subject is instructed to gaze at a dot in the center of the pattern during display. The pattern stimulator is operated at about two reversals per second. Patient having field defects or amblyopia may shift their center of gaze into the good visual field. So in order to offset this, a 1° to 2° blank strip may be inserted on either side of the fixation point during partial field stimulation (Chiappa, 1983).

2.4.4 Interpretation

Abnormalities of VEPs have been described in many disorders of the optic nerve, chiasma and retrochiasmatic visual pathways. The VEP is considered abnormal when the latency of P100 wave is outside the boundaries established for normals, or the P100 is absent. The most frequent abnormality is characterized by normal amplitude but prolonged latency of N70 and P100, but a prolonged latency may sometimes be associated with decreased amplitude. The most sever abnormality is an absent VEP (Celesia and Tobimatsu, 1990).

Monocular VEP abnormality

This abnormality suggests a conduction defect in the left/right visual pathway anterior to the optic chiasm. Although demyelinating disease is the most common aetiology for such a finding, various other possibilities cannot be excluded e.g. retinal disease and compressive lesions of the optic nerve (Poon's, 2003a).

In patients with small monocular delays in N70 and P100, it is useful to look at the intereye latency difference. A latency difference between the two eyes greater than 10 msec is clearly indicative of pathology on the side with the longer latency (Celesia and Tobimatsu, 1990).

Binocular VEP abnormality

These abnormalities suggest conduction defects in the visual pathways bilaterally. However, because of the binocular nature of the findings, the lesion location (retina, optic nerve, tracts or radiations) cannot be determined (Poon's, 2003a).

2.4.5 Pitfalls

Check size of 27 seconds of visual angle may result in normal P100 latency in a patient with cortical blindness; smaller checks (i.e. 20 seconds of visual angle or less) should be used to demonstrate the abnormality. If cortical blindness is suspected, large checks should not be used (Bodis-Wollner, 1977).

In conditions such as retinal disease or refractory errors, the amplitude may be smaller and, at very small check sizes, the latency may increase. For this reason proper refraction is of great importance (Chiappa, 1990).

2.5 Factors affecting VEP

Factors which affect VEP are either technical and / or subject factors.

2.5.1 Technical factors

2.5.1.1 Screen luminance

A decrease in brightness results in delaying P100 i.e. increase in its latency (Halliday et al., 1973). Stochard et al., 1979 showed that the pupillary diameter has an effect on retinal illumination and thus also on P100 latency.

2.5.1.2 Degree of contrast

Reduction in the degree of contrast between the black and white squares of checkerboard pattern increases P100 latency and reduces the amplitude (Mackay and Jeffreys, 1973).

2.5.1.3 Size of the stimulating pattern

A decrease of the size of the stimulating pattern (degree of visual angle) results in a reduction of the amplitude of the response (Asselman et al., 1975).

2.5.1.4 Check size

Smaller checks give the highest amplitude responses (Leserve and Romand, 1972).

2.5.1.5 Electrode placement

Ipata et al., 1997 assessed interhemispheric visual transfer of information in humans. Estimates of interhemispheric transfer time ranged between 5.77 and 12.54 msec, depending upon the type of component and the location of the electrode sites. More anterior locations yielded shorter values and overall transfer time tended to be 7 msec shorter for the N70 component than for the P100 component.

2.5.1.6 Stimulus rate

When the rate of pattern reversal is increased, changes in P100 latency is noticed. Increasing the rate beyond 8 per second transforms the evoked responses into a steady state evoked potential (a long train of repetitive wave with a sinusoidal appearance) (Stockord et al., 1979).

2.5.2 Subject factors

2.5.2.1 Age

There is an increase in the latency for subjects of ages starting from the end of the second decade onwards. This increase amounts to 2 msec per decade (Celesia and Daly, 1977). However, Stochard et al., 1979 found no change in P100 latency for subjects of age until the fifth decade. Then, the latency increases at a rate of 2 msec per decade.

2.5.2.2 Sex

Females have usually shorter P100 latency than males. This may be due to difference in the head size (Stockard et al., 1979). However, Shearer and Dustman, (1980) reported no such difference.

2.5.2.3 Visual acuity

Changes in visual acuity markedly affect P100 amplitude. In visual acuity lower than 6 / 18, no latency changes is observed but the amplitude is reduced (Fitzgerald et al., 1980). Diminution of visual acuity has a greater effect on latency using smaller checks (giving visual angle 12) than larger checks (giving visual angle 48). (Sokol et al., 1981).

2.5.2.4 Body temperature

No significant change in P100 latency results by raising body temperature in normals (Matthews et al., 1979). Also, little effect on P100 latency is noticed in patients having multiple sclerosis.

2.5.2.5 Physiological changes of serum glucose level

Sannita et al., 1995 evaluated the correlation between amplitude and latencies of the pattern-reversal VEP and serum glucose level in healthy volunteers. Pattern VEP and serum glucose levels were obtained at 2-hour intervals during an 8-hour experimental session. At serum glucose concentrations within the physiological range of variability (55-103 mg/dL), the P100 latency increased with increasing serum glucose level, with a 6.9% estimated latency difference between lower and higher glucose concentrations.

2.5.2.6 Medications

2.5.2.6.1 Carbamazepine

Certain drugs, such as carbamazepine, prolong VEPs. The effects of carbamazepine monotherapy on VEPs were studied in epileptic children by Yuksel et al., 1995. Pattern-reversal VEPs were determined before administration of the antiepileptic drugs and after 1 year of therapy. The VEP amplitude showed no consistent changes after 1 year of therapy, but VEP P100 latencies were significantly prolonged after 1 year of carbamazepine therapy. The conclusion was that carbamazepine slows down central impulse conduction.

2.5.2.6.2 Lithium

Previous reports in the literature have suggested that lithium medication does not affect the VEP to flash stimulation. It was predicted that this would not be true for pattern reversal stimulation. Seven patients had their pattern evoked potential measured using a 42' check to fractional pattern displacement of 1/4, 1/2, 3/4 and Full Square. The VEP was measured before, 1 week after and 5 weeks after the commencement of lithium medication. The results show that there is a significant increase in both the N70-P100 and P100-N145 amplitudes when the 'before lithium' sessions are compared to 'after lithium.' Seven normal subjects matched for the age and sex of the patient group were tested twice, once as a 'control' and a further 5 weeks after this. No significant differences were found in the 'control' sessions between patient and normal groups although a significant difference in both the N70-P100 and P100-N145 amplitude after the treatment of the patient group with lithium was found (Fenwick and Robertson, 1983).

2.5.2.6.3 Levodopa

Pattern visual evoked potentials (PVEPs) were recorded at three luminance levels and five different check sizes in a group of 16 control subjects before and after the oral administration of levodopa. At the lower luminance levels, significant decrease in PVEP latencies were found. For PVEPs the latency changes occurred only at small check sizes. No changes were observed in control experiments without levodopa administration. These results are in agreement with a VEP delay found in Parkinson's disease and with a VEP latency increase in rats after dopamine depletion (Gottlob et al., 1989).

2.6 Clinical applications of VEP

Clinical usefulness of VEPs includes the following

- More sensitive than MRI or physical examination in prechiasmatic lesions.
- Objective and reproducible test for optic nerve function.
- Abnormality persists over long periods of time.
- Inexpensive as compared with to MRI.
- Under certain circumstances, may be helpful to positively establish optic nerve function in patients with subjective complaint of visual loss; normal VEP excludes significant optic nerve or anterior chiasmatic lesion (Leslie et al., 2002).

With abnormal VEP, some of the differential diagnostic considerations are as follows

- Optic neuropathy.
- Optic neuritis.

- Toxic amblyopia.
- Glaucoma.
- Leber's hereditary optic neuropathy.
- Retrobulbar neuritis.
- Ischemic optic neuropathy.
- Multiple sclerosis.
- Tumors compressing the optic nerve e.g. Optic nerve gliomas, meningiomas, craniopharyngiomas, giant aneurysms and pituitary tumors (Andrew et al., 2002).

2.6.1 VEP in Optic neuritis

Prolongation of P100 latency is the most common abnormality and usually represents an optic nerve dysfunction. VEP is clearly more sensitive than physical examination in detecting optic neuritis. Elvin et al., 1998 used Doppler ultrasonography, MRI and VEP measurements to study abnormal optic nerve function. VEP assessments were performed in 16 patients. Patients with impairment of visual acuity and a prolonged VEP initially had a more swollen nerve and increased flow resistance in the affected optic nerve. Statistically significant side-to-side differences were found in the optic nerve diameter and in the resistance to flow in the central retinal artery between the affected and unaffected eyes.

2.6.2 VEP in Multiple Sclerosis

Visual evoked potentials have become widely accepted in diagnostic schemes for the assessment of multiple sclerosis. It has been shown that a deviation in latency is a better criterion than a deviation in amplitude, since amplitude varies widely among subjects, whereas evoked potential latency remains restricted rather to a narrow range (McDonald and Brans, 1992).

VEPs has the ability to reveal the presence of a clinically silent lesion in the visual pathway in a patient having signs of demyelination evident in other parts of the CNS, thus confirming the diagnosis of multiple sclerosis (Russel et al., 1991).

In multiple sclerosis, P100 absolute latency may be increased unilaterally or a significant interocular difference may occur (Cutler et al., 1985). Moreover, broad response of P100 latency and abnormal shape of NPN was found in majority of multiple sclerosis patients (Glaser, 1990).

In a review of 180 patients with multiple sclerosis 73 % had abnormal VEPs; more importantly, VEPs were abnormal in 54 % of patients without any symptoms or signs referable to the visual system. Such patients are often in the early stages of the disease, when diagnosis is difficult even with modern neuroimaging techniques (Halliday et al., 1977). MRI demonstrated high-signal lesions in 84-88 % of symptomatic patients, whereas VEPs were abnormal in 100% of cases (Kojima et al., 1990).

Brigell et al., 1994 described the pattern VEP using standardized techniques. They concluded that the peak latency of pattern-reversal VEP is a sensitive measure of conduction delay in the optic nerve caused by demyelination. Pattern-reversal VEPs were recorded from 64 healthy subjects and 15 patients with resolved optic neuritis. The results showed that the N70 and P100 peak latencies and N70-P100 interocular amplitude difference were sensitive measures of resolved optic neuritis.

2.6.3 Flash VEP in Cerebral stroke

Ipata et al., 1997 studied left-right asymmetry of flash VEPs in patients after stroke. The VEP amplitude was smaller over the ischemic hemisphere than over the intact hemisphere. This finding indicates that the left-right asymmetry in VEPs of patients after brain damage may be a result of changes in the conductivity of the volume conductor, due to the ischemic region between the source and the electrodes.

2.6.4 Pattern-reversal VEP in classic and common migraine

Shibata et al., 1997 recorded pattern-reversal VEP to transient checkerboard stimulus in 19 patients with migraine with visual aura (i.e. classic migraine), 14 patients with migraine without aura (i.e. common migraine) in the interictal period, and 43 healthy subjects. Latencies and amplitudes of pattern-reversal VEPs in each group were analyzed. In patients with classic migraine, P100 amplitude was significantly higher than in healthy subjects, whereas latencies of pattern-reversal VEPs did not differ significantly. No significant differences were noted in latency between the common migraine group and healthy subjects or in latencies and amplitudes of pattern-reversal VEP between the classic migraine and common migraine groups. These results suggest that patients with classic migraine may have hyperexcitability in the visual pathway during interictal periods and that the increased amplitude of pattern-reversal VEPs after attacks may be due to cortical spreading depression.

2.6.5 VEP in adrenoleukodystrophy

Adrenoleukodystrophy is an X-linked metabolic disorder with very long-chain fatty acid (VLCFA) accumulation and multifocal nervous system demyelination, often with early involvement of the visual pathways. Kaplan et al., 1993 found that pattern-reversal VEPs were abnormal in 17% of patients with adrenoleukodystrophy; no evidence indicated that reduction of VLCFA levels improved or retarded visual pathway demyelination.

2.6.6 functional disorders

In malingering and hysterical visual loss normal VEP usually suggests continuity of the visual pathways ruling out disease up until area 17 but does not exclude fully cortical blindness in such cases (Bodis-Wollner, 1977).

2.6.7 VEPs in retinopathies and maculopathies

Diseases of the retina, especially diseases affecting the macular region, are associated with abnormal VEPs. In maculopathies, simultaneous recording of pattern Electroretinogram (ERG) and VEPs may be diagnostically useful in differentiating between involvement of the macula and optic nerve. In maculopathies and retinopathies involving the macular region, pattern ERG are absent or have a prolonged b-wave latency. The retinocortical time remains within the normal boundaries, indicating that the P100 delay occurs at the retinal level. In optic nerve diseases VEPs may be absent or prolonged, but pattern ERG are normal; the retinocortical time is thus prolonged, indicating that the pathology is postretinal (Celesia and Kaufman, 1985).

In patients with retinopathies the latency of P100 was found to be prolonged by a mean of 19.6 msec with a range of 6 to 39 msec. Delays in latency that exceeded the limits of normality by more than 45 msec usually indicate optic nerve dysfunction especially in multiple sclerosis (Lennerstrand, 1982).

3. Brainstem Auditory Evoked Potentials (BAEPs)

3.1 Introduction

On applying auditory stimulus to one ear, activation of peripheral and central auditory pathways occurs. Brain stem auditory evoked potentials (BAEPs) are the electrical activities resulting from the activation of the eighth nerve, cochlear nucleus, tracts and nuclei of the lateral lemniscus and inferior colliculus (Chiappa, 1983).

Brain stem auditory evoked potential recording is a physiological technique which can be used to evaluate the auditory pathway. It has the advantage of not requiring a voluntary response by the patient and occurring during sleep (Stephen, 1983).

3.2 Description and origin of BAEPs (Figure 2,3)

Clinical stimuli delivered to one or both ears evoke seven submicrovolt vertex-positive waves that appear at the human scalp in the first 10 msec after each stimulus (Picton et al., 1974). They are named according to their sequence in roman letters (from I to VII) (Chiappa et al., 1978).

Wave (I)

This wave is generated from the auditory portion of the eighth cranial nerve, probably from the proximal portion of that nerve just lateral to the brain stem in contact with the spiral ganglia. It is a prominent initial upgoing peak in the ipsilateral ear recording channel. It is important as a reference point for interwave latency measurement (Rowe III, 1978). Patients who have only central nervous system problems should have a preserved wave I. Conversely, patients who have a significant peripheral hearing impairment may have a very poor formed or absent wave I, but may have relatively normal waves II-V (Nuwer et al., 1994).

Wave I can sometimes be seen to have two separate components. The first, earlier component is present and higher in amplitude especially during high intensity, high pitched stimulation. This component should be used for scoring whenever it is present. The second, slightly later lower amplitude component of wave I, is present at a more wide range of stimulus intensities and pitch (Matsuoka et al., 1994).

Waves (II)

This wave may be generated near or at the cochlear nucleus (Row III, 1978). A portion of it can come from the eighth nerve fibers around the cochlear nucleus, and this part of II can be preserved despite brain stem death. Wave II is poorly defined in some adults and most neonates. It sometimes appears as a small peak along the downgoing slope of the wave I. At other times, it merges into the upgoing slope of wave III. It is more often prominent on the contralateral channel recording, where it has a slightly prolonged latency compared to the ipsilateral channel, sometimes fusing with wave III into an M-shaped II-III complex (Aminoff et al., 1994).

Wave (III)

This wave is probably generated from the lower pons as the pathway travels through the superior olive and trapezoidal body (Row III, 1978). The nuclei or fiber tracts that are most responsible for generating this potential are unknown and may be multiple.

Wave III is usually a prominent peak and is followed by a prominent III trough. In the contralateral channel wave III often appears smaller and earlier than on the ipsilateral channel, because its amplitude is similar at the vertex and contralateral ear (Goodin et al., 1994).

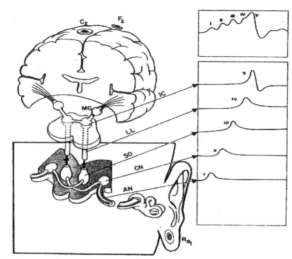

Figure 93. Auditory evoked response studies. AN = auditory nerves; CN = cochlear nuclei; SO = superior olives; LI = lateral lemnisci; IC = inferior colliculi; MG = medial geniculates.

Fig. 2. Anatomical-electrophysiological correlation of BAEP *(Poon's, 2003b).*

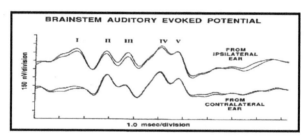

Fig. 3. Normal components of BAEP *(Nuwer et al., 1994).*

Waves (IV) and (V)

Contribution to these two potentials probably includes generators in the upper pons or lower midbrain, in the lateral lemniscus and the inferior colliculus. There are conflicting reports about whether these peaks are generated in the ipsilateral or contralateral brain stem, but the preponderance of evidence favors a contralateral brain stem generator site for wave V (Starr et al., 1994).

These peaks may fuse together into a IV-V complex on the ipsilateral recording channel. This complex can vary between: (a) two peaks which are close but still visibly separate, and (b) a single peak which is completely fused as a tall and wide pyramid. There are also various intermediate stages of trapezoid-shaped figures which represent the partial fusion of the two peaks. On the contralateral recording channel the IV and V peaks tend to be separated more from each other with wave IV being slightly earlier and wave V being slightly later. Comparison of ipsilateral and contralateral peaks can be helpful for distinguishing which peak or shoulder to score as wave V. The wave V is generally followed by a large V trough. Sometimes wave VI appears before the bottom of this trough, and then wave VI can be confused with wave V if the reader is not careful. The fusion of wave VI into a IV-V-VI complex occurs more often when a 10-30 Hz low filter is used for recording (Nuwer et al., 1994).

The typical IV-V complex has a shape of a somewhat inflated pyramid or trapezoid. The base of this complex should be more than 1.5 msec across. A peak narrower than this is usually a wave IV alone. Wave V is usually most prominent at an intermediate intensity of stimulation. As this stimulus intensity increases further beyond that point, the identification of wave V can actually become more difficult. It is often helpful to have the technician reduce the intensity of stimulation to identify wave V. Wave V is a robust peak that is present despite moderately low intensities of stimulation (and often even despite high frequency hearing impairment, or other types of peripheral auditory changes). Wave V and especially the V trough are often the last deflections to disappear when the stimulus intensity is gradually decreased to threshold (Matsuoka et al., 1994).

Overall there are several ways to help identify wave V when its identity is unclear: the typical contralateral splitting of the IV-V complex; the wide base of a IV-V complex and the preservation of wave V at lower stimulus intensities (Aminoff et al., 1994).

Waves (VI) and (VII)

Are not found in all normal subjects. They are generated in medial geniculate body and auditory radiation from the thalamus to temporal cortex respectively (Row, 1980).

The most constant and most important waves, from the clinical point of view, are waves I, III, V (Rosenhall et al., 1985). Their measurements include absolute latency (stimulus to peak) and interpeak latency (time interval between the peaks). The clinical interpretation is based on the interpeak latencies. Absolute amplitudes are extremely variable in normal subjects (Chiappa, 1983).

3.3 Normal limits and the clinical correlation of changes

There are 5 principle features used to assess routine BAEPs

3.3.1 I-V interpeak interval

This is the primary feature for most BAEP interpretations. It represents conduction from the proximal eighth nerve through pons and into the midbrain. It can be slowed in a variety of disorders, including focal damage (demyelination, ischemia, tumors), or diffuse problems (degenerative disorders, post-hypoxic damage, etc.) (Starr et al., 1994).

A typical upper limit of normal for the I-V interpeak interval is 4.5 msec. That limit is slightly lower for young women and slightly higher for older men. Normal right-left asymmetries for the I-V interpeak interval should be at most 0.5 msec. For full-term infants, the I-V interpeak interval should be less than 5.4 msec (Goodin et al., 1994).

3.3.2 I-III interpeak interval

This interpeak interval represents conduction from the eighth nerve across the subarachnoid space, into the core of the lower pons. The I-III interpeak interval can be increased in any diffuse process that affects the whole I-V interpeak interval. This I-III portion of the pathway is susceptible to a tumor, inflammation or other disorders especially affecting the proximal portion of the eighth nerve, or the ponto-medullary junction where the eighth nerve enters the brain-stem, or impairments in the lower pons around the superior olive or trapezoidal body. Acoustic neuromas or other cerebello-pontine angle tumors can cause a delay at the juncture. Infarction can cause an interruption or a delay here too, although the classical

Wallenberg syndrome is usually too caudal to affect this segment. Inflammation in the subarachnoid space can also increase this I-III interpeak interval (subarachnoid hemorrhage, meningitis and Guillain-Barre syndrome) (Aminoff et al., 1994).

The upper limit of normal for the I-III interpeak interval is about 2.5 msec. The acceptable right-left asymmetry of this interval is less than 0.5msec. An excessively long interpeak interval I-III cannot be considered unless there is an accompanying prolongation of the I-V interpeak interval (Matsuoka et al., 1994).

3.3.3 III-V interval

This interval reflects conduction from the lower to the upper pons and possibly into the midbrain. There is not yet complete agreement about whether this III-V interpeak interval represents conduction along the ipsilateral or contralateral brain-stem, compared to which ear is stimulated. The preponderance of evidence favors a contralateral brain-stem site (Nuwer et al., 1994).

The typical upper limit of normal for a III-V interpeak interval is about 2.4 msec. A right-left asymmetry for these intervals should be less than 0.5 msec. An excessively long III-V interpeak interval is not considered abnormal unless either the I-V interval or the V/I amplitude ratio is also abnormal (Goodin et al., 1994).

3.3.4 V/I amplitude ratio

Absolute amplitudes of BAEP peaks vary widely among normal subjects. In addition, several technical factors influence the absolute amplitudes of BAEP peaks. To reduce this normal intersubject variability, a ratio of amplitudes is usually calculated. For this ratio, the amplitude of IV-V complex is divided by the amplitude of the wave I. The IV-V complex is measured from the highest point of the complex to the trough of the V peak. When V is completely separated from IV, the V amplitude is used In place of the IV-V amplitude. When wave VI is found lying part way down the descending slope of wave V, then the amplitude is measured to the trough following wave VI. The wave I amplitude is measured from the top of the highest part of wave I to the bottom of the trough of I. If wave II is riding on the descending slope of I, then wave I amplitude is measured to the succeeding trough of the wave II (Starr et al., 1994).

The amplitude ratio should be between 50% and 300%. These numbers vary between laboratories and they are especially affected by filter setting changes. When the V/I amplitude ratio is less than 50%, then the IV-V peaks are too small. In that case, suspicion is raised of some central impairment which has diminished the amplitude of the IV-V even if it may have not increased I-V interpeak interval. This is useful criterion for abnormality, especially when the IV-V peaks are so low that they are difficult to distinguish from background noise. Then the record may be interpreted as abnormal because of such low amplitude central peaks, even if the latencies cannot be precisely defined. For full-term infants, the lower limit for V/I is 30% (Goodin et al., 1994).

When the V/I amplitude ratio is greater than 300%, wave I is usually considered to be too small. This raises the suspicion of some peripheral hearing impairment, especially of a high frequency or a sensorineural hearing loss (Aminoff et al., 1994).

3.3.5 Presence of wave I-V

The wave I-V all are seen in most normal individuals. Occasional normal subjects have a wave IV that is so merged into a IV-V complex that it cannot be distinguished as a separate peak, unless extra traces are run at different stimulus rates and intensities. Such a merging of wave IV into a IV-V complex is considered to be a normal variant. Wave II can also be difficult to distinguish when testing some normal subjects. Upon changing stimulus intensities, rates and phase, wave II can be distinguished in essentially all normal subjects. However wave II can appear to be missing at the specific rates and intensities used for simple clinical BAEPs, and this would be considered a normal variant (Matsuoka et al., 1994).

When all waves I-V are absent the BAEP is abnormal, although the cause is usually peripheral (Technical problems must also be considered). It is also abnormal to record a wave I, but not succeeding waves. Finally, it is abnormal if wave I and III are present but IV-V is absent. These roles for the absence of peaks are predicted upon the assumption that technically good quality records have been obtained. The record should be considered technically unsatisfactory if moderate or large amount of background noise are present in the tracing, rather than being interpreted as showing an absence of important peaks (Nuwer et al., 1994).

Waves VI, VII, VIII can normally be present or absent or asymmetrical in latency or amplitude, without any apparent clinical correlation. The main reason for knowing their existence is to prevent confusion with the earlier important waves (Starr et al., 1994).

3.3.6 Absolute latency measurements
The absolute latency measurements of wave I, III and V can be occasionally of clinical value. This is particularly so when some peaks are absent. For example, the absolute latency of wave V can be compared against normal limits when there is no waves I-IV. The absolute latency of wave V is normally less than 6.4 msec. The right-left asymmetry of the wave V absolute latency is normally 0.5 msec or less. Absence of waves I-IV with delayed wave V may be due to a hearing loss. When waves I, III and V are all present, the standard means of interpretation is by the interpeak intervals (Goodin et al., 1994).

The absolute latency of wave I can be used as part of the assessment of hearing. The wave I is often seen around 1.75 msec, but may be seen up to 2.2 msec in some normal subjects. The right-left asymmetry of the wave I absolute latencies is normally 0.4 msec or less. Wave I latency delays or asymmetry suggest a hearing impairment, rather than brain-stem dysfunction (Aminoff et al., 1994).

3.3.7 Reference Values of BAEP (Tandon and Krishna, 1990)

Wave	Mean	Range
Wave I	1.62	1.26-1.98
Wave II	2.80	2.23-3.37
Wave III	3.75	3.24-4.26
Wave IV	4.84	4.15-5.53
Wave IV/V	5.27	4.61-5.93
Wave V	5.62	4.93-6.31
I-III	2.63	
III-V	2.31	
I-IV/V	4.32	

3.4 Principles of recording of BAEPs
3.4.1 Technical details

The test can be performed under sedation or under general anesthesia; Filter band pass 100-3000 Hz; Standard broadband click stimulation is used on the ear tested; Monoaural stimulation is used; The click intensity should be 60-70 dB above click perception threshold;

The contralateral ear receives masking noise of 30- to 40-dB lesser intensity; The first 10 ms are averaged, and 2-4000 responses may be averaged; At least 2 separate trials should be performed (Leslie et al., 2002).

3.4.2 Stimulation procedures

In neurological practice a sound (Click) generated by pulses through headphones is used as an auditory stimulus. The hearing threshold is determined and the click is applied at an intensity 30,40,50 or 60 decibel (dB) above that hearing threshold. The stimulated ear (in monoaural stimulation) is called ipsilateral ear, the other is the contralateral one (Starr et al., 1976).

To avoid stimulation of the contralateral ear by bone and air conduction on applying the click to the ipsilateral ear, the former should be masked by noise at an intensity of 30 to 40 dB less than of the click stimulus (Leslie et al., 2002).

3.4.3 Electrode montage

The recording montage is at least, and usually, a 2-channel montage channel 1 is ipsilateral ear to vertex and channel 2 is contralateral ear to vertex. The recording electrodes are located, one for each ear lobule and a third electrode is located on the scalp at the vertex at Cz position of 10-20 international system (Stockard et al., 1979a and Leslie et al., 2002).

3.4.4 Interpretation (Poon's, 2003b)

3.4.4.1 Abnormal I-III interpeak latency (IPL): This abnormality suggests the presence of a conduction defect in the brain-stem auditory system between the eighth nerve close to the cochlea and the lower pons.

3.4.4.2 Abnormal III-V IPL: This abnormality suggests the presence of a conduction defect in the brain-stem auditory system between the lower pons and the midbrain.

3.4.4.3 I absent & III-V is normal: Wave I (the eighth nerve activation potential) could not be recorded. This is usually due to a peripheral hearing disorder. Because of this, the state of conduction in the brain-stem auditory pathway between peripheral eighth nerve and lower pons could not be determined. Lower pons to midbrain conduction was normal.

3.4.4.4 IV or V absent or of abnormally low amplitude: This abnormality suggests the presence of a conduction defect in the brain-stem auditory system rostral to the lower pons.

3.4.4.5 Absent II, III, IV and V with normal I: This abnormality indicates a significant lack of function in brain-stem auditory tracts.

3.5 Factors affecting BAEPs

Factors which affect BAEPs are either technical and / or subject related factors

3.5.1 Technical factors

3.5.1.1 Intensity of the stimulus (click)

The intensity of the click stimulus affects the amplitude and absolute latencies of BAEPs peaks. Stockard et al., 1979 reported that absolute latencies increase and amplitudes diminish with decreasing intensity by about 0.03 msec/dB.

Chiappa, (1983) found that waves II, IV and VI diminish more quickly than waves I, III,V with decreasing intensity and also reported that the constancy of the interpeak latency is more reliable in neurologic applications than the use of absolute latency.

3.5.1.2 Rate of the stimulus

Increasing click rate results in increased absolute latency of all BAEPs waves and decrease in the amplitude of most of them. Interpeak latencies increase slightly at higher rates (Stockard et al., 1978 & 1979). Stockard et al., 1980b added that, using rates higher than 30 per second will often worsen pre-existing abnormalities in the BAEP. Some studies used higher rates to reveal the abnormalities. However, Chiappa et al., 1979 mentioned that increasing click rate from 10/second to only 30/second has no value.

3.5.1.3 Stimulus mode

Binaural stimulation produces higher amplitude waves III, IV, V at all stimulus intensities than monoaural stimulation and, because of the monoaural contribution to wave I but binaural contribution to wave IV and V, binaural stimulation logically produces a higher V/I amplitude ratio than monoaural stimulation at a given stimulus intensity. Binaural stimulation should be avoided in routine clinical applications because monoaural abnormalities are common in neurologic disease and may otherwise be masked by the response from the normal ear (Stockard et al.,1978). Separate monoaural stimulation of each ear also allows for comparison of interaural asymmetries in interpeak latency (IPL) and thus may indicate abnormality even when BAEPs from each ear are within normal limits when considered separately (Berlin and Hood, 1984).

3.5.1.4 Filter setting

Filter settings affect relative amplitudes more than interpeak latencies and, in diagnostic applications, should remain fixed at the values used when collecting each laboratory's normative data. The ideal bandpass for clinical purposes is probably 100 to 3,000 Hz or higher. A low frequency filter of much less than 100 Hz allows EMG, EEG and other signals into the average, and a cutoff much higher than 100 Hz distorts the low-frequency BAEP components. A high frequency cutoff of at least 3,000 Hz is necessary to resolve the highest-frequency components of BAEP; settings of less than 1,000 Hz increase the apparent latencies of the BAEPs and decrease their resolution. Increases in high-pass filter above 100 Hz markedly reduce V/I amplitude ratio because of the longer duration of wave V than I. High pass-filtering at 30 Hz or lower is needed in audiologic BAEP applications (Stockard et al., 1978).

3.5.1.5 Site of reference

Using the electrode applied to the contralateral ear as a reference produces a decrease in the II-III interpeak latency and increase the IV-V interpeak latency. Peak latencies of waves II and V are increased when the electrode applied to the contralateral ear is used as a reference in comparison to the use of electrode applied to the ipsilateral ear (Stokard et al., 1978).

De Montes et al., 2002 concluded that BAEP obtained with reference to Cz and Fz are ideal for interpretation, since there is greater constancy, global amplitude and morphological clarity of the first five deflections and less morphological complexity of the other waves.

3.5.2 Subject factors

3.5.2.1 Age

Below the age of 2 years, interpeak latencies are prolonged relative to adult values (Starr et al.,1976). By the age of 2 years, the ranges for adults are reached, the absolute latencies of wave I, III, V increase by 0.1-0.2 msec with age. However, the I-V interpeak latency remains the same (Rosenhall et al., 1985). One obvious explanation for the age-related latency shift is progressive myelination of the auditory tract in infants (Tarantino et al., 1988).

The effects of age on the brain-stem auditory evoked potentials were studied on 156 healthy subjects with ages ranging from 18 to 76 years. There was a small progressive prolongation in the peak latency with increasing age, particularly peak V. Although a correlation between the age and the I-III interval was not observed, there was also a small increase with age in the interpeak latencies of III-V and I-V (Chu, 1985).

Since age effects on central conduction time in the acoustic pathway are still debated, brainstem auditory evoked potentials were recorded in normoacoustic subjects, with no history of neurologic or otologic pathology. Linear regression has been used for statistical analysis. Data obtained show an age-related prolongation of latency values which is particularly marked for wave I, while other waves (particularly wave III) do not show a significant change. Thus, IPL values do not increase with increasing age: in particular IPLs I-II and I-III decrease, showing a negative "r" value, and IPLs I-V and II-V (which is to be considered the true "central conduction time" through the acoustic pathway) do not show a significant change. These data seem to demonstrate that the aging process is essentially a peripheral phenomenon which does not involve the central part of the acoustic pathway (Costa et al., 1990).

Brainstem auditory evoked response (BAER) was recorded in children from birth to 6 years and adults to study the development of wave amplitude. The amplitudes of all BAER waves increased with age, the greatest changes occurring during early infancy. Adult values were reached at 6 months of age for wave I and 2 years for wave V. The two waves continued to increase above the adult values until the highest amplitude value was reached at 3 years for wave I and 5 years for wave V. Subsequently, the amplitudes decreased towards the values in adults. The V/I amplitude ratio, which was slightly lower than the adult value shortly after birth, decreased during the first year of life and reached the minimum value between 1 and 4 years. Thereafter, it increased towards the adult value. Throughout the maturational stages the ratio was smaller than in adults. The amplitude of wave V was relatively stable and its variation was much smaller than those of wave I and V/I amplitude ratio (Jiang et al., 1993).

3.5.2.2 Sex

Females have shorter interpeak latencies than males. This may be explained by shorter corresponding segments of the auditory pathway due to smaller brain size. However, no difference could be detected before the age of 8 years (Stochard et al., 1979).

Sex differences in the amplitudes and latencies of the auditory brain stem potential (BAEP) were investigated using 3 levels of intensity and 3 stimulus presentation rates. The females displayed consistently larger BAEPs for waves IV, V, VI and VII than the males. The only latency differences which reached significance over all the intensities and rates occurred for wave V. The females showed significantly shorter wave V latencies than the males. Since hearing losses and individually determined click thresholds were comparable between the two groups tested, the exact sources of the uneven distribution of amplitude and latency effects are in question. Differences in the relative distances of the anatomical generators are considered in accounting for the sex differences. Because the precise origin of the sex differences cannot be stated with certainty, attempts to develop normative data for the BAEP should consider the possible influences of sex differences (Michalewski et al., 1980).

3.5.2.3 Hearing disorders

Peripheral hearing disorders give a similar effect on BAEP as decreasing stimulus intensity i.e. the absolute latencies of all waves are increased but no change of the interpeak latencies (Chiappa, 1983).

In patients with sensorineural hearing loss, Coats and Martin, 1977 found an abrupt increase in the latency of wave I at 50 to 60 dB, 4 to 8 kHz hearing loss; this abrupt increase in wave I peak latency was not paralleled by a similar increase in wave V latency, thus the I-V interpeak latencies in these subjects were shorter than in those with normal audiograms.

3.5.2.4 Body temperature

A decrease in body temperature leads to increase in both the absolute and interpeak latencies (Picton et al.,1982).

3.5.2.5 Hypoglycemia

Kern et al., 1994 studied the effects of insulin-induced hypoglycemia on the auditory brainstem response (ABR) in humans. ABRs were examined in healthy men during euglycemia and after 20 minutes and 50 minutes of steady-state hypoglycemia of 2.6 mM induced with insulin. Hypoglycemia increased interpeak latencies III-V and I-V, whereas changes in the latency of wave I were not significant.

3.5.2.6 Medications

3.5.2.6.1 Barbiturate

BAEPs are not affected significantly by barbiturate doses sufficient to render the EEG "flat" (i.e. isoelectric) or by general anesthesia (although it was reported that BAEP has been lost with combined lidocaine and thiopental infusion) (Garcia-Larrea et al., 1988).

3.5.2.6.2 Nicotine (smoking)

Reports of tobacco-induced electrocortical activation have frequently indicated that this effect is mediated via nicotine's action on sub-cortical structures. Twelve regular smokers were tested on two separate sessions involving sham or real smoking. On each session, BAEPs were recorded during a baseline period and immediately after smoking. BAEPs, recorded from Cz, were elicited by presentation of 1,000 monaural, rare fraction click stimuli. Latency and amplitudes of peak components I, III and V were assessed and analyzed. No significant effects were observed for latency measures or for amplitudes of peaks I and III. A significant effect was observed for peak V with tobacco resulting in larger amplitudes relative to sham smoking. Peak V reflects activity from upper pontine-lower midbrain sites (Knott, 1987).

3.5.2.6.3 Aminophylline

To determine the neurophysiological effects of aminophylline on apnea of prematurity, the BAEPs of 30 apnoeic infants and 34 age matched controls were evaluated and compared. After six days of treatment with aminophylline, the brain stem conduction time (interpeak latency of I-V) in apnoeic infants decreased compared with controls of a similar postconceptional age. The mean latencies of the peaks and interpeaks of all waves except wave I were significantly lower in the apnoeic infants after than before receiving aminophylline. No significant differences were found in the latencies of BAEPs between the apnoeic infants who responded and those who did not respond to aminophylline treatment. These results suggest that aminophylline may enhance conduction along central auditory pathways and stimulate the regulatory effect on the respiratory centre of the brain stem (Chen et al.,1994).

3.6 Clinical applications of BAEPs
BAEPs are very resistant to alteration by anything other than structural pathology in the brainstem auditory tracts. Disorders of the peripheral vestibular system do not affect BAEP. Thus, patients who had labyrinthine diseases (i.e. Ménière's disease, labyrinthitis, vestibular neuronitis) had no BAEP interwave latency abnormalities using the limits employed for clinical neurological purposes (Garcia-Larrea et al., 1988).
Brainstem auditory evoked potentials have obtained widespread clinical application in assessing neurologic and audiologic problems. These have maximal clinical utility in evaluating comatose patients, in patients with suspected demyelinating disorders, posterior fossa tumors, or in audiologic evaluation, especially in infants. They are also used for intraoperative monitoring of eighth-nerve and brainstem function during different types of posterior fossa surgery (Markand, 1994).
ABR audiometry is considered an effective screening tool in the evaluation of suspected retrocochlear pathology. However, an abnormal ABR suggestive of retrocochlear pathology indicates the need for MRI or CT scanning. In general, ABR exhibits a sensitivity of over 90% and a specificity of approximately 70-90% (Schmidt et al., 2001).

3.6.1 BAEPs in multiple sclerosis (MS)
An abnormal response may be seen with higher frequency in symptomatic patients; however, a positive test may be recorded in the absence of clinical brainstem symptomatology. BAEPs should be considered if the clinical symptom implicates a lesion outside the brain stem. In this case an abnormal BAEPs would further support the diagnosis of MS. If, however, the clinical sign (e.g., diplopia) points to the brain stem, BAEPs abnormality is merely confirmatory. In various studies about 20% of the population tested for a second lesion have an abnormal BAEPs and about half of these go on to develop MS in the next 1-3 years (Kjaer, 1987).
Purves et al., 1981 reported pattern-shift VEPs to be abnormal in 45%, SSEP abnormal in 35%, and BAEP in 14% of patients without brainstem signs. Combining all 3 modalities, 97% of patients with definite MS, 86% of patients with probable MS, and 63% of patients with possible MS had abnormal findings on at least one of these tests. Similar findings were reported by Ferrer et al., 1993. Kjaer, 1987 reported 38% abnormal BAEPs in patients with silent lesions, while 50% of these patients had an abnormal VEPs and only 13% an abnormal SEP.
Brain-stem auditory evoked responses (BAERs) were examined in 178 patients with multiple sclerosis (MS) and compared to the frequency of abnormalities in visually evoked responses (VERs) and in CSF electrophoresis. In clinically definite MS, BAERs were abnormal in 61% and a significant relationship was noted between disability due to MS and the frequency and severity of BAER abnormalities. In suspected MS, BAERs showed evidence of a second lesion in 14% whereas VERs indicated a second lesion in 24%.

Abnormal BAERs in patients with suspected MS with brain-stem signs were significantly associated with the presence of ataxia. In progressive possible MS, abnormal BAERs were found in 49% but indicated a second lesion in 35% of patients and were significantly related to the duration of illness. In progressive possible MS, abnormal VERs but not abnormal BAERs, were significantly associated with the presence of cerebrospinal fluid (CSF) oligoclonal IgG banding. Normal BAERs in association with clinical brain-stem abnormalities were found in 24% of patients with clinically definite MS, 50% with suspected MS and 33% with progressive possible MS (Hutchinson et al., 1984).

Furthermore, Lehmann and Soukos, 1982 examined patients with certain, probable and possible MS using checkerboard VEP and click-BAEP and concluded that VEPs were clearly more useful than BAEPs in the early diagnostics of MS, however in occasional cases, BAEPs might contribute to the early diagnosis.

Chiappa, 1990 found that the BAEP is positive in 21% of clinically unsuspected cases. Most authors have concluded that BAEP yields the smallest percentage of patients, but it still adds to the detection rate because it is abnormal in a different subset of patients.

3.6.2 CNS tumors

3.6.2.1 Cerebellopontine angle lesions

BAEP may be abnormal when audiometry fails to disclose a lesion. The characteristic findings are increased I-V and increased I-III interpeak latencies ipsilateral to the lesion. Bilateral prolongation of latencies and interpeak latencies may be seen. Gordon and Cohen, 1995 evaluated the efficacy of auditory brainstem response (ABR) as a screening test for small acoustic neuromas by performing a prospective trial to determine the diagnostic sensitivity of brainstem auditory evoked response (BAER) in these tumors. Randomly selected patients with surgically proven acoustic neuromas underwent preoperative BAER tests within 2 months of surgery. A test result was considered abnormal when the interaural I-V interpeak latency difference was greater than 0.2 ms, the absolute wave V latency was abnormally prolonged, or waveform morphology was abnormal or absent. 87.6% Of the tested patients, had an abnormal BAER and 12.4% had completely normal waveforms and wave latencies. Patients with tumors greater than 2 cm in total diameter had abnormal BAER results. Patients with tumors 1.6-2 cm / 1-1.5 cm / 9 mm or smaller, 86% / 85% / 69% had abnormal BAERs respectively. These data show that BAER sensitivity decreases with decreasing tumor size. Therefore, MRI scanning is the preferred study because the accuracy for detection of tumor smaller than 1 cm through BAER is 70%. Nevertheless, BAER is useful in patients who have implanted medical devices (e.g., pacemakers) that prevent MRI scanning.

3.6.2.2 Meningomyelocele

The brainstem auditory evoked potentials (BAEPs) of twenty-seven meningomyelocele (MMC) patients were analyzed and compared with the results of a normal population. The longest wave V or I-V interpeak latencies were seen in patients with shunted hydrocephalus and cranial nerve defects. The shortest wave V and I-V interpeak latencies were found in patients without hydrocephalus. However, these latencies of MMC patients were significantly longer than the latencies of a normal population. It is assumed that I-V interpeak latency prolongation in MMC patients, which is related to the severity of the clinical signs of the Arnold Chiari malformation, is mostly due to an elongation of the brainstem (Lutschg et al., 1985).

It is difficult to estimate the accurate onset of symptoms clinically resulting from Chiari II malformation. Brainstem auditory evoked potentials (BAEPs) may be a useful method in the selection of potential candidates for surgery. BAEPs were studied in asymptomatic infants under 6 months of age with meningomyelocele (MMC). Both the wave latencies and interpeak latencies (IPLs) gradually became shorter during the first 6 months of life in asymptomatic infants with MMC. In particular, shortening of the III-V IPLs and the I-V IPLs was observed from 1 to 4-6 months of age in these infants. These may be characteristic parameters of central auditory function (III-V IPLs) and global auditory function (I-V IPLs). Maturation of brainstem function as viewed by BAEPs in asymptomatic infants with MMC was delayed when compared to data in normal neonates and infants. These data on asymptomatic infants with MMC could potentially be a good reference for selecting the modalities of treatment in infants with symptomatic Chiari II malformation (Fujii et al., 1996).

Taylor et al., 1996 studied BAER in infants with meningomyelocele to determine whether EPs reflect early neurological status and whether BAER have prognostic value in neurological outcome. The infants, aged 1 day to 3 months, were tested while still in hospital after the meningomyelocele repair. Normal BAEPs were found in 41% of patients while abnormal BAEPs were found in all infants studied who had symptomatic Arnold-Chiari malformation. So, BAEPs showed a positive predictive value of 88% and accuracy of 84% in predicting central neurological sequelae.

3.6.3 Brainstem stroke

Brainstem stroke syndromes are primarily determined by clinical criteria. There are few diagnostic procedures which are of benefit for the evaluation of brainstem ischemic events. Brainstem auditory evoked responses are important electrophysiologic technique for assessing brainstem function. The response is variable; some lesions cause abnormal latencies while some do not (Tsuda et al., 1995).

To evaluate the use of BAERs in patients with brainstem ischemic events, 35 individuals with recent brainstem strokes, selected by strict clinical criteria, were evaluated with BAERs. The initial BAER was abnormal in 22 of 35 patients (63%). When the clinical course and site of the lesion are correlated with the BAER results. An unstable course, characterized by progression or remission and relapse, was present in 19/35 (54%) of patients, and 15/19 (79%) of these individuals had an initially abnormal BAER. The other 16 brainstem stroke patients with a stable clinical course had an initially abnormal BAER in 7 instances (44%). This difference is statistically significant at the $P = 0.04$ level. The principal sites of ischemia were mesencephalic in 11/35, pontine in 13/35 and medullary in 11/35. The association of an abnormal BAER with an unstable clinical course seemed independent of the site of the lesion, However, of the 9 deaths that occurred, all were in patients with mesencephalic or pontine lesions, and 8 of these individuals had an initially abnormal BAER. Abnormal BAERs in patients with brainstem ischemic lesions correlate with an unstable clinical course. Furthermore, individuals with ponto-mesencephalic infarction and abnormal BAERs have an especially poor prognosis. The BAER may be of prognostic value in the early evaluation of patients with brainstem ischemic strokes (Stern et al., 1982).

Brain stem auditory evoked potentials were studied in patients with the lateral medullary (Wallenberg's) syndrome. The observed changes included: prolongation of the interpeak latencies from wave I-V and III-V; prolongation of the interaural latency difference for wave V; splitting or absence of wave III and the presence of a broad partly fused wave III-V complex. This study showed that BAEP can be used to confirm the diagnosis of this syndrome and ascertain the site of the lesion (Elwany,1985).

A study of brainstem auditory evoked potentials was carried out in subjects suffering from vertebrobasilar TIA in order to obtain a comparative evaluation of cortical-subcortical functions. The obtained data demonstrate a delay of peak III of the BAEPs in patients with previous vertebrobasilar TIA. These data show that the study of the BAEPs is useful in evaluating the damage produced by anoxia (Benna et al., 1985).

3.6.4 Respiratory insufficiency following encephalitis
Schwarz et al., 1996 showed prolonged interpeak latencies (I-III, I-V, III-V, IV-V) and delayed absolute latencies of waves II, III, V, and I, at least on one side, in the BAEP. The auditory pathways are near the respiratory control centers in the brain stem; therefore, the electrophysiologic abnormalities of wave III and the IV-V complex may be a reflection of the disturbed central control of ventilation.

3.6.5 Prediction of posttraumatic coma in children
BAEP studies were performed within 72 hours of admission in children with severe head injury in order to predict the outcome of posttraumatic coma. Outcomes were categorized as brain death or survival. On first assessment, 40% of comatose children had normal BAEP. About 78% survived and 22% deteriorated and died. 32% 0f children had abnormal findings; 69% of them improved and survived, whilst 31% deteriorated and died. All children who did not have recordable BAEP died. These data suggest that BAER is a useful test in predicting neurological outcome in this setting (Butinar and Gostisa, 1996).

3.6.6 Comatose patient
BAEP can be done while the patient is sedated. It can be used as a prognostic indicator. Survival is unlikely in the absence of BAEP. The brain-dead patient has invariably abnormal BAEPs either the absence of all waveforms or the presence of wave I and the absence of all subsequent waveforms (Goldie et al., 1981).

3.6.7 Intraoperative monitoring
ABR, often used intraoperatively with electrocochleography, provides early identification of changes in the neurophysiologic status of the peripheral and central nervous system. This information is useful in the prevention of neurotologic dysfunction and the preservation of postoperative hearing loss. For many patients with tumors of cranial nerve (CN) VIII or the cerebellopontine angle, hearing may be diminished or completely lost postoperatively, even when the auditory nerve has been preserved anatomically.

Typical uses of intraoperative auditory brainstem response

- **Monitoring cochlear function directed at hearing preservation**

Cerebellopontine angle tumor resection (acoustic neuroma surgery); Vascular decompression of trigeminal neuralgia; Vestibular nerve section for the relief of vertigo; Exploration of the facial nerve for facial nerve decompression; Endolymphatic sac decompression for Ménière's disease.

- **Monitoring brainstem integrity**

Brainstem tumor resection; Brainstem aneurysm clipping or arteriovenous malformation resection (Kileny et al., 1988).

3.6.8 Screening of hearing in newborns

Several clinical trials have shown automated auditory brainstem response (AABR) testing as an effective screening tool in the evaluation of hearing in newborns, with a sensitivity of 100% and specificity of 96-98%. When used as a threshold measure to screen for normal hearing, each ear may be evaluated independently, with a stimulus presented at an intensity level between 35-40 dB. Click-evoked ABR is highly correlated with hearing sensitivity in the frequency range from 1000-4000 Hz. AABRs test for the presence or absence of wave V. No operator interpretation is required (Oudesluys-Murphy et al., 1996).

4. Conclusion

The VEP is preferable in optic nerve and anterior chiasmatic lesions, while MRI is clearly superior in retrochiasmatic disease. Note that the VEP is nonspecific as to the underlying etiology and pathology (Andrew et al., 2002).

The most common uses of BAEP are in MS and in acoustic neuroma. It is a useful screening test, with limitations; MRI scanning may be preferable when a small lesion is under consideration. Increased I-III interpeak latency indicates a lesion from CN VIII to the superior olivary nucleus, while increased III-V interpeak latency suggests a lesion from the superior olivary nucleus to the inferior colliculus ipsilateral to the ear stimulated. Intraoperative monitoring during cerebellopontine angle tumor surgery may be helpful in aiding the surgeon to preserve as much function as possible (Gordon and Cohen, 1995).

Involvement of CNS sensory pathways in hereditary motor and sensory neuropathies has been reported by Carroll et al and Jones et al. However, at that time molecular genetic diagnosis was not yet available and their finding could not be linked to a particular gene defect. Jones et al speculated that the abnormalities might be due to a dying back phenomenon of the affected peripheral nerves. On the other hand, Scaioli et al failed to show central nervous system involvement in patients with Charcot-Marie-Tooth (CMT). Recently, evidence for involvement of the central acoustic pathway was obtained by measuring BAEPs in patients with CMT1X with Cx32 mutations. However, no other CNS pathways were examined in this study (for example, VEPs or transcortical magnetic stimulation measurements) and it remained unclear whether the disorder would also affect structures other than the acoustic pathway.

Bähr et al and Tony et al found that, not only acoustic but also visual and central motor pathways are affected, suggesting a much larger central nervous system involvement than has been presumed from clinical examinations, in which such widespread central nervous system abnormalities have not been reported to date. These findings underscore the necessity of a careful analysis of CNS pathways in patients with CMT and Cx32 mutations. Thus, screening for Cx32 mutations seems to be important in patients with a peripheral neuropathy and abnormalities in motor and sensory central nervous system pathways.

5. References

Aminoff M, Nuwer MR, Goodin D, Matsuoka S and Starr A (1994): IFCN recommended standards for brain-stem auditory evoked potentials. Report of an IFCN committee. Electroencephalography and clinical neurophysiology, February, 91:12-17.

Andrew SB, Leslie H and Francisco T (2002): Clinical Utility of Evoked Potentials. e Medicine, Neurology, Electroencephalography and evoked potentials, May, 30:1-8.

Arden GB, Efaulkner DJ and mair C (1977b): The visual evoked potential in healthy subjects. In: evoked potential in clinical testing edited by A.M. Hallday. Churchill Livingstone New York (first edition), Pp. 72-100.

Asselman P, Chadwick DW and Marsden CD (1975): Visual evoked responses in the diagnosis and management of patients suspected of multiple sclerosis. Exp. Brain Res., Vol. 98: Pp. 261.

Bähr M, Andres F, Timmerman V, Nelis M E, Van Broeckhoven C, Dichgans J (1999): Central visual, acoustic, and motor pathway involvement in a Charcot-Marie-Tooth family with an Asn205Ser mutation in the connexin 32 gene. J Neurol Neurosurg Psychiatry;66:202-206.

Baumgartner J and Epstein CM (1982): Voluntary alteration of visual evoked potential. Ann. Neurol., 12:476.

Benna P, Bianco C, Costa P, Piazza D and Bergamasco B (1985): Visual evoked potentials and brainstem auditory evoked potentials in migraine and transient ischemic attacks. Cephalgia. May;5 Suppl., 2:53-58.

Berlin C and Hood L (1984): Asymmetries in evoked potentials. Hearing Science. San Diego, CA: College-Hill Press. Pp. 73-85.

Berson EL (1994): Visual function testing: Clinical correlations. J. Clin. Neurophysiol., 11:472-481.

Blumhardt LD and Halliday AM (1979): Hemisphere contributions to the composition of the pattern evoked potential waveform. Exp. Brain Res. Vol. 36:53-69.

Bodis-Wollner I, Atkin A, Raab E and Wolkstein M (1977): Visual association cortex and vision in man: Pattern-evoked occipital potentials in a blind boy. Science Nov 11; 198(4317): 629-631.

Brigell M, Kaufman DI and Bobak P (1994): The pattern visual evoked potential. A multicenter study using standardized techniques. Doc. Ophthalmol., 86(1):65-79.

Butinar D and Gostisa A (1996): Brainstem auditory evoked potentials and somatosensory evoked potentials in prediction of post-traumatic coma in children . Pflugers Arch; 431(6 Suppl 2): Pp. 289-290.

Carroll WM, Jones SJ, Halliday AM. Visual evoked potential abnormalities in linked Charcot-Marie-Tooth disease and comparison with Friedreich's ataxia. J Neurol Sci 1983;61:123–33.

Celesia GG (1988): anatomy and physiology of visual evoked potential and electroretinograms. Neurol.Clin., 6:657-665.

Celesia GG and Daly RE (1977): Visual electroencephalographic computer analysis (VECA). Neurology, 27:637-641.

Celesia GG and Kaufman D (1985): Pattern ERGs and visual evoked potentials in maculopathies and optic nerve diseases. Invest. Ophthalmol. Vis. Sci., 26:726.

Celesia GG and Tobimatsu S (1990): Electroretinograms to flash and to patterned visual stimuli in retinal and optic nerve disorders. In Desmedt JE (ed): visual evoked potentials. Elsevier, Amsterdam. Pp.45.

Chen YJ, Liou CS, Tsai CH and Yeh TF (1994): Effect of aminophylline on brainstem auditory evoked potentials in preterm infants. Arch. Dis. Child Fetal Neonatal Ed. Jul., 71(1):Pp. 20-23.

Chiappa KH (1982): Evoked potential in clinical medicine. In clinical neurology edited by AB Baker and LH Baker, JB Lippincott, Philadelphia.

Chiappa KH (1983): Evoked potential in clinical medicine. Edited by KH Chiappa and Con Yiannikas Raven press. New York (1st. ed.).

Chiappa KH (1988): The use of evoked potential in clinical practice with special reference to the diagnosis of multiple sclerosis. In: Evoked Potentials in Clinical Medicine. Chiappa KH, Ravin Press New York Second edition. 1-92.

Chiappa KH (1990): Evoked Potentials in Clinical Medicine. 2nd ed. New York: Raven Press; 37-171, 196-197.

Chiappa KH, Choi S and Young RR (1978): The results of new method for the registration of human short latency somatosensory evoked responses. Neurology, 28:385.

Chiappa KH, Gladston KJ and Young RR (1979): Brainstem auditory evoked responses: Studies of waveform. Arch. Neurol., 36:81-87.

Chiappa KH, Martin JB and Young RR (1987): Diagnostic Methods In Neurology: Disorders of the central nervous system. In Harrison's principles of internal medicine edited by JB Martin Mc Graw-Hill, Inc. Hamburg, Pp. 1913-1921.

Chu NS (1985): Age-related latency changes in the brainstem auditory evoked potentials. Electroencephalogr. Clin. Neurophysiol. Nov., 62(6): 431-436.

Coats AC and Martin JL (1977): Human auditory nerve action potentials and brainstem evoked responses: Effects of audiogram shape and lesion location. Arch. Otolaryngol., 103:105.

Costa P, Benna P, Bianco C, Ferrero P and Bergamasco B (1990): Aging effects on brainstem auditory evoked potentials. Electromyogr. Clin. Neurophysiol. Dec., 30(8):495-500.

Cutler JR, Aminoff MJ and Zawadzki M (1985): Evaluation of patients with multiple sclerosis by evoked potentials and magnetic resonance imaging. Ann. Neurol., 20:645-648.

De Montes C, Manjn M and Viuales M (2002): Morphological study of brainstem auditory evoked potentials. the effect of the position of the reference electrode. Rev. Neurol. Jan 1;34(1):84-88.

Elvin A, Andersson T and Soderstrom M (1998): Optic neuritis. Doppler ultrasonography compared with MR and correlated with visual evoked potential assessments . Acta Radiol. May, 39(3):243-248.

Elwany S (1985): Brainstem auditory evoked potentials in patients with the lateral medullary (Wallenberg's) syndrome. ORL J Otorhinolaryngol Relat. Spec., 47(2):90-94.

Erwin CW (1980): Pattern reversal evoked potentials. Am. J. EEG technol., 20:161-184.

Fenwick PB and Robertson R (1983): Changes in the visual evoked potential to pattern reversal with lithium medication. Electroencephalogr. Clin. Neurophysiol. May., 55(5):538-545.

Ferrer S, Jimenez P, Mellado L and Thieck E (1993): Clinical correlations and evoked potentials in 29 cases of definitive multiple sclerosis. Rev Med Chil Oct; 121(10): 1154-1160.

Fitzgerald PF, Picton TW, Maru J and Wolfe RG (1980): Pattern reversal visual responses. Proceedings from 1st. international workshop and symposium on evoked potentials, Milan.

Fujii M, Tomita T, McLone DG, Grant JA and Mori K (1996): Natural course of brainstem auditory evoked potentials in infants less than 6 months old with asymptomatic meningomyelocele. Pediatr. Neurosurg. Nov., 25(5):227-232.

Garcia-Larrea L, Artru F and Bertrand O (1988): Transient drug-induced abolition of BAEPs in coma. Neurology Sep., 38(9):1487-1489.

Glaser JS (1990): Topical diagnosis: prechiasmal visual pathways. Ophthalmology. 91:255-262.

Goldie WD, Chiappa KH and Young RR (1981): Brainstem auditory and short-latency somatosensory evoked responses in brain death. Neurology Mar., 31(3):248-256.

Goodin D, Nuwer MR, Aminoff M, Matsuoka S and Starr A (1994): IFCN recommended standards for brainstem auditory evoked potentials. Report of an IFCN committee. Electroencephalography and clinical neurophysiology, February; 91:12-17.

Gordon ML and Cohen NL (1995): Efficacy of auditory brainstem response as a screening test for small acoustic neuromas. Am. J. Otol. Mar., 16(2):136-139.

Gottlob I, Weghaupt H, Vass C and Auff E (1989): Effect of levodopa on the human pattern electroretinogram and pattern visual evoked potentials. Graefes. Arch. Clin. Exp. Ophthalmol., 227(5):421-427.

Halliday AM (1982): The Visual EP in clinical testing. Halliday AMI (ed.), Churchill Livingstone, London, (first edition), Pp. 71-120.

Halliday AM, Butler SR and Paul R (Eds) (1987): Visual potential. A textbook of Clinical Neurology. A. Wiley Medical Publication Pp. 348-367.

Halliday AM, Halliday E and Kriss A (1976): The pattern-evoked potential in compression of the anterior visual pathways. Prog. Brain Res. 99:357-374.

Halliday AM, Mc Donald WI and Mushin J (1977): Visual evoked potentials in patients with demyelinating disease . In Desmedt JE (ed): Visual evoked potentials in man: New Developments. Clarendon Press, Oxford. Pp. 438.

Halliday AM, Mconald WI and Mushin J (1973): Delayed pattern responses in optic neuritis in relation to visual acuity. Trans. Ophthalmo. Soc. UK vol. 93:315-324.

Harter MR and White CT (1968): Effects of contour sharpness and check size on visually evoked cortical potentials. Vision Res., 8:Pp. 701-711.

Hutchinson M, Blandford S, Glynn D and Martin EA (1984): Clinical correlates of abnormal brain-stem auditory evoked responses in multiple sclerosis. Acta Neurol. Scand. Aug., 70(2):90-95.

Ikeda H, Nishijo H and Miyamoto K (1998): Generators of visual evoked potentials investigated by dipole tracing in the human occipital cortex. Neuroscience Jun., 84(3):723-739.

Ipata A, Girelli M and Miniussi C (1997): Interhemispheric transfer of visual information in humans: The role of different callosal channels. Arch. Ital. Biol. Mar., 135(2):169-182.

Jiang ZD, Zhang L, Wu YY and Liu XY (1993): Brainstem auditory evoked responses from birth to adulthood: development of wave amplitude. Hear. Res. Jun., 68(1):35-41.

Jones SJ, Carroll WM, Halliday AM. Peripheral and central sensory conduction in Charcot-Marie-Tooth disease and comparison with Friedreich's ataxia J Neurol Sci 1983;61:135-48.

Kaplan PW, Tusa RJ and Shankroff J (1993): Visual evoked potentials in adrenoleukodystrophy: a trial with glycerol trifoliate and Lorenzo oil. Ann. Neurol. Aug., 34(2):169-174.

Kern W, Kerner W and Pietrowsky R (1994): Effects of insulin and hypoglycemia on the auditory brainstem response in humans. J. Neurophysiol. Aug., 72(2):678-683.

Kileny PR, Niparko JK and Shepard NT (1988): Neurophysiologic intraoperative monitoring: I. Auditory function. Am. J. Otol. Dec., 9 Suppl: 17-24.

Kimura J (1985): Abuse and misuse of evoked potentials. Arch. Neuro. 48:78-80.

Kjaer M (1987): Brainstem auditory and visual evoked potentials in multiple sclerosis. Acta Neurol. Scand. Jul., 62(1):14-19.

Knott VJ (1987): Acute effects of tobacco on human brain stem evoked potentials. Addict. Behav., 12(4):375-379.

Kojima S, Hirayama K, Kakisu Y and Adachi E (1990): Magnetic resonance imaging in optic nerve lesions with multiple sclerosis. No To Shinkei, 42:1191.

Kriss A (1980): Setting up an evoked potential laboratory. In evoked potentials in clinical testing edited by AN Halliday (First edition), Churchill Livingstone, New York. Pp. 10-45.

Lehmann D and Soukos I (1982): Visual evoked potentials and click-evoked brainstem potentials in early diagnosis of multiple sclerosis: statistics. Nervenarzt.. Jun., 53(6):327-332.

Lennerstrand G (1982): Delayed visual evoked cortical potentials in retinal disease. Acta Ophthalmol., 60:497.

Leserve N and Romand A (1972): Effects of the diminution of the pattern and density of contrast on evoked potentials. Electroenceph. Clin. Neurophysiol., 35:239-247.

Leslie H, Andrew SB and Francisco T (2002): Clinical Utility of Evoked Potentials. e Medicine, Neurology, Electroencephalography and evoked potentials, May, 30:1-8.

Lutschg J, Meyer E, Jeanneret-Iseli C and Kaiser G (1985): Brainstem auditory evoked potentials in meningomyelocele. Neuropediatrics, Nov., 16(4):202-204.

Mackay DM and Jeffreys DA (1973): Visual evoked potentials and visual perception in man. In: Handbook of sensory physiology. Vol. VII/3 part B. Edited by R Jung Springer, New York, Berlin, Heidelberg. Pp. 647-678.

Markand ON (1994): Brainstem auditory evoked potentials. J. Clin. Neurophysiol. May., 11(3):319-342.

Matsuoka S, Nuwer MR, Aminoff M, Goodin D and Starr A (1994): IFCN recommended standards for brain-stem auditory evoked potentials. Report of an IFCN committee. Electroencephalography and clinical neurophysiology, February; 91:12-17.

Matthews WB, Read DJ and Pountney E (1979): Effects of raising body temperature on visual and somatosensory evoked potentials in patients with multiple sclerosis. J. Neurol. Neurosurg. Psychiatry., 42:250-255.

McDonald WI and Brans D (1992): The ocular manifestations of multiple sclerosis. Abnormalities of the visual system. J. Neurol. Neurosurg. Psychiatry, 55:747-752.

Michalewski HJ, Thompson LW, Patterson JV, Bowman TE and Litzelman D (1980): Sex differences in the amplitudes and latencies of the human auditory brainstem potential. Electroencephalogr. Clin. Neurophysiol. Mar., 48(3):351-356.

Nicholson G, Corbett A. Slowing of central conduction in X-linked Charcot-Marie-Tooth neuropathy shown by brain stem auditory evoked responses. J Neurol Neurosurg Psychiatry 1996;61:43-6.

Nuwer MR, Aminoff M, Goodin D, Matsuoka S and Starr A (1994): IFCN recommended standards for brainstem auditory evoked potentials. Report of an IFCN committee. Electroencephalography and clinical neurophysiology, February., 91:12-17.

Oudesluys-Murphy AM, Van Straaten HL and Bholasingh R (1996): Neonatal hearing screening. Eur. J. Pediatr. Jun., 155(6):429-435.

Phelps ME, Mazziotta JC, Kuhl DE, Nuwer M, Packwood J and Engel J (1981): Tomographic mapping of human cerebral metabolism. Visual stimulation and deprivation. Neurol., 31:517-529.

Picton TW, Hillyard SA, Krauzs HI and Galambos R (1974): Human auditory evoked potentials: I. Evaluation of components. Electroencephalogr. Clin. Neurophysiol. 36:179-190.

Picton TW, Stapells DR and Combell KB (1982): Auditory evoked potentials from the human choclea and brainstem. J. Otolaryngol. Supp 9:1-14.

Poon's M (2003a): Visual Evoked Potentials. Michael Poon's Shrine of Neurology, 12 March, Pp. 1-5.

Poon's M (2003b): Brainstem Auditory Evoked Potentials. Michael Poon's Shrine of Neurology, 14 May., Pp.1-3.

Purves SJ, Low MD and Galloway J (1981): A comparison of visual, brainstem auditory, and somatosensory evoked potentials in multiple sclerosis. Can. J. Neurol. Sci. Feb., 8(1):15-19.

Richard-Caton (1875): The electric currents of the brain. Br. Med. J.,2: 278.

Rosenhall ULF, Bjorkman G, Pederson K and Kall A (1985): Brainstem auditory evoked potentials in different age groups. Electroenceph. Clin. Neurophysiol. Vol 62:426-430.

Row MJ (1980): The brainstem auditory evoked response (BAER) in patients with vertigo. Electroencephalogr. Clin. Neurophysiol., 49:45.

Row MJ III (1978): Normal variability of the brainstem auditory evoked responses in young and old adult subjects. Electroenceph. Clin. Neurophysiol. 44:428-459.

Russel MH, Murray IJ, Metcalfe RA and Kulikowski L (1991): The visual defect in multiple sclerosis and optic neuritis. Prog. Brain Res., 144, 2419-2435.

Sannita WG, Fatone M and Garbarino S (1995): Effects of physiological changes of serum glucose on the pattern-VEP of healthy volunteers. Physiol. Behav. Nov., 58(5):1021-1026.

Scaioli V, Pareyson D, Avanzini G, et al. F response and somatosensory and brainstem auditory evoked potential studies in HMSN type I and II. J Neurol Neurosurg Psychiatry 1992;55:1027-31.

Schmidt RJ, Sataloff RT and Newman J (2001): The sensitivity of auditory brainstem response testing for the diagnosis of acoustic neuromas. Arch. Otolaryngol. Head & Neck Surg., 127(1):19-22.

Schwarz G, Litscher G and Rumpl E (1996): Brainstem auditory evoked potentials in respiratory insufficiency following encephalitis. Int. J. Neurosci. Feb., 84(1-4):35-44.

Shagass C (1976): Evoked brain potential in man. In: Generally RG and Gabay S (eds). Biological foundations of psychiatry. New York: Raven Press. Pp. 199-253.

Shearer DE and Dustman RE (1980): The pattern reversal evoked potential, The need for laboratory norms. Am. J. EEG Technol., 20:185-200.

Shibata K, Osawa M and Iwata M (1997): Pattern reversal visual evoked potentials in classic and common migraine. J. Neurol. Sci. Feb., 12; 145(2):177-181.

Sokol S (1980): Visual evoked potential. In electrodiagnosis in clinical neurology edited by M. Aminoff. Churchill Livingstone, New York, Pp. 348-378.

Sokol S, Moskowitz A and Towle LE (1981): Age related changes in the latency of the visual evoked potential. Influence of check size. Electroenceph. Clin. Neurophysiol., 51:559-562.

Starr A, Allen A and Don M (1976): Effect of click rate on the latency of auditory brainstem response in man. Ann. Otol., 86:186-195.

Starr A, Nuwer MR, Aminoff M, Goodin D and Matsuoka S (1994): IFCN recommended standards for brainstem auditory evoked potentials. Report of an IFCN committee. Electroencephalography and clinical neurophysiology, February., 91:12-17.

Stephen W (1983): Brainstem auditory evoked potentials. American Academy of Neurology, Annual course 209:35-52.

Stern BJ, Krumholz A, Weiss HD, Goldstein P and Harris KC (1982): Evaluation of brainstem stroke using brainstem auditory evoked responses. Stroke. Sep-Oct.,13(5):705-711.

Stockard JJ, Hughes JF and Sharbrough FW (1979): Visually evoked potentials to electronic pattern reversal. Latency variations with gender, age technical factors. Am J EEG 19:171-204.

Stockard JJ, Stockard JE and Sharbrough FW (1978): Non pathological factors influencing brain stem auditory evoked potential. Amer. J. EEG Technol. 18:117-209.

Stockard JJ, Stockard JE and Sharbrough FW (1980b): Brainstem auditory evoked potentials in neurology: Methodology interpretation clinical application. In: Electrodiagnosis in clinical neurology edited by Aminoff. Churchill Livingstone, New York Pp. 370-413.

Tandon OP and Krishna SV (1990): Brainstem auditory evoked potentials in children a normative study. Indian Pediatr. Jul.,27(7):737-740.

Tarantino V, Stura M and Vallarino R (1988): Development of auditory evoked potentials of the brainstem in relation to age. Pediatr. Med. Chir. Jan-Feb.,10(1):73-76.

Taylor MJ, Boor R and Keenan NK (1996): Brainstem auditory and visual evoked potentials in infants with myelomeningocele. Brain Dev. Mar-Apr., 18(2): 99-104.

Tony Wu, Hung-Li Wang1, Chun-Che Chu, Jia-Ming Yu2, Jeng-Yeou Chen3, Chin-Chang Huang (2004): Clinical and Electrophysiological Studies of a Family with Probable X-linked Dominant Charcot-Marie-Tooth Neuropathy and Ptosis. Chang Gung Med J Vol. 27 No. 7

Tsuda H, Katsumi Y and Nakamura M (1995): Cerebral blood flow and metabolism in Lafora disease. Rinsho. Shinkeigaku. Feb., 35(2):175-179.

Yiannikas C and Walsh JC (1983): The variation of the pattern shift visual evoked response with the size of the stimulus field. Clin. Neurophysio., 55:427-436.

Yuksel A, Sarslan O and Devranoglu K (1995): Effect of valproate and carbamazepine on visual evoked potentials in epileptic children. Acta. Paediatr. Jpn. Jun., 37(3):358-361.

EMG and Evoked Potentials in the Operating Room During Spinal Surgery

Induk Chung and Arthur A. Grigorian

Georgia Neurosurgical Institute and Mercer University School of Medicine, Macon, GA, USA

1. Introduction

EMG is an important clinical electrodiagnostic tool to assess function of neuromuscular tissue. It assesses spinal motor nerve roots and determines correct placement of hardware in surgical procedures, including cervical, thoracic, and lumbosacral spinal decompression, instrumentation, and fixation of spinal deformity. Evoked potentials provide information on vascular compromise of the spinal cord and nerves. Hence, concurrent recordings of EMG and evoked potentials can assess function integrity of the spinal cord and nerve more accurately. In this chapter, we will discuss application of EMG and evoked potentials in spinal surgery.

2. EMG recording techniques in the operating room (OR)

2.1 Recording electrodes

Surface, intramuscular, and subdermal needle electrodes are used to record EMG activity in the OR. Surface electrodes may not be used because of their inability to detect neurotonic discharges in spine surgery (Skinner et al., 2008). In addition, sweat causes electrodes to detach from the skin, preventing stable recording during lengthy surgery (Chung, unpublished data). Both intramuscular and subdermal needle electrodes are sufficient to detect neurotonic discharges (Skinner et al., 2008). Intramuscular needle electrodes may have an advantage to record EMG activity when the subcutaneous tissue is thick. Subdermal needle electrodes (13 mm length and 0.4 mm diameter) are generally used to record EMG in the OR, and we also routinely use subdermal needle electrodes in our practice.

2.2 Recording parameters

EMG is a simple and reliable technique which does not interfere with the surgical procedure. It is important to use proper recording parameters to achieve EMG recordings to obtain high signal-to-noise ratio. Recommended parameters of routine free-run EMG are low-frequency filter (LFF) of 20-30 Hz, high frequency filter (HFF) of 1-3 KHz, a gain of 500-5,000, a sensitivity of 50-500 µV, and a sweep speed of 10-200 msec per division (Toleikis et al., 2000; Bose et al., 2002; Chung et al., 2009). LFF of greater than 50 Hz and HFF of less than 3 KHz should be avoided. Impedance of subdermal needle electrodes is recommended to be less than 5 KΩ, for impedance greater than 5 KΩ may mask real EMG activity. If impedance of all electrodes is too high, ground electrode should be replaced. If a particular electrode gives high impedance, the electrode should be replaced.

2.3 Muscle group selections and electrode placement

EMG in spinal surgery should cover all nerve roots at risk innervated by surgical levels. In routine EMG, depending on the surgical levels and number of channels available, bipolar electrodes (an active and a reference) are placed subdermally over the belly of each muscle group of interest. Electrodes should be placed ~1 cm apart with care and secured with tape to prevent dislodgement. EMG should be recorded from the bilateral muscle groups to increase specificity of nerve root activation. If fewer channels are available in the monitoring equipment, an active electrode is placed in one muscle and a reference electrode is placed in other muscle. Multiple nerve roots can be monitored with this montage, but it may be difficult to identify specific nerve root at risk. Table 1 indicates representative muscle groups to be recorded during spinal surgery (Leppanen, 2008).

Cervical	Muscle
C2, C3, C4	Trapezius, Sternomastoid (spinal portion of the spinal accessory nerve)
C5, C6	Deltoid, Biceps
C6	Triceps, Extensor Carpi Radialis
C7	Flexor Carpi Radialis
C8, T1	Abductor Pollicis Brevis, Abductor Digiti Minimi
Thoracic	
T5, T6	Upper Rectus Abdominis
T7, T8	Middle Rectus Abdominis
T9, T10, T11	Lower Rectus Abdominis
T12	Inferior Rectus Abdominis
Lumbar	
L2, L3, L4	Vastus Medialis, Adductor Magnus
L4. L5, S1	Vastus Lateralis, Tibialis Anterior
L5, S1	Proneous Longus, Gastrocnemius
Sacral	
S1, S2	Gastrocnemius
S2, S3, S4	External anal sphincter

Table 1. Representative muscle groups innervated by the cervical, thoracic, lumbar, and sacral nerve roots.

3. EMG recording

3.1 Neuromuscular junction (NMJ) recording

Blockade of NMJ significantly attenuates motor activity. Short acting muscle relaxants may be used to facilitate intubation, but long acting muscle relaxants should be avoided. If pre-existing nerve root injury should be identified, succinylcholine, an NMJ blocking agent, is recommended to use. However, succinylcholine should not be used for patients with malignant hyperthermia (Minahan et al., 2000).

There are electrical stimulation techniques to monitor status of NMJ, and these are single twitch, train-of-four (TOF) twitch ratio, tetanus, post-tetanic stimulation, and pulse or double burst technique (Leppanen, 2008). TOF twitch ratio is routinely used during surgery. Electrical stimulation (stimulation frequency of 1 Hz, duration of 300~500 msec, and intensity of 10~40 mA) is delivered to a peripheral nerve 4 times, and 4 resulting compound muscle action potentials (CMAPs) are recorded. TOF is monitored from the thenar eminence following stimulation of the median nerve, the abductor pollicis brevis following stimulation of the ulnar nerve at the wrist, the tibialis anterior following stimulation of the peroneal nerve at the knee, or the abductor hallucis following stimulation of the posterior tibial nerve. It is recommended that TOF should be monitored in a muscle of the extremity where EMG activity is being monitored (Minahan et al., 2000; Leppanen, 2008). Four of four twitch ratio is obtained if less than 75% of NMJ is blocked. Three of four twitch ratio is obtained with 75% blockade, 2 of 4 with 80% blockade, and 1 of 4 with 90% blockade. No twitch is obtained if 100% of NMJ is blocked (Leppanen, 2008). It is not desirable to use muscle relaxants during surgical procedures where direct stimulation of pedicle screws and nerve roots are required (Minahan et al., 2000).

3.2 Free-run EMG

The dorsal and ventral roots spit into rootlets and minirootlets. The nerve root is susceptible to mechanical injury at the area that the split is present. The axons at this point are enclosed by a thin root sheath and cerebrospinal fluid meninges, but lack epineurim and perineurim. Hypovascularity at the junction of the proximal and middle 1/3 of the dorsal and ventral roots place nerve roots more susceptible to injury (Berthold et al., 1984). Intraoperative free-run EMG is utilized to detect motor nerve root compromise during decompression for spinal stenosis and spondylosis, correction of spinal deformity, radiculopathy secondary to disc herniation, and removal of tumor involving neural tissue in anterior and posterior surgical approaches (Holmes et al., 1993; Beatty et al., 1995; Maguire et al., 1995; Welch et al., 1997; Balzer et al., 1998; Toleikis et al., 2000; Bose et al., 2002; Chung et al., 2011).

To determine any pre-existing nerve root injury, baseline EMG recording is made before surgery starts. EMG recording is then made continuously throughout the surgical procedure. Pre-existing nerve root injury will be shown as spontaneous activity with low amplitude and periodic activity, whereas a normal free-run EMG response is absence of activity. If small amplitude, low frequency, or isolated discharge occurs at times which do not correlate with surgical manipulation of nerve roots, the EMG may not be pathologic. Mechanically elicited activity is characterized as polyphasic or a burst pattern consisting of single or nonrepetitive asynchronous potentials (Fig. 1A). Tonic or train activity consisting of multiple or repetitive synchronous discharges may last for several minutes (Fig. 1B). Burst potentials are associated with direct nerve trauma such as tugging, displacement, free irrigation, electrocautery, and application of soaked pledgets, but may not be associated with neural insult. Train activity is related to sustained traction and compression of nerve roots, and it is more associated with neural injury. When these patterns occur, the surgeon should be notified and corrective maneuver should occur. Audio and visual signal recognitions are available in most monitoring equipment. For communication with the operating surgeon, it is recommended to use audio signal through loud speakers for immediate feedback.

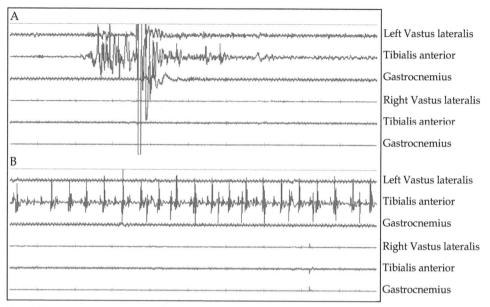

Fig. 1. Free-run EMG. EMG activity was recorded from the vastus lateralis, tibialis anterior, and gastrocnemius muscles during posterior spinal decompression. Bursts (A) and prolonged trains (B) of EMG activity are present in the left tibialis anterior muscle during decompression of nerve roots. Sensitivity 100 μV, time base 2 sec.

3.3 Stimulated EMG
3.3.1 Monitoring segmental motor nerve root function

Segmental nerve root monitoring involves monitoring of function of the motor unit axon. This is achieved by recording free-run and electrically stimulated EMG activity from the muscle fibers of the motor units. When EMG activity is recorded with needle electrodes, the activity recorded may be the result of activation of only a few motor units innervating that muscle. Other motor units may be activated, but this activation will go undetected because of the location of the recording electrodes. A monopolar EMG needle records the summated activity of 9 to 17 muscle fibers (Leppanen, 2008).

Motor nerve root stimulation technique is applied when motor axons and non-neural tissue (tumor, scar) should be identified and differentiated between motor and sensory roots. When scar tissue is present from previous surgical procedures, electrical stimulation can identify where the motor axons lie within the scar tissue. The direct nerve root stimulation technique is also used to determine a degree of decompression of compressed nerve roots. A nerve root is stimulated using an insulated ball-tip probe, and a reference needle electrode placed around the site of incision. The current (duration of 0.1 msec, frequency of 1-3 Hz) is gradually increased until stimulus evoked EMG responses or CMAPs are recorded from the muscle innervated by the nerve root. Stimulation threshold should not be greater than several milliamperes for uninjured motor nerve roots when neural tissue is directly stimulated. If tumor or scar is stimulated and threshold is greater than this value, viable neural tissue lies within the tumor or scar or no neural tissue is involved (Holland et al., 1998; Leppanen, 2008).

3.3.2 Evaluation of pedicle screws

3.3.2.1 Pedicle screw stimulation technique

Electrophysiological pedicle screw stimulation technique has been developed to assess whether the screws have been placed within the pedicle bone. The principle of the pedicle screw stimulation technique is that the electrical resistance of bone is higher than that of surrounding fluid and soft tissue. If an implanted pedicle screw is completely surrounded by bone, the screw is electrically shielded and electrical stimulation of the screw will fail to activate the nerve (Fig. 2A). However, if there is a breach in the medical wall of the pedicle, a low resistance pathway is formed between the screw and the adjacent tissue (Fig. 2B and C). Application of electrical current to the screw will result in stimulation of the nerve root and a subsequent muscle contraction, which is recorded as a CMAP. Constant current or constant voltage stimulations can be used, and constant current stimulation appears less variable than constant voltage stimulation. For direct screw stimulation, monopolar, cathodal, constant current stimulation (duration of 0.2 msec, frequency of 1~3 Hz) is delivered using an insulated ball-tip probe, and the anodal reference needle electrode is placed in or around the site of incision. The current is gradually increased until CMAPs are elicited (Leppanen, 2008).

3.3.2.2 Evaluation of lumbosacral pedicel screws

Spinal instrumentation technique with pedicle screws and rods has long been used correct spinal instability and deformity, for it provides rigidity for the vertebral motion segment. However, incorrect placement of screws results in considerable radicular pain or postoperative neurological deficits (Matsuzaki et al., 1990; West et al., 1991). Although intraoperative fluoroscopy or postoperative radiography guide screw placement, these image studies may not detect functional integrity of pedicle screws. For instance, pedicle screw stimulation technique was 93% sensitive, whereas radiography was 63% sensitive to detect drill bits and screws that had breached the cortex (Maguire et al., 1995). Pedicle screw stimulation could detect incorrect screw placement in 8 out of 90 patients that was not identified on radiograph (Glassman et al., 1995). With 102 pedicle screws placed in 18 patients, 7 mA was delivered to test correct placement of screws. Electrophysiological evidence of a perforation was seen in 13% of the patients, but palpation or visualization could not detect this perforation (Calancie et al., 1994).

It appears that there is close correlation between the intensity of screw stimulation to elicit CMAPs and the risk for neurological injury associated with the screw placement. A stimulation threshold of 10~15 mA was associated with adequate screw position in 512 pedicle screws implanted to 90 patients, but exploration of the pedicle was recommended. A stimulation threshold of greater than 15 mA indicated adequate screw position. A threshold of 5~10 mA was used as an indicator of abnormal thresholds (Glassman et al., 1995). With 3,409 pedicle screws placed in 662 patients, a threshold of 7~10 mA was associated with pedicle breach or a slight medial exposure of the screw. With threshold of 5~7 mA, there was a 58% likelihood that the screw should be removed and redirected. A stimulation threshold of less than 5 mA was associated with a significant cortical perforation and direct contact with a nerve root (Toleikis et al., 2000). A stimulus threshold of less than 6 mA correlated with misplaced drill bits and screws that breached the cortex in 144 screws and 95 drill bits tested in 29 patients (Maguire et al., 1995).

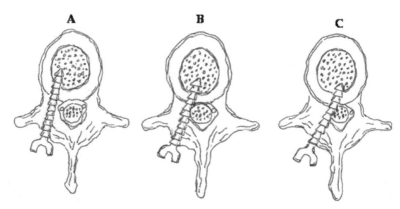

Fig. 2. Placement of pedicle screws. Screws are placed within the pedicle (A), close to the medical wall of the pedicle (B), or breach the cortex to make a direct contact with a nerve root (C).

Fig. 3 is a representative trace of CMAPs following stimulation of a pedicle screw. CMAPs were recorded mostly from the right vastus lateralis and tibialis anterior muscles with a stimulation threshold of 17 mA, indicating that the pedicle screw was placed securely within the pedicle bone.

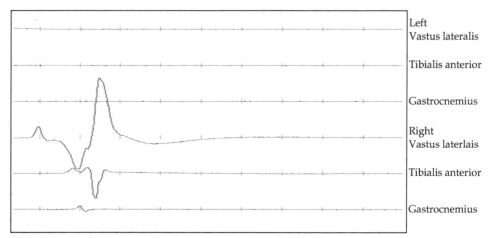

Fig. 3. CMAPs were elicited following electrical stimulation of the pedicle screw. EMG was recorded from the bilateral vastus lateralis, tibialis anterior, and gastrocnemius muscles. Current (duration of 0.2 msec, frequency of 1 Hz) was slowly increased to right L4 pedicle screw head via monopolar ball-tip probe. CMAPs were recorded mostly from the right vastus lateralis and tibialis anterior muscles at the current threshold of 17 mA. Sensitivity 200 µV, timebase 0.1 sec.

3.3.2.3 Evaluation of cervical pedicle screws

C5 nerve root palsy is most commonly attributed to direct nerve root injury secondary to manipulation or traction of the nerve root and a segmental spinal cord injury secondary to ischemia. Free-run EMG monitoring could detect potential injury to single nerve root (Fan et al., 2002; Bose et al., 2004; Hillbrand et al., 2004; Khan et al., 2006). Simulated EMG technique for posterior cervical screws is also a useful tool to guide screw placement. Djurasovic and colleagues (2005) tested the lateral mass and pedicle screws (122 lateral mass screws and 25 C7 pedicle screws) implanted in 26 patients. A stimulation threshold of 15 mA provided a 99% positive predictive value (89% sensitivity and 87% specificity) that the screw was within the lateral mass or pedicle. A stimulation threshold of 10~15 mA provided a 13% predictive value (66% sensitivity and 90% specificity) that the screw was within the lateral mass or pedicle. A stimulation threshold of less than 10 mA provided a 100% predictive value that the screw was malpositioned (70% sensitivity and 100% specificity).

3.3.2.4 Evaluation of thoracic pedicle screws

Placement of thoracic pedicle screws is a considerable technical challenge because of the smaller pedicle size (Cinotti et al., 1999). The risk of misplacement of screws in the thoracic spine ranged between 16% and 41% even with careful probing of the pedicle wall (Vaccaro et al., 1995; Xu et al., 1999). Simulation threshold values did not seem to reflect whether the screws were correctly positioned nor predict postoperative outcomes associated with the screw placement (Danesh-Clough et al., 2001). With 87 thoracic pedicle screws placed in 22 patients, 81 screws had a stimulus threshold >11 mA and 6 screws had thresholds ≤11 mA, of which 3 showed cortical breakthrough. However, new postoperative neurologic complications did not result in any of the 22 patients (Shi et al., 2003). Two hundred and nine thoracic pedicle screws were placed in 29 patients. Five of 6 screws penetrated cortical bone in one patient, but no new postoperative neurologic deficit, visceral injuries, or pedicle screw instrumentation failure was developed in this patient (Kuntz et al., 2004). Six hundred and seventy-seven thoracic pedicle screws were placed in 92 patients, and 27 screws had a stimulation threshold of <6.0 mA and 6 of 27 screws had medial wall perforations. There were no new postoperative neurologic deficits or radicular chest wall complaints (Raynor et al., 2002). One hundred and sixteen thoracic pedicle screws were placed in 7 patients. There were medical wall defects in 19 screws, and average stimulus thresholds of these pedicle screws were 19.8±5.3 mA. Eight of these 19 screws had thresholds 25~30 mA (Donohue et al., 2008).

4. Evoked potentials

Free-run and stimulated EMG can detect injury to neural tissue during surgical manipulations. However, the same technique fails to detect malpositioned thoracic pedicle screws and predict postoperative outcomes. Literature indicates that evoked potential monitoring assesses integrity of the spinal cord and nerve roots and improve clinical efficacy of EMG monitoring.

4.1 Somatosensory evoked potential (SSEPs) and recording technique

SSEP is an evoked response generated from nerve tracts and nuclei in the brain after peripheral nerve stimulation. Typically, the median or ulnar nerves at the wrist is stimulated to acquire SSEPs from the upper extremities and the posterior tibial nerve at the ankle or the peroneal nerve at the fibular head to acquire SSEPs from the lower extremities. The ascending sensory volley enters the spinal cord through dorsal nerve roots at several segmental levels and ascends to the sensory cortex. SSEPs are mediated by primarily through the dorsal column (Nuwer, 1999) or dorsal spinocerebellar tracts (York,

1985). SSEPs are used to assess the functional status of somatosensory pathways during surgical procedures which affect peripheral nerve or plexus (Prielipp et al., 1999; Chung et al., 2009), spinal cord (deformity correction, traumatic spinal fracture, tumor removal, Duffau, 2008), and brain (carotid endarterectomy, aneurysm repair, Friedman et al., 1991; Lam et al., 1991).

For upper extremity SSEP recordings, cortical (C3, C4 of the international 10-20 system, reference to Fz) and subcortical SSEPs (cervical spinous process, reference to Fz) are monitored upon alternate stimulation of the median or ulnar nerve at the wrist (stimulation intensity of ~20 mA, stimulation frequency of 3.1 Hz, stimulation duration of 0.5 msec) through surface electrodes (Fig. 4, left panel). For lower extremity SSEP recordings, cortical (Cz, reference to Fz) and subcortical SSEP (cervical spinous process, reference to Fz) are monitored upon alternate stimulation of the posterior tibial nerve at the ankle or peroneal nerve at the popliteal fossa (stimulation intensity of ~30 mA, stimulation frequency of

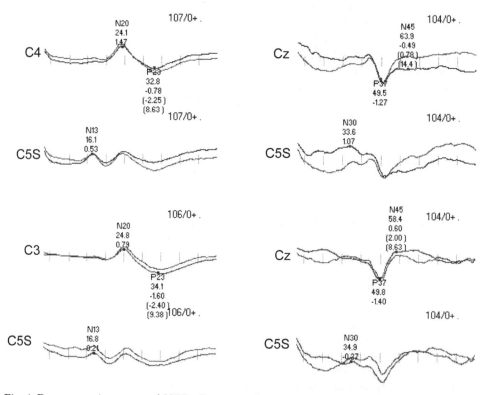

Fig. 4. Representative traces of SSEPs. Traces on the left column are upper-extremity SSEPs recorded from C3, C4 for cortical response and C5 spinous process for subcortical response following alternate stimulation of the ulnar nerve at the wrist (Timebase 50 msec). Lower-extremity SSEPs are shown in the right column. SSEPs were recorded from Cz and C5 spinous process following alternate stimulation of the posterior tibial nerve at the ankle (Timebase 100msec). The number of averaged samples, latency (msec), and amplitude (µV) are indicated in the trace. Parentheses indicate interpeak latency and interpeak amplitude.

3.1 Hz, a stimulation duration of 0.5 msec) through surface electrodes (Fig. 4, right panel). A few hundreds of samples (sampling rate of 8 kHz) are required to average to increase a signal-to-noise ratio. Signals were amplified (gain of 5,000~20,000) and filtered (LFF of 30 Hz, HFF of 300 Hz,). Impedance of electrodes should be ~5 KΩ. All of these electrical connections are grounded at patient's shoulder (Balzer et al., 1998; Chung et al., 2009).

4.2 Motor evoked potentials (MEPs) and recording technique

MEPs assess functional integrity of the anterolateral column of the spinal cord. MEPs provide information about long tract function, segmental interneurons, and anterior gray matter function. Epidural stimulation of the spinal cord and transcranial electrical (TES) or magnetic stimulation (TMS) of the motor cortex of the brain are the techniques used to obtain MEPs. TES is the most favorite technique utilized in the OR (McDonald, 2002, 2006). TES technique involves eliciting CMAPs after transcranial electrical stimulation of motor area at 1~2cm anterior to C3 and C4, referenced to C4 and C3 (Calalncie et al., 1998; Chung et al., 2011) or C1 and C2, reference to C2 and C1 (Bose et al., 2004; Drake et al., 2010). For electrical stimulation, an internal or external stimulator can be used. Some monitoring equipment has its own internal stimulator. An external cortical stimulator is also used for this purpose. Digitimer™ D185 Multipulse stimulator (Digitimer Ltd., Welwyn Garden City, UK) is the only FDA approved stimulator for this clinical use. It has capabilities to control inter-stimulation interval (ISI) and stimulation intensity up to 1,000 volts. Multipulse stimulation technique (4~6 repetitive stimulations and ISI of 1~2 msec) is usually applied (Calalncie et al., 1998; Bose et al., 2004; Drake et al., 2010; Chung et al., 2011). Stimulation thresholds range between a few hundreds and several hundreds of volts to elicit CMAPs depending on pathophysiological status of the spinal cord, depth of anesthesia, and bone thickness. Evoked CMAPs are recorded from the muscles of upper and lower extremities as indicated in Table 1.

Representative traces of MEPs are shown in Fig. 5. After TES, evoked CMAPs were recorded from the muscles of upper and lower extremities during placement of thoracic pedicle screws. Stable CMAPs were present in all the muscles during pedicle screw placement, and the patient did not develop new postoperative complication. We have been routinely testing MEPs during all cervical and thoracic spine surgery for the past over ten years, and the presence of stable MEPs is the most reliable indicator to assess cervical and thoracic spinal cord and nerve root function, instead of stimulation of mass and pedicle screws (Chung, unpublished data).

There are safety concerns to test MEPs for patients. High voltage transcranial electrical stimulation causes jaw movement, resulting in tong laceration and mandibular fracture in 0.2% of the patients undergoing TES. Bite blocks should be placed to prevent these complications. MEPs should not be tested for patients with pre-existing history of seizure, intracranial injury, or presence of intracranial metal implants (McDonald, 2002, 2006).

4.3 Dermatomal somatosensory evoked potentials (DSSEPs) and recording technique

Researchers have demonstrated that SSEPs increase specificity of EMG during lumbosacral (Holmes et al., 1993; Balzer et al., 1998; Chung, unpublished data) and anterior spine surgery (Chung et al., 2011). However, one can argue that SSEPs can not detect injury in a single nerve root because multiple nerve roots contribute to generate SSEPs. Dermatomal somatosensory evoked potentials (DSSEPs) are suggested to use when assessing function of individual nerve roots. Stimulation is achieved with paired patch paste skin electrode placed 3-4 cm apart at dermatomal sites such as L3 at anterior mid-thigh, L4 at medial

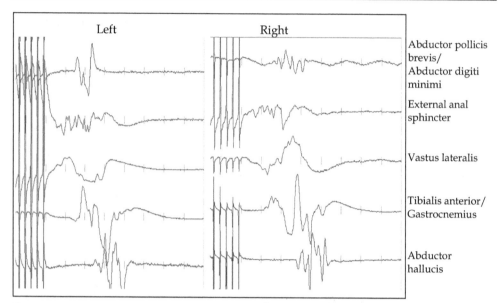

Fig. 5. MEPs were obtained after transcranial electrical stimulation (325V, ISI of 2 msec, 5 repetitive pulse trains). CMAPs were recorded from the abductor pollicis brevis/abductor digiti minimi, external anal sphincter, vastus laterlais, tibialis anterior/gastrocnemius, and abductor hallucis muscles bilaterally. Timebase 100 msec, 100msec, vertical scales 50-200 µV.

midcalf, L5 at the dorsum of the foot, and S1 at the lateral aspect of the foot. Responses are recorded from cervical spinous process. Recording parameters are stimulation intensity of ~40 mA, duration of 0.3 msec, frequency of 5.1 Hz, LFF of 30 Hz, and HFF of 1 KHz. Each trial usually consists of 500 samples (Tsai et al., 1997). Clinical efficacy of intraoperative DSSEPs appears controversial. DSSEPs are sensitive to detect nerve root compression and mechanical manipulation, but insensitive to nerve root decompression. DSSEPs can detect a misplaced pedicle screw only when the screw directly contacts and mechanically injures a nerve root (Toleikis, 1993). DSSEPs are difficult to record and often require averaging ~500 samples to increase a signal-to-noise ratio, indicating that DSSEPs can not detect mechanical insult immediately. Even with averaging more samples, Tsai and colleagues (1997) could obtain baseline in only 57.6% of the patients. Hence, it is suggested that DSSEPs may be an adjunct to improve the sensitivity and specificity for detecting individual nerve injury when free-run and/or stimulated EMG is concurrently recorded.

4.4 Clinical efficacy of SSEPs and MEPs

Research for over the past three decades supports that SSEPs can detect and prevent spinal cord injury in cervical and thoracic, lumbosacral spinal surgeries. No quadriplegia resulted in a group of 100 patients with SSEP monitoring, compared with 8 quadriplegic patients from a group of unmonitored 218 patients (Epstein et al., 1993). Five patients with persistent SSEP changes were associated with postoperative motor deficit among 20 patients undergoing cervical and thoracic intramedullary cervical cord tumor removal (Kearse et al., 1993). SSEPs could detect ischemia in 44 out of 210 patients undergoing anterior cervical surgery. With simultaneous monitoring of SSEPs and EMG during posterior lumbar spinal fusion, bursts and trains of EMG activity were associated with a concurrent decrease in amplitudes of SSEPs (Chung, unpublished data).

However, SSEPs may not be sensitive to predict postoperative clinical status in anterior cervical spine surgery. Significant SSEP amplitude changes were observed in 33 out of 191 patients, and 50% of the patients developed postoperative neurological deterioration in anterior and/or posterior cervical spinal surgery (May et al., 1996). In a study with 871 patients undergoing anterior cervical deformity surgery, 26 patients had significant SSEP changes, and only 5 patients had postoperative neurological deficit (Leung et al., 2005). In 508 patients undergoing anterior cervical discectomy and fusion (ACDF) with corpectomy, 8 patients had postoperative deficits with preserved SSEPs (Khan et al., 2006). Seven patients developed new postoperative neurological deficit with preserved SSEPs in 758 patients undergoing ACDF. SSEPs showed 35% sensitivity and 100% specificity to predict postoperative neurological functions (Chung et al., 2011). A retrospective study with 1,055 patients demonstrated that SSEPs had a sensitivity of 52% and a specificity of 100% to predict postoperative neurological status in cervical spine and spinal cord surgery (Kelleher et al., 2008). Quadriparesis and paraplegia still resulted in patients with preserved SSEPs in anterior cervical fusion (Ben-David et al., 1987; Bose et al., 2004; Smith et al., 2007; Taunt et al., 2005).

Simultaneous monitoring of SSEPs and MEPs has proven that MEP monitoring is more reliable than SSEP monitoring to predict postoperative motor deficits. Hillbrand and colleagues (2004) reported that 12 out of 427 patients undergoing cervical surgery had substantial or complete MEP loss. Ten patients restored MEPs with surgical intervention, and did not develop new postoperative deficit. Two patients with persistent MEP loss developed new postoperative motor weakness. This study claimed that MEP monitoring showed 100% sensitivity and 100% specificity to predict postoperative neurological status, whereas SSEP monitoring had 25% sensitivity and 100% specificity (Hillbrand et al, 2004). Six patients with persistent MEP loss had new postoperative deficits, whereas significant SSEP loss without MEP changes observed in 2 patients did not have postoperative deficit in 69 intracranial and spinal surgeries (Weinzierl et al., 2007). MEPs were also more sensitive than SSEPs for detection of ischemia. MEPs were lost due to fluctuating blood pressure, and an increase in the mean arterial pressure above 90 mmHg restored them in 1 patient, but SSEPs were preserved during the entire surgical course in this patient (Wee et al., 1989). MEPs were superior to SSEPs for detection and prediction of postoperative neurological status. Whereas MEPs showed 100% sensitivity and 77% specificity, SSEPs had 35% sensitivity and 100% specificity to predict postoperative neurological outcomes in 758 patients receiving ACDF (Chung et al., 2011).

5. Anesthesia

Although EMG is minimally sensitive to anesthesia, muscle relaxants should not be used during EMG recordings (Minahan et al., 2000). Evoked potentials, especially MEPs are highly sensitive to anesthesia, but monitoring was still feasible with propofol/fentanyl/nitrous oxide and partial neuromuscular blocking agents. In animal studies, inhalant anesthetics significantly increased onset latency and amplitudes of MEPs (Haghighi et al., 19990a, 1990b, 1996). Under general anesthesia with fentanyl/propofol/nitrous oxide, 20% and 40~60% nitrous oxide attenuated MEPs by 40~60% and 50~70%, respectively (vanDongen et al., 1999), and 66% of nitrous oxide completely abolished MEPs

(Zentner & Ebner, 1989). Narcotics were also shown to depress MEPs. Following administration of equipotent intravenous bolus of fentanyl, alfentanil, or sufentanil, amplitudes of MEPs were decreased to 34%, 43%, and 53% of baseline values, respectively (Thees et al., 1999). Total intravenous anesthetic or TIVA technique comprising remifentanil with minimally depressive agents such as ketamine and etomidate improved MEP recordings (Ghaly et al., 1999, 2001). Compared with sufentanil or fentanyl, remifentanil infusion could always produce stable MEPs with faster emergence (Chung, unpublished data).

6. Conclusion

Free-run and stimulated EMG assesses spinal motor nerve roots and determines correct placement of hardware in cervical, thoracic, and lumbosacral spinal surgeries. Because SSEPs and MEPs provide additional information on functional integrity of the spinal cord and nerves, SSEPs and MEPs together with free-run and stimulated EMG should provide more accurate assessment of spinal cord and nerve function during spinal surgery.

7. References

Balzer, JR.; Rose, RD.; Welch, WC.; Sclabassi, RJ. (1998) Simultaneous somatosensory evoked potential and electromyographic recordings during lumbosacral decompression and instrumentation. *Neurosurgery* 42:1318-1324

Beatty, RM.; McGuire, P.; Moroney, JM.; Holladay, FP. (1995) Continuous intraoperative electromyographic recording during spinal surgery. *J Neurosurg* 82:401-405

Ben-David, B.; Haller, G.; Taylor, P. (1987) Anterior spinal fusion complicated by paraplegia. A case report of a false-negative somatosensory evoked potential. *Spine* 12:536-539

Berthold, CH.; Carlstedt, T.; Coeneliuson, O. 1984. Anatomy of the root at the central-peripheral transitional region, In: *Peripheral neuropathy*, Dyck PJ, Thomas PK, Lambert EH, Bunge R (Eds.), pp 156-170, W. B. Saunders, Philadelphia.

Bose, B.; Sestokas, AK.; Schwartz, DM. (2004) Neurophysiological monitoring of spinal cord function during instrumented anterior cervical fusion. *Spine J* 4:202-207

Bose, B.; Wierzbowski, LR.; Sestokas, AK. (2002) Neurophysiologic monitoring of spinal nerve root function during instrumented posterior lumbar spine surgery. *Spine* 27:1444-1450

Calancie, B.; Harris, W.; Broton, JG.; Alexeeva, N.; Green, BA. (1998) "Threshold-level" multipulse transcranial electrical stimulation of motor cortex for intraoperative monitoring of spinal motor tracts: description of method and comparison to somatosensory evoked potential monitoring. *J Neurosurg* 88:457-470

Calancie, B.; Madsen, P.; Lebwohl, N. Stimulus-evoked EMG (1994) monitoring during transpedicular lumbosacral spine instrumentation: Initial clinical results. *Spine (Phila Pa 1976)* 19:2780-2786

Chung, I.; Glow, JA.; Dimopoulos, V.; Walid, S.; Smisson, HF.; Johnston, KW., et al (2009) Upper-limb somatosensory evoked potential monitoring in lumbosacral spine surgery: a prognostic marker for position- ulnar nerve injury. *Spine J* 9:287-295

Chung, I.; Glow, JA.; Grigorian, AA.; Smisson, HF.; Johnston, KW.; Robinson, JS. (2011) Clinical efficacy of intraoperative somatosensory and motor evoked potential monitoring during anterior cervical discectomy and fusion (ACDF): A review of 758 cases. Submitted to *Global Spine J*

Cinotti, G.; Gumina, S.; Ripani, M.; Postacchini ,F. (1999) Pedicle instrumentation in the thoracic spine. A morphometric and cadaveric study for placement of screws. *Spine (Phila Pa 1976)* 15; 24:114-119

Danesh-Clough, T.; Taylor, P.; Hodgson, B.; Walton, M. (2001) The use of evoked EMG in detecting misplaced thoracolumbar pedicle screws. *Spine (Phila Pa 1976)* 26:1313-1316

Djurasovic, M.; Dimar, JR.; Glassman, SD.; Edmonds, HL.; Carreon, LY. (2005) A prospective analysis of Intraoperative electromyographic monitoring of posterior cervical screw fixation. *J Spinal Disord Tech* 18:515-518

Donohue, M.; Murtagh-Schaffer, C.; Basta, J.; Moquin, RR.; Bashir, A.; Calancie, B. (2008) Pulse-train stimulation for detecting medical malpositioning of thoracic pedicle screws. Spine 33:E378-385

Drake, J.; Zeller, R.; Kulkarni, AV.; Strantzas, S.; Holmes, L. (2010) Intraoperative neurophysiological monitoring during complex spinal deformity cases in pediatric patients: methodology, utility, prognostication, and outcome. *Childs Nerv Syst* 26:523-544

Duffau, H. (2008) Intraoperative neurophysiology during surgery for cerebral tumors, In: *Intraoperative monitoring of neural function*, Nuwer, MR. (Ed.), pp 491-507, Elsevier, ISBN 978-0-444-51824-8, ISBN 1567-4231, Amsterdam, The Netherlands

Epstein, NE.; Danto, J.; Nardi, D. (1993) Evaluation of intraoperative somatosensory-evoked potential monitoring during 100 cervical operations. *Spine* 18:737-747

Fan, D. & Schwartz, DM.(2002) Intraoperative neurophysiologic detection of iatrogenic C5 nerve root injury during laminectomy for cervical compression myelopathy. *Spine* 22:2499-2502

Friedman, WA.; Chadwick, GM.; Verhoeven, FJ.; Mahla, M.; Day, AL. (1991)Monitoring of somatosensory evoked potentials during surgery for middle cerebral artery aneurysms. *Neurosurgery* 29:83-88

Ghaly, RF.; Lee, JJ.; Ham, JH.; Stone, JL.; George, S.; Raccforte, P. (1999) Etomidate dose-response on somatosensory and transcranial magnetic induced spinal motor evoked potentials in primates. *Neurol Res* 21:714-720

Ghaly, RF.; Ham, JH.; Lee, JJ. (2001) High-dose ketamine hydrochloride maintains somatosensory and magnetic motor evoked potentials in primates. *Neurol Res* 23:881-886

Glassman, DS.; Dimar, JR.; Puno, RM.; Johnson, JR.; Shields, CB.; Linden, RD. (1995) A prospective analysis of Intraoperative electromyographic monitoring of pedicle screw placement with computed tomographic scan configuration. *Spine* 20:1375-1379

Haghighi, SS.; Green, KD.; Oro, JJ.; Drake, RK.; Kracke, GR. (1990) Depressive effect of isoflurane anesthesia on motor evoked potentials. *Neurosurgery* 26:993-997

Haghighi, SS.; Madsen, R.; Green, KD.; Oro JJ.; Kracke GR. (1990) Suppression of motor evoked potentials by inhalation anesthetics. *J Neurosurg Anesthesiol* 2:73-78

Haghighi, SS.; Sirintrapun, SJ.; Keller, BP.; Oro, JJ.; Madsen, R. (1996) Effect of desflurane anesthesia on transcortical motor evoked potentials. *J Neurosurg Anesthesiol* 8:47-51

Hillbrand, AS.; Schwartz DM.; Sethurman, V.; Vaccaro, AR.; Albert, TJ. (2004) Comparison of transcranial electric motor and somatosensory evoked potential monitoring during cervical spine surgery. *J Bone Joint Surg* 86:1248-1253

Holland, NR.; Lukaczyk, TA.; Kostuik, JP. (1998) A comparison of the stimulus thresholds required to evoke myogenic response from normal and chronically compressed nerve roots: implications for intraoperative testing during transpedicular instrumentation. *Spine* 23:224-227

Holmes, JT. & Chappuis, JL. (1993) Monitoring of lumbosacral nerve roots during spinal instrumentation. *Spine* 18:2059-2062

Kearse, LA, Jr.; Lopez-Bresnahan, M.; McPeck, K.; Tambe, V. (1993) Loss of somatosensory evoked potentials during intramedullary spinal cord surgery predicts postoperative neurologic deficits in motor function. *J Clin Anesth* 5:392-398

Kelleher, MO.; Tan, G.; Sarjeant, R.; Fehlings, MG. (2008) Predictive value of intraoperative neurophysiological monitoring during cervical spine surgery: a prospective analysis of 1055 consecutive patients. *J Neurosurg Spine* 8:215-221

Khan, MH.; Smith, PN.; Balzer, JR.; Crammond, D.; Welch, WC.; Gerszten, P. et al. (2006) Intraoperative somatosensory evoked potential monitoring during cervical spine corpectomy surgery: experience with 508 cases. *Spine* 15:E105-113

Kuntz, C,; Maher, C.; Levine, N.; Kurokawa, R. (2004) Prospective evaluation of thoracic pedicle screw placement using fluoroscopic imaging. *J Spinal Disord Tech* 17:206-214

Lam, AM.; Lam, AM.; Manninen, PH.; Ferguson, GG.; Nantau, W. (1991) Monitoring electrophysiologic function during carotid endarterectomy: a comparison of somatosensory evoked potentials and conventional electroencephalogram. *Anesthesiology* 75:15-21

Leppanen, RE. (2008) Intraoperative monitoring of segmental nerve root function with free-run and electrically triggered electromyography and spinal cord function with reflexes and F-responses. In: *Position Statement by American Society of Neurophysiological Monitoring*, pp 1-46

Leung, YL.; Grevitt, M.; Henderson, L.; Smith, J. (2005) Cord monitoring changes and segmental vessel ligation in the "at risk" cord during anterior spinal deformity surgery. *Spine* 30:1870-1874

Maguire, J.; Wallace, S.; Madiga, R.; Leppanen, R.; Draper, V. (1995) Evaluation of intrapedicular screw position using intraoperative evoked electromyography. *Spine* 20:1068-1074

May, DM.; Jones, SJ.; Crockard, A. (1996) Somatosensory evoked potential in cervical surgery: identification of pre- and intraoperative risk factors associated with neurological deterioration. *J Neurosurg* 85:566-573

Matsuzaki, H.; Toiyama, Y.; Matsumoto, F.; Hoshino, M.; Kiuchi, T.; Toriyama, S. (1990) Problems and solutions of pedicle screw plate fixation of lumbar spine. *Spine* 15:1159-1165

McDonald, DB. (2002) Safety of intraoperative transcranial electrical stimulation motor evoked potential monitoring. *J Clin Neurophysiol* 19:416-429

McDonald, DB. (2006) Intraoperative motor evoked potential monitoring: overview and update. *J Clin Neurophysiol* 20:347-377

Minahan, RE.; Riley, III LH.; Lukacyk, T.; Cohen, DB.; Kostuik, JP. (2000) The effect of neuromuscular blockade on pedicle screw stimulation thresholds. *Spine* 25:2526-2530

Naito, M.; Owen, JH.; Bridwell, KH.; Sugioka, Y. (1992) Effects of distraction on physiologic integrity of the spinal cord, spinal cord blood flow, and clinical status. *Spine* 17:1154-1158

Nuwer, MR. (1999) Spinal cord monitoring. *Muscle Nerve* 2:620-1630

Prielipp, RC.; Morell, RC.; Walker, FO.; Santos, CC.; Bennett, J.; Butterworth, J. (1999) Ulnar nerve pressure: influence of arm position and relationship to somatosensory evoked potentials. *Anesthesiology* 91:345-354

Raynor, BL.; Lenke, LG.; Kim, Y.; Hanson, DS.; Wilson-Holden, TJ.; Bridwell, KH., et al. (2002) Can triggered electromyograph thresholds predict safe thoracic pedicle screw placement? *Spine (Phila Pa 1976)* 27:2030-2035

Sebastián, C.; Raya, JP.; Ortega, M.; Olalla, E.; Lemos, V.; Romero, R. (1997) Intraoperative control by somatosensory evoked potentials in the treatment of cervical myeloradiculopathy. *Eur Spine J* 6:316-323

Shi, YB.; Binette, M.; Martin, WH.; Pearson, JM.; Hart, RA. (2003) Electrical stimulation of intraoperative evaluation of thoracic pedicle screw placement. *Spine* 28:595-601

Skinner, SA.; Transfeldt, EE.; Savik, K. (2008) Surface electrodes are not sufficient to detect neurotonic discharges: observations in a porcine model and clinical review of deltoid electromyographic monitoring using multiple electrodes. *J Clin Monit Comput* 22:131-139

Smith, PN.; Balzer, JR.; Khan, MH.; Davis, RA.; Crammond, D.; Welch, WC., et al. (2007) Intraoperative somatosensory evoked potential monitoring during anterior cervical discectomy and fusion in nonmyelopathic patients - a review of 1,039 cases. *Spine J* 7:83-87

Taunt, CJ.; Sidhu, KS.; Andrew, SA. (2005) Somatosensory evoked potential monitoring during anterior cervical discectomy and fusion. *Spine* 30:1970-1972

Tew, JM Jr. & Mayfield, FH. (1976) Complications of surgery of the anterior cervical spine. *Clin Neurosurg* 23:424-434

Thees, C.; Scheufler, KM.; Nadstawek, J.; Pechstein, U.; Hanisch, M.; Juntke, R., et al. (1999) Influence of fentanyl, alfentanil, and sufentanil on motor evoked potentials. *J Neurosurg Anesthesiol* 11:112-118

Thompson, JP. & Rowbotham, DJ. (1996) Remifentanil-an opioid for the 21st century. *Br J Anaesth* 76:341-343

Toleikis, JR.; Carlvin, AO.; Shapiro, DE.; Schafer, MF. (1993) The use of dermatomal evoked responses during surgical procedures that use intrapedicular fixation of the lumbosacral spine. *Spine* 18:2401-2407

Toleikis, JR.; Skelly, JP.; Carlvin, AO.; Toleikis, AC.; Bernard, TN.; Burkus, KJ., et al. (2000) The usefulness of electrical stimulation for assessing pedicle screw placements. *J Spinal Disorders* 13:283-289

Tsai, RYC.; Yang, R.; Nuwer MR.; Kanim, LEA.; Delamarter, RB.; Dawson EG. (1997) Intraoperative dermatomal evoked potential monitoring fails to predict outcome from lumbar decompression surgery. *Spine* 17:1970-1975

Ueta, T.; Owen, JH.; Sugioka, Y. (1992) Effects of compression on physiologic integrity of the spinal cord on circulation, and clinical status in four different directions of compression: posterior, anterior, circumferential, and lateral. *Spine* 17:S217-S226

Vaccaro, AR.; Rizzolo, SJ.; Balderston, RA.; Allardyce, TJ.; Garfin, SR.; Dolinskas, C., et al. (1995) Placement of pedicle screws in the thoracic spine. Part II: An anatomical and radiographic assessment. *J Bone Joint Surg Am* 77:1200-1206

van Dongen, EP.; ter Beek, HT.; Schepens, MA.; Morshuis, WJ.; de Boer, A.; Aarts, LP., et al. (1999) Effect of nitrous oxide on myogenic motor potentials evoked by a six pulse train of transcranial electrical stimuli: a possible monitor for aortic surgery. *Br J Anesth* 82:323-328

Wee, AS. & Ashley, RA. (1989) Cortical somatosensory evoked potentials during acute hemorrhagic hypotension. *Eur Neurol* 29:284-286

Weinzierl, MR.; Reinacher, P.; Gilsbach, JM.; Rohde, V. (2007) Combined motor and somatosensory evoked potentials for intraoperative monitoring: intra- and postoperative data in a series of 69 operations. *Neurosurg Rev* 30:109-116

Welch, WC.; Rose, RD.; Balzer, JR.; Jacobs, GB. (1997) Evaluation with evoked and spontaneous electromyography during lumbar instrumentation: a prospective study. *J Neurosurg* 87:397-402

West, JL III.; Ogilvie, JW.; Bradford, DS. (1991) Complications of the variable screw plate pedicle screw fixation. *Spine* 16:576-579

Xu, R.; Ebraheim, NA.; Shepherd, ME.; Yeasting, RA. (1999) Thoracic pedicle screw placement guided by computed tomographic measurements. *J Spinal Disord* 12:222-226

York, DH. (1985) Somatosensory evoked potentials in man: differentiation of spinal pathways responsible for conduction from forelimbs vs. hindlimb. *Prog Neurbiol* 25:1-25

Zentner, J. & Ebner, A. (1989) Nitrous oxide suppresses the electromyographic response evoked by electrical stimulation of the motor cortex. *Neurosurgery* 24:60-62

Extraction and Analysis of the Single Motor Unit F-Wave of the Median Nerve

Masafumi Yamada and Kentaro Nagata
Kanagawa Rehabilitation Institute,
Kanagawa Rehabilitation Center,
Japan

1. Introduction

The matrix type multielectrodes have been proved to be useful for getting the information of motor unit (MU) properties (Monster et al., 1980; Reucher et al., 1987; Yamada et al., 1987; Masuda and Sadoyama, 1988; Kleine et al., 2000; Gazzoni et al., 2004). By this electromyography (EMG) technique, we can obtain many essential properties of MU that could not be obtained by conventional surface EMG and/or needle EMG. One of them is the waveform property of motor unit action potential (MUAP) which is enabled by extracting the single propagating MUAP. Another is the two-dimensional location of motor end-plates. There have been many applications of multichannel surface EMG for measuring voluntary muscle activities, but few for evoked EMG responses. However, recent studies have demonstrated the applications of the multichannel surface EMG for the measurement of muscle fiber conduction velocities (MFCVs) (Metani et al., 2005) , for the estimation of firing thresholds (Yamada, 2004), and for the motor unit number estimate (MUNE) (Blok et al., 2005; van Dijk et al., 2008).

The F-wave represents a long latency response detected from a muscle following stimulation of a peripheral nerve at supramaximal intensity. The F-waves are produced by antidromic activation of motor neurons. The latency and the waveform of the F-wave change with each stimulus. The F-wave studies are widely used in clinical neurophysiology as a quantitative estimation method of the objective pathological changes. The F-waves that consist of a single MUAP occur also with submaximal stimulation. Low intensity stimulation could increase the probability of the single MU F-wave (Komori et al., 1991; Doherty et al., 1994; Stashuk et al., 1994; Yamada, 2004), and reduce the discomfort of the subjects. Therefore, different MUAPs can be readily analyzed by classifying F-waves. Many studies concerned with the single MU F-wave were performed for the estimation of the conduction velocity of nerve fibers (Doherty et al., 1994; Felice, 1998; Wang et al., 1999) and the MUNE (Stashuk et al., 1994; Hara et al., 2000). The conventional surface EMG technique was used in these studies, and there were few applications of multichannel surface EMG for F-wave studies.

In a previous study, we investigated the classification and analysis of multichannel bipolar F-waves (Yamada et al., 2007). It is difficult to detect deep MUs from the bipolar EMG. So, in the present study, the thenar MUs F-waves were investigated by extracting single MU F-waves from monopolar multichannel surface EMG signals. By increasing the number of processing data measured under different stimulus conditions, many single MU F-waves could be extracted, and the properties of F-waves and MUs could be analyzed successfully. Then we could find the single MU F-waves with the same waveform but different latencies.

2. Methods

2.1 Subjects and measurements

The subjects were 6 men, aged $22-60$ years (mean±S.D., 30.2±14.9 years). None of them had a history of neurological disorders. All subjects gave informed consent prior to participation in the study. The subject sat comfortably on a chair with his right hand supinated. The right median nerve was stimulated at the wrist and the evoked responses were recorded from the thenar muscles with a matrix-type multielectrode. The multielectrode was composed of 32 silver electrodes (8x4 array), 1 mm in diameter, which were arranged on a silicone rubber board (thickness 2 mm) at 4 mm distance in both directions (Fig. 1). This electrode was fixed by bandages with the eight electrode arrays in parallel with the muscle fibers. A small diameter of electrode and a short distance of electrodes enabled the extraction of single MUAP from surface EMG signals. The use of a semi-solid type electrode paste enabled to measure EMG signals for a long period. A reference electrode and a ground electrode, both conventional Ag/AgCl electrodes, were attached to the bone of the dorsal hand. The block diagram of the multichannel surface EMG system is shown in Fig. 2.

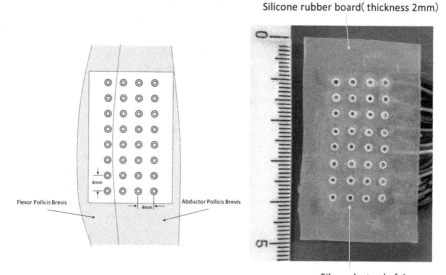

Fig. 1. Thirty-two channel matrix-type multielectrode. Each electrode (1mm in diameter) is arranged on a silicone rubber board at 4 mm distance in both directions.

The 32 channel monopolar evoked potentials (8x4 array) were amplified through a bandwidth of 10-1000 Hz (gain 30dB). The amplified evoked signals were sampled at 10kHz with 16-bit resolution. The stimulation was squarewave pulse of 0.2 ms duration and frequency of 5 Hz or less. The high stimulus rate may cause muscle fatigue, and may change the shape of MUAP. Therefore the low stimulus frequency was selected for recording consecutive evoked responses. The stimulation strength was set to submaximal, approximately 40-80 % of the supramaximal stimulation. Each of the record length was 50ms, and 300 consecutive evoked responses were recorded. Changing the stimulation intensity, several sessions of 300 evoked responses were recorded. The bipolar potentials were obtained by calculating the difference between the monopolar potentials of two adjacent electrodes placed along the muscle fibers.

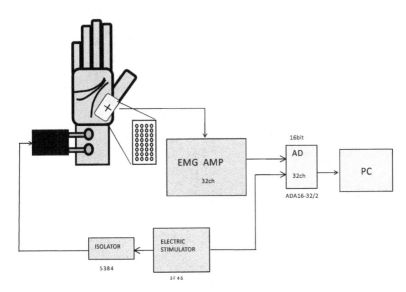

Fig. 2. Block diagram of the multichannel surface EMG system.

As in the case of bipolar signals (Yamada, 2004; Yamada et al., 2007), the origin of the F-wave could be also evaluated by the distribution pattern of monopolar MUAPs. It is presumed that the MUs whose center arrays estimated at array 1 and array 2 are originated from the abductor pollicis brevis (APB), and those estimated at array 3 and array 4 are originated from the flexor pollicis brevis (FPB). In Fig. 3(A), the distribution of 32 channel monopolar evoked potentials recorded in a thenar muscle is shown. This MU is originated from the APB muscle. Fig. 3(B) shows 8 channel records of the center array (array 1).

2.2 Classification of F-waves
The outline of the classification of F-waves is shown in Fig. 4. All channels evoked responses are digitally high-pass filtered in order to remove the late components of the M-waves with a drift filter which barely affects the waveform parameters of the F-waves. The superimposed traces in Fig. 5 show 10 sequentially evoked responses of one electrode array. Although the M-waves are almost uniformed, the F-waves show various patterns. When the evoked response contains the F-wave, the center of the MU in transverse section (center array) is evaluated by the sum of the peak-to-peak amplitude of F-waves in each electrode array. Then we select the records (latency 20-45 ms) in the array for the classification process.

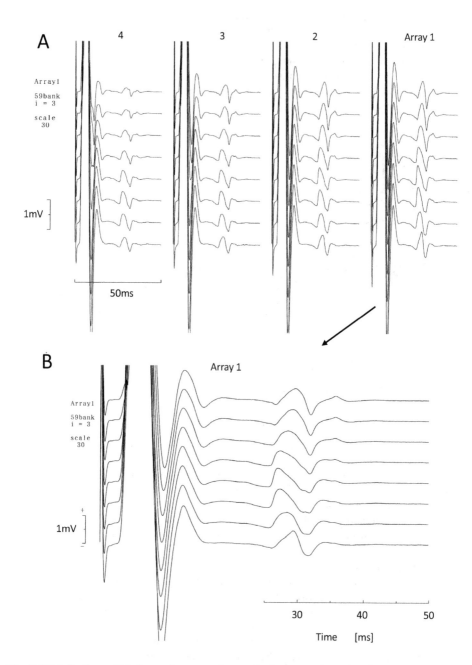

Fig. 3. Distribution of 32 channel monopolar evoked potentials in the thenar muscles at submaximal stimulation (A). Expanded 8 channel monopolar potentials of the center array (B). The signals were digitally high-pass filtered with a drift filter.

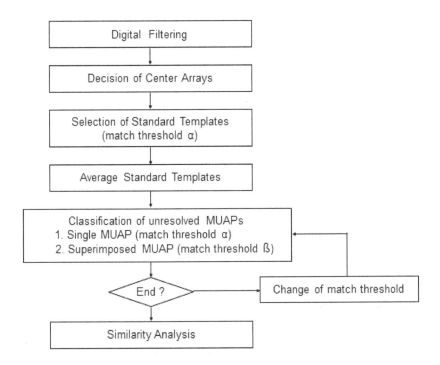

Fig. 4. Flow chart of the classification of F-waves.

Eight channel MUAP waveforms in its center array are classified using a template-matching method based on the least-square error criterion where an initial match threshold α is set to 5% of the objective area value typically. If the F-wave and templates do not match, the waveforms on both sides of the center array are also estimated, because the decision of center arrays is critical and not always proper. After this procedure, the standard templates are selected by the decision rule dependent on the identified number of the corresponding template, and the average waveforms are computed for the next procedure. The group of F-waves, which is not identified as one of the standard templates, is repeatedly classified into an averaged standard template or 2-3 combinations of them by the same method in the selection of standard templates. The match threshold β in case of superposition is initially set to lower than α (typically 4.5% of the objective area value), because high thresholds tend to lead to incorrect combinations of standard templates. After having thresholds α and β gradually increased, the unresolved F-waves are repeatedly processed. By these procedures, the single MU F-waves are classified. Five sessions of recordings measured at different stimulus intensities were processed to extract many single MUs. Fig. 6 shows 38 single MU F-waves extracted and classified from the thenar muscles of a subject.

2.3 Estimation of F-wave parameters
The amplitude of a single MUAP was evaluated from measuring the largest peak-to-peak amplitude in 8 channel MUAP waveforms in its center array, and the latency was obtained

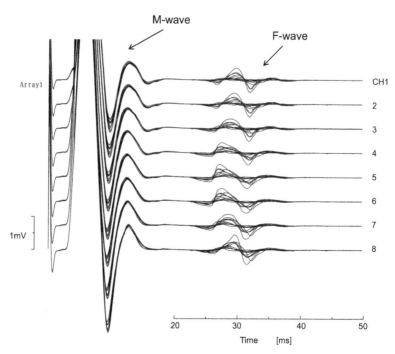

Fig. 5. Superimposed 10 evoked responses of one electrode array.

from measuring the fastest onset of MUAP in the array. In the case of MUAPs showing propagating time delays, the MFCV was calculated from the time delay of a single pair of MUAPs in the array. The MUAPs in the region of the motor end-plates band indicated non-linear propagating time delays, and we estimated the conduction velocity in the area a small distance on either side of the band, where the conduction velocity was uniform along the length of the muscle. The muscle fiber conduction velocities of all classified MUAPs, excepting superimposed ones, were computed according to the above considerations, and other parameters were estimated automatically as well.

Statistical analysis was carried out for F-wave parameters. The correlation coefficients among amplitudes, latencies and MFCVs were calculated in each subject. The level of statistical significance was set at $p < 0.05$.

2.4 Detection of single MU F-waves with the same waveform but different latencies

From these classified F-waves, the F-waves with the same waveform but different latencies (latency differences above 0.5 ms) were searched using 8 channel and 32 channel similarity values between the two averaged F-waves.

In the case of similarity values higher than 0.8, the comparison of two F-waves was performed by examining 8 channel propagation patterns of MUAPs in its center array and 32 channel distribution patterns of MUAPs in a superimposed form and in an averaged form. In addition, bipolar waveforms were also compared for reference. The F-wave analysis is planned to execute interactively, or automatically. At present, the operator is required in some processes to obtain reliable and accurate results.

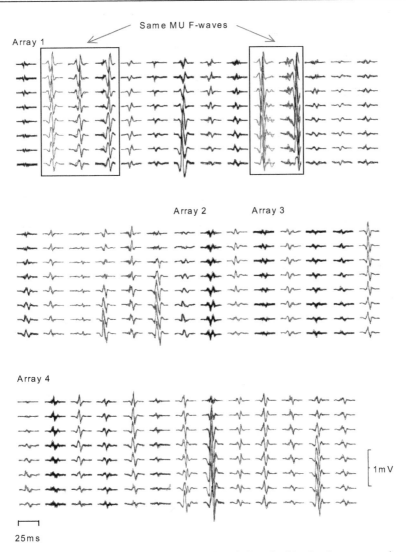

Fig. 6. Thirty-eight single MU F-waves extracted and classified in the thenar muscles of one subject. Two APB MUs with the same waveform but different latencies are shown in the top traces.

3. Results

Single MU F-waves were classified by using the template-matching method. The classification results and estimated F-wave parameters of thenar MUs in 6 normal subjects are shown in Table 1 and Fig. 7. The mean F-wave persistence (occurrence rate) was high (88.8%), and a total of 7724 F-waves were detected in the evoked responses. The numbers of MUs extracted from 5 sessions of data (1500 responses) were increased by 75-116%

Subjects	F-wave (n=1500)	MU			
		n(APB+FPB) (FPB)	Amplitude Mean ± SD. (mV)	Latency Mean ± SD. (ms)	MFCV Mean ± SD. (m/s)
1	1376(91.7%)	38(18)	0.367±0.304	28.07±2.08	5.369±1.065(11)
2	1279(85.3%)	41(22)	0.179±0.130	27.20±1.63	5.425±1.096(2)
3	1413(94.2%)	35(10)	0.317±0.222	25.99±2.95	6.200±0.000(3)
4	1080(90.0%)*	30(6)	0.142±0.107	25.30±0.97	3.832±1.331(5)
5	1236(82.4%)	31(15)	0.250±0.188	26.20±2.25	4.112±1.020(10)
6	1340(89.3%)	26(3)	0.183±0.186	27.90±1.23	4.753±1.56(3)
Total	7724(88.8%)	201(74)	0.251±0.222	26.74±2.25	4.800±1.237(35)

*n=1200

Table 1. Classification results for the F-waves in 6 normal subjects: the numbers of F-waves, the numbers of MUs and the estimated MU parameters.

(mean±S.D., 92±15%) compared with those from the maximum sessions (300 responses). The numbers of MU in 6 subjects were 38, 41, 35, 30, 31 and 26, respectively. The total of 201 thenar MUs were extracted from the F-wave data.

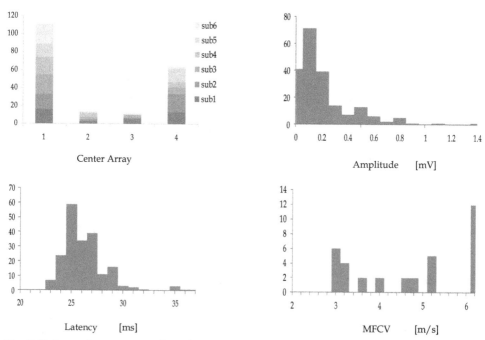

Fig. 7. Estimated parameters of single MU F-waves: Center array, Amplitude, Latency and MFCV.

The numbers of MUs originated from the APB and FPB were 127 (63.2%) and 74 (36.8%). In 5 out of 6 subjects, the numbers of APB MUs were larger than those of FPB MUs. Fig. 6(a) shows the histogram of the center arrays of 201 MUs. Thirty-eight single MU F-waves classified in a subject are shown in Fig. 7. This example shows 20 APB MUs and 18 FPB MUs. The mean peak-to-peak amplitudes, latencies, and MFCVs were 0.251±0.222 mV, 26.74±2.25 ms and 4.80±1.24 m/s. The long latencies greater than 30 ms were detected in 11 MUs (5 subjects). The numbers of MUs in which MFCVs could be evaluated in 6 subjects were 11, 2, 4, 5, 10 and 3, respectively. The total was 35 MUs (17.4%). The significant correlations were not found between amplitudes, latencies and MFCVs in all subjects.

An example of single MU responses (FPB MU) with the same waveform but different latencies is shown in Fig. 8. The latencies of the two responses were (a) 25.7 ms and (b) 36.1 ms, and the latency difference was 10.4 ms. The similarity values for 8 channel and 32 channel signals were high, namely 0.91 and 0.90 respectively.

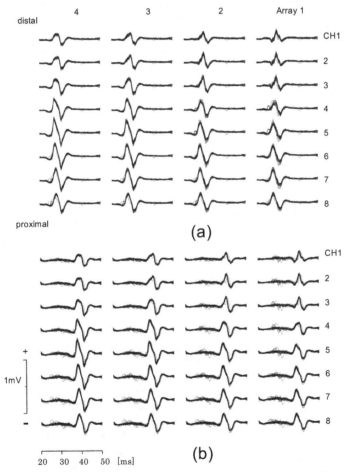

Fig. 8. Distributions of 32 channel MUAPs with the same waveform but different latencies. The latencies were (a) 25.7 ms and (b) 36.1 ms, and the latency difference was 10.4 ms.

The single MU F-waves with the same waveform but different latencies were detected in 5 out of 6 subjects, the total number was 12 MUs (8 APB MUs and 4 FPB MUs, 6%). The estimated F-wave parameters of these MUs are summarized in Table 2.

The latency differences of the two responses ranged 0.9 to 10.4 ms (mean 2.82±3.22 ms), and half of them were around 1 ms. There was no significant relationship between the stimulus intensities and the latencies in these MUs. Figs. 9(a) and 9(b) show the examples of the single MU F-waves (a: FPB MU, b: APB MU) with 0.9 ms and 1.2 ms latency differences. One of the MUs with 3 different latencies (APB MU, 26.3, 29.4 and 32.2 ms) is shown in Fig. 10(a)-(c). The waveforms in Fig. 10(b) differ slightly from those in Figs. 10(a) and 10(c), because the F-waves in Fig. 10(b) are overlapped by the FPB MU with small amplitude MUAPs. These results were confirmed by the distribution and propagation patterns of the MUAPs.

Subject	Array	Amplitude (mV)	Latency 1 (ms)	Latency 2 (ms)	Latency 3 (ms)	Similarity (8CH)	Similarity (32CH)
1	1	1.08	24.0	33.5(9.5)		0.96	0.95
	1	0.57	26.3	29.4(3.1)	32.2(5.9)	0.94	0.91
2	4	0.18	23.9	26.0(2.1)		0.92	0.83
	1	0.68	24.4	25.3(0.9)		0.86	0.89
	4	0.53	24.8	26.0(1.2)		0.90	0.87
	4	0.56	25.7	36.1(10.4)		0.91	0.90
3	1	0.12	25.3	26.3(1.0)		0.87	0.89
	2	0.21	25.7	27.0(1.3)		0.81	0.79
	1	0.26	25.7	27.0(1.7)		0.82	0.72
4	4	0.41	24.8	26.0(1.2)		0.94	0.94
	1	0.19	24.8	26.6(1.8)		0.85	0.83
5	1	0.12	27.1	28.0(0.9)		0.88	0.93
Mean		0.41±0.29	25.2±0.95	28.0±3.23 (2.82±3.22)		0.89±0.05	0.87±0.07

Table 2. Estimated parameters of single MU F-waves with the same waveform but different latencies.

4. Discussion

The F-wave persistence in monopolar recordings was high compared with that in bipolar signals, because it is thought that the deep MUs, which could not be detected from bipolar waveforms, might be detectable from monopolar waveforms. Accordingly, the numbers of MUs that were extracted and classified from evoked responses were increased than those in the previous study (Yamada et al., 2007). In the case of bipolar signals, the noise and interference are lower than those in the monopolar signals. Then, the MUAPs can be classified precisely, and the superimposed MUAPs can be decomposed into its constituent MUAPs. On the other hand, in the case of monopolar signals, the decomposition processing of superimposed MUAPs had a little problem with the classification accuracy.

By using the distribution and propagation patterns of the MUAPs measured by the multichannel surface EMG technique, the single MU F-waves could be extracted and

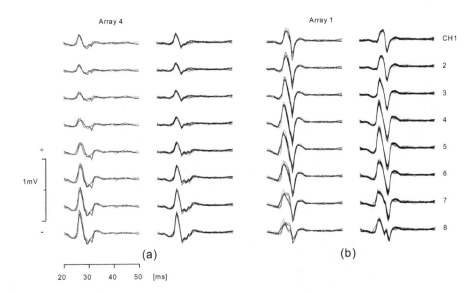

Fig. 9. Single MU F-waves (a: FPB MU, b: APB MU) with 0.9 ms and 1.2 ms latency differences.

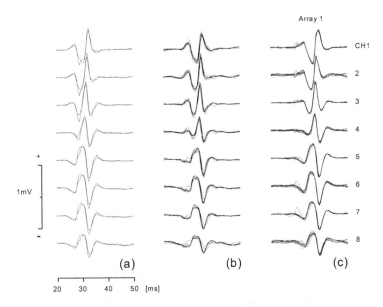

Fig. 10. Single MU F-waves with 3 different latencies ((a) 26.3 ms, (b) 29.4 ms and (c) 32.2 ms). The latency differences were (b)-(a) 3.1 ms and (c)-(a) 5.9 ms.

classified precisely, and the origin of the F-wave is evaluated easily. In the case of bipolar signals, the extracted numbers of APB MUs were larger than those of FPB for all the subjects, and most of the MUs (84.5%) were originated from the APB muscle (Yamada et al., 2007). In this study, 127 APB MUs (63.2%) were extracted from monopolar signals. These results suggest that the number of APB MU is greater than that of FPB MU.

The F-wave amplitude and persistence were increased with increasing the stimulus intensity (Yamada et al., 2007; Fisher et al., 2008). On the other hand, low intensity stimulation increased the probability of single MU F-wave (Komori et al., 1991; Doherty et al., 1994; Shefner, 2001; Yamada et al., 2007). By investigating in detail the relationship between stimulus intensity and the properties of the extracted MUs, it seems that the experimental conditions of stimulus intensity and the combination of intensities, from which more MUs can be extracted, may be determined.

The latency of F-wave is useful to detect alterations in peripheral nerves (Fisher, 1992; Panayiotopoulos and Chroni, 1996; Toyokura and Murakami, 1997; Nobrega et al., 2001). Moreover the latency varies in each MU, so this parameter is useful for classifying individual F-waves. By using the multichannel surface EMG technique, the latency may be measured precisely than other methods, because the locations of motor end-plates, where the MUAPs begin to propagate along muscle fibers in both directions, are readily identified in the two-dimensional plane (Yamada et al., 1991; Yamada, 2004).

The single MU responses with the same waveform but different latencies were detected in 12 MUs out of 201 extracted MUs (6%). Though the latency differences of the two single MUAPs ranged 0.9 to 10.4 ms (Table 2), many of the differences were around 1 ms (50%). In these examples, it suggests that the prolonged latencies occurred due to synaptic delays in the spinal interneuronal network. The synaptic delay is usually of about 0.5 ms (Guyton and Hall, 1996). Therefore, in the case of one interneuron in the pathway, the time delay will be about 1 ms. The long-latency reflexes (LLRs) can be elicited by electric stimulation of the median nerve at the wrist during voluntary contraction of the thenar muscles (Upton et al., 1971; Conrad et al., 1977; Deuschl et al., 1989; Burke et al., 1999). As shown in Figs. 8 and 10 (10.4 ms, 3.1, 5.9 ms), it was confirmed that single MUAP LLRs with prolonged latencies were included in F-wave data. In the present study, the record length was set to 50 ms. By using a longer record length, single MUAP LLRs with longer latencies may be detected further.

In the MUNE by the F-wave method, the same MUs with prolonged latencies should be excluded from the calculation of the mean MUAP. In particular, the MUs with long latencies, which were due to supraspinal or transcortical pathways, should not be included in the MUNE process, because they will affect the MUNE values more sensibly than in the case of small latency differences.

5. Conclusions

The extracted number of single MU F-waves could be increased by increasing the number of processing data measured under different stimulus conditions, then the properties of many MUs could be analyzed easily, and we could find the single MU responses with the same waveform but different latencies. The similarity analysis was useful to search the same waveform pair from many pairs of single MU responses. It is suggested that the prolonged latencies occurred due to spinal interneuronal pathways, in the case of large differences in latencies, supraspinal pathways, or transcortical pathways.

6. References

Blok, JH.; van Dijk, JP.; Zwarts, MJ. & Stegeman, DF. (2005). Motor unit action potential topography and its use in motor unit number estimation, *Muscle Nerve*, Vol.32, pp. 280-291

Burke, D.; Hallet, M.; Fuhr, P. & Pierrot-Deseilligny, E. (1999). H reflexes from the tibial and median nerves. In Recommendations for the Practice of Clinical Neurophysiology: guidelines of the International Federation of Clinical Neurophysiology. *Electroenceph. Clin. Neurophysiol.* (Suppl. 52), pp. 259-262

Conrad, B.; & Aschoff, JC. (1977). Effects of voluntary isometric and isotonic activity on late transcortical reflex components in normal subjects and hemiparetic patients. *Electroencephalogr. Clin. Neurophysiol.*, Vol.42(1), pp. 107-116

Deuschl, G.; Ludolph, A.; Schenck, E. & Lücking, CH. (1989). The relations between long-latency reflexes in hand muscles, somatosensory evoked potentials and transcranial stimulation of motor tracts, *Electroencephalogr. Clin. Neurophysiol.*, Vol.74, pp. 425-430

Doherty, TJ.; Komori, T.; Stashuk, DW.; Kassam, A. & Brown, WF. (1994). Physiological properties of single thenar motor units in the F-response of younger and older adults, *Muscle Nerve*, Vol.17, pp. 860-872

Felice, KJ. (1998). Nerve conduction velocities of single thenar motor axons based on the automated analysis of F waves in amyotrophic lateral sclerosis. *Muscle Nerve*, Vol.21, pp. 756-761

Fisher, MA. (1992). AAEM Minimonograph #13: H reflexes and F waves: physiology and clinical indications, *Muscle Nerve*, Vol.15, pp. 1223-1233

Fisher, MA.; Zhu, JQ.; Uddin, MK. & Grindstaff, P. (2008). Submaximal stimulation and f-wave parameters, *J. Clin. Neurophysiol.*, Vol.25, No.5, pp. 299-303

Gazzoni, M.; Farina, D. & Merletti, R. (2004). A new method for the extraction and classification of single motor unit action potentials from surface EMG signals, *J Neuroscience Methods*, Vol.136, pp. 165-177

Guyton, AC. & Hall, JE. (1996). *Human Physiology and Mechanisms of disease*, 6th ed., Saunders, Philadelphia , USA

Hara, Y.; Akaboshi, K.; Masakado, Y. & Chino, N. (2000). Physiologic decrease of single thenar motor units in the F-response in stroke patients, *Arch. Phys. Med. Rehab.*, Vol.81, pp. 418-423

Kleine, BU.; Schumann, NP. Stegeman, DF. & Scholle, HC. (2000). Surface EMG mapping of the human trapezius muscle: the topography of monopolar and bipolar surface EMG amplitude and spectrum parameters at varied forces and in fatigue, *Clin. Neurophysiol.*, Vol.111, pp. 686-693

Komori, T.; Watson, BV. & Brown, WF. (1991). Characteristics of single 'F' motor units at different stimulus intensities, *Muscle Nerve, Vol.*14 pp. 875

Masuda, T. & Sadoyama, T. (1988). Topographical map of innervation zones within single motor units measured with a grid surface electrode, *IEEE Trans. biomed. Engng.*, Vol.BME-35, pp. 623-628

Metani, H.; Tsubahara, A. Hiraoka, T.; Aoyagi, Y. & Tanaka, Y. (2005). A new method using F-waves to measure muscle fiber conduction velocity (MFCV), *Electromyogr. Clin. Neurophysiol.*, Vol.45, pp. 245-253

Monster, AW.; Pittore, J. & Barrie, W. (1980). A system for the rapid acquisition of surface potential maps of human skeletal muscle motor units, *IEEE Trans. biomed. Engng.* Vol.BME-27, pp. 110-112

Nobrega, JAM.; Manzano, GM. & Monteagudo, PT. (2001). A comparison between different parameters in F-wave studies, *Clin. Neurophysiol.*, Vol.112, pp. 866-868

Panayiotopoulos, CP. & Chroni, E. (1996). F-waves in clinical neurophysiology: a review, methodological issues and overall value in peripheral neuropathies, *Electroencephalogr. Clin. Neurophysiol.*, Vol.101, pp. 365-374

Reucher, H.; Rau, G. & Silny, J. (1987). Spatial filtering of noninvasive multielectrode EMG: Part I- Introduction to measuring technique and applications, *IEEE Trans. biomed. Engng.* Vol.BME-34, pp. 98-105

Shefner, JM. (2001). Motor unit number estimation in human neurological diseases and animal models, *Clin. Neurophysiol.*, Vol.112, pp. 955-964

Stashuk, DW.; Doherty, TJ.; Kassam, A. & Brown, WF. (1994). Motor unit number estimates based on the automated analysis of F-responses. *Muscle Nerve* Vol.17, pp881-890

Toyokura, M. & Murakami, K. (1997). F-wave study in patients with lumbosacral radiculopathies, *Electromyogr. Clin. Neurophysiol.*, Vol.37, pp. 19-26

Upton, ARM.; McComas, AJ. & Sica, REP. (1971). Potentiation of «late» responses evoked in muscles during effort, *J Neurol. Neurosurg. Psychiatry.*, Vol.34, pp. 699-711

van Dijk, JP.; Blok, JH.; Lapatki, BG.; van Schaik, IN.; Zwarts, MJ. & Stegeman, DF. (2008). Motor unit number estimation using high-density surface electromyography, *Clin. Neurophysiol.*, Vol.119, pp. 33-42

Wang, FC.; de Pasqua, V. & Delwaide, PJ. (1999). Age-related changes in fastest and slowest conducting axons of thenar motor units. *Muscle Nerve,* Vol.22, pp.1022-1029

Yamada, M.; Kumagai, K. & Uchiyama, A. (1987). The distribution and propagation pattern of motor unit action potentials studied by multi-channel surface EMG, *Electroencephalogr. clin. Neurophysiol.* Vol.67, pp. 395-401

Yamada, M.; Kumagai, K. & Uchiyama, A. (1991). Muscle fiber conduction velocity studied by the multi-channel surface EMG. *Electromyogr. Clin. Neurophysiol.*, Vol.31, pp. 251-256

Yamada, M. (2004). Comparison of F-waves and motor unit action potentials activated during voluntary contraction. *Electromyogr Clin Neurophysiol,* Vol.44, pp. 29-34

Yamada, M.; Nakazawa, T.; Kyoso, M. & Ishijima, M. (2007). Single motor unit F-waves in the thenar muscles studied by the multichannel surface EMG, *Electromyogr. Clin. Neurophysiol.*, Vol.47, pp. 43-48

4

Combination of Transcranial Magnetic Stimulation with Electromyography and Electroencephalography: Application in Diagnosis of Neuropsychiatric Disorders

Faranak Farzan[1], Mera S. Barr[1],
Paul B. Fitzgerald[2] and Zafiris J. Daskalakis[1]
[1]*Centre for Addiction and Mental Health,
University of Toronto, Toronto*
[2]*Monash Alfred Psychiatry Research Centre,
The Alfred and Monash University School of Psychology and Psychiatry, Melbourne*
[1]*Canada*
[2]*Australia*

1. Introduction

Transcranial magnetic stimulation (TMS) is a non-invasive brain stimulation technique that allows for in vivo examination of cortical processes. In 1985, Barker et al. introduced TMS as a tool for investigating the functional state of the motor pathways in patients with neurological disorders as well as in healthy human subjects (Barker et al., 1985). It was shown that a single TMS pulse applied to the motor cortex could activate cortical tissues associated with the hand or leg muscles and this activation could elicit a motor evoked potential (MEP) at the periphery captured through electromyography (EMG) recordings. The amplitude, area, latency and duration of this TMS induced MEP could then be used to investigate the integrity of the corticospinal pathways and the activation threshold of human motor cortex. Since this discovery, the combination of single and multi-pulse TMS with peripheral EMG recordings has allowed for examining various other processes in the human motor cortex such as excitability, plasticity, cortico-cortical connectivity, as well as the interaction between excitatory and inhibitory cortical processes. The integration of EMG with TMS has, therefore, offered a valuable tool for assessment of pathological processes that underlie neurological and psychiatric disorders such as Parkinson's disease, dystonia, stroke, Alzheimer's disease, schizophrenia, and depression.

The combination of paired pulse TMS with EMG recordings, for example, permits altering the excitability of the motor cortex and observing the effect of this alteration on subsequent stimulation. In paired pulse TMS, the first TMS pulse (conditioning stimulus) inhibits or facilitates the MEP response to the second TMS pulse (test stimulus). The nature and the strength of this modulatory effect depend on the intensity of the conditioning stimulus and the latency (i.e. interstimulus interval (ISI)) at which it is delivered with respect to the test stimulus. It has been demonstrated that the TMS induced modulation of MEPs are selectivity impaired in several neurological conditions (e.g. schizophrenia, Alzheimer's disease) when compared to the measures obtained in the age- and sex-matched healthy subjects. In this regard, the TMS induced MEP modulation has been associated with the activation and interaction between specific inhibitory and excitatory mechanisms at the cortical level, which provides insight on the specific cortical processes that may underlie the neuropsychopathology of such disorders. However, evidence for the cortical origin of MEP modulation is relatively scarce and has often been collected from rather invasive procedures such as epidural recordings in patients with implanted electrodes and by demonstrating that MEP modulation is not due to the refractoriness of the corticospinal tract.

In recent years, it has become possible to combine TMS-EMG with simultaneous electroencephalography (EEG) recordings. The combination of TMS with EEG, however, has not been easy. Simultaneous EEG recording during TMS stimulation was previously unattainable because of the technological shortcomings of EEG amplifiers that would saturate for a long duration due to the large artifact produced by the magnetic stimulation. For example, application of a single TMS pulse would result in artifact lasting for several seconds after the pulse. Such long lasting artifact blocked the window of time during which neurophysiological processes such as cortical inhibition occur. Through advances in EEG amplifier technology, researchers have conducted series of studies to examine TMS paradigms in the motor cortex through simultaneous EEG and EMG recordings and in non-motor regions of the cortex through EEG recordings.

The integration of EEG recordings with TMS-EMG will generate important neurophysiological leads in both the healthy and diseased states. First, it allows for non-invasive examination of the origin and the mechanisms through which MEPs are modulated. For example, using the TMS-EEG technology we have recently examined the EEG substrate of the MEP modulation induced by the paired pulse paradigm long interval cortical inhibition (LICI). In LICI, a conditioning stimulus precedes the test stimulus by 100 ms and suppresses the amplitude of the MEP response to the test stimulus by about 50% (Daskalakis et al., 2002a; Valls-Sole et al., 1992), a processes which is thought to be mediated by the activity of cortical GABAergic inhibitory interneurons and more specifically the activation of $GABA_B$ receptors (McDonnell et al., 2006; Sanger et al., 2001). Through concurrently recording MEP and EEG responses, we were able to show that the LICI induced suppression of MEPs at the periphery is positively correlated with the suppression of cortical evoked potentials at the site of TMS stimulation, therefore, providing further evidence for the cortical origin of the MEP modulation in the LICI paradigm (Daskalakis et al., 2008).

A second advantage of online EEG recording is the possibility to evaluate the effects of electromagnetic induction on cortical oscillatory activity in order to identify the cortical oscillations that more closely underlie the TMS induced MEP generation and modulation. Indeed, we have recently demonstrated that following LICI application to the motor cortex, cortical oscillations in the frequency range of 1 Hz to 30 Hz are significantly suppressed, while higher frequencies (e.g. gamma oscillations (30-50 Hz)) are not affected (Farzan et al., 2009). Identifying the cortical oscillatory activities that underlie TMS induced MEP modulation may provide further insight into the neurophysiology of the human motor cortex and would be valuable in improving the diagnostic and therapeutic strategies in several neuropsychiatric disorders.

Furthermore, a major advantage of combined TMS-EMG and EEG is the possibility to evaluate the cortico-cortical connectivity between motor cortices. Functional connectivity between cortical regions (e.g. left and right motor cortices) can be more easily probed through measuring the propagation of TMS induced cortical responses across cortical mantles, as opposed to evaluating the modulation of the peripheral activity. In this regard, we have recently demonstrated that by monitoring the propagation of TMS induced cortical evoked potentials from the site of stimulation to the contralateral motor area, it may be possible to evaluate the extent of cross talk between the left and right motor areas in healthy subjects at rest (Voineskos et al., 2010). The propagation of TMS induced cortical activity can be also investigated during various motor tasks. Such cortical indices would be of great value in several clinical populations, first for understanding the underlying pathology, for example by comparing the topographical map of signal propagation in stroke patients compared to healthy subjects, and second for optimizing more individually tailored treatment approaches.

One of the most important features of the TMS-EEG combination, however, is the ability to study the neurophysiology of non-motor regions of the cortex where a peripheral response may not be available. For example, examining the modulatory effect of LICI in the prefrontal cortex would enhance our understanding of the inhibitory mechanisms in a cortical area that is more closely associated with the pathophysiology of psychiatric disorders such as schizophrenia and depression. Indeed, using TMS-EEG technology, we have been able to demonstrate selective differences between the modulations of gamma oscillations in the dorsolateral prefrontal (DLPFC) of patients with schizophrenia in comparison to both healthy subjects and patients with bipolar disorder (Farzan et al., 2010a). This is while no deficits were observed in the MEP modulation or modulation of the cortical oscillations in the motor cortex. Therefore, TMS-EEG-EMG combination offers the possibility to monitor subtle changes in the non-motor regions of the cortex which previously were not available through examinations of the peripheral responses.

In this chapter, we provide a brief overview of the past, present and the future status of the TMS-EMG-EEG research. First, we provide a description of the working principle of TMS. We proceed by introducing commonly used TMS-EMG paradigms while providing evidence for the cortical mechanisms that are thought to be involved in the generation and modulation of the TMS evoked MEPs in each TMS paradigm. Then, the way in which TMS-EMG and EEG can be integrated are described along with examples of recent findings which illustrate the validity, reliability and thus the power of combined measurements. Finally, we highlight the application of these techniques in healthy and diseased states, and conclude by briefly discussing the future directions for the TMS-EMG-EEG research.

2. Examining motor pathways through cortical stimulation

2.1 In vitro and animal studies

In vivo examination of the mammalian motor pathways can be traced back to electrical stimulation of the motor cortex of cats under anesthesia (Adrian & Moruzzi, 1939). In these studies, electric shocks were delivered to an exposed area of the cat motor cortex and the potential changes in the pyramidal tracts were recorded through thin wire electrodes inserted into the dorsal surface of the medulla (Adrian & Moruzzi, 1939). Such direct recordings from the pyramidal tracts demonstrated that the stimulation of the motor area results in an excitatory response followed by a period of complete inactivity of the pyramidal tract (Adrian & Moruzzi, 1939). In subsequent experiments, it was further shown that the excitatory response lasted up to 20 ms which was succeeded by a silent period that would last about 200 ms (Krnjevic et al., 1964). It was also shown that the repetitive application of electrical stimulation with a frequency of 5 to 10 pulses per second (i.e. 5-10 Hz) would prolong the duration of the inhibitory period (Adrian & Moruzzi, 1939), while at higher stimulation frequencies (e.g. 20-50 Hz) convulsive firing would be generated followed by even a longer period of inhibition. This long lasting inhibitory phase, which was unlikely to be a result of the refractory period that lasts only about 4 ms, was associated with activation of cortical GABAergic inhibitory interneurons (Krnjevic et al., 1964). Similarly, later in vitro stimulation of human neocortical slices demonstrated similar findings (McCormick, 1989). In this regard, the intracellular recordings from the human temporal lobe slices showed three distinct response phases: an initial fast excitatory post synaptic potential (EPSP) followed by a fast inhibitory post synaptic potential (IPSP) and finally a slow IPSP (McCormick, 1989). It has been suggested that glutamate may underlie the initial EPSP and pharmacological assessments have associated the fast inhibitory response with activation of $GABA_A$ receptors and the second slow acting response with activation of $GABA_B$ receptors (McCormick, 1989).

2.2 Cortical stimulation in humans

Transcranial electrical stimulation (TES) can be regarded as the first technique that permitted the focal stimulation of the human motor cortex by the placement of external electrodes on the scalp (Merton & Morton, 1980). In TES, the electrical stimulation is delivered through a set of two electrodes, one positioned over the motor cortex, and the other 4 cm anterior to the first electrode. Merton and Morton demonstrated that TES applied to the motor cortex through these electrodes could generate a MEP at the periphery that could be captured through EMG recordings. It has been suggested that the activation of cortex through TES is similar to the direct electrical stimulation of the exposed motor cortex of non-human primates (for a review see (Day et al., 1989)). However, TES is a painful procedure, owing to the dissipation of a significant amount of current over the skin before it reaches the brain tissue. For example, to evoke a peripheral response a capacitor that is charged up to 2000 V has to be discharged within a very short time of about 10 µs. As such, TES is mostly used to examine motor pathways in patients with spinal cord injuries and it is often administered during anesthesia. Since the introduction of TMS in 1985, it has now become possible to non-invasively examine the excitability of the motor pathways in awake healthy humans.

2.2.1 Working principles of TMS

Activation of neurons through TMS technique is based on the Faraday's law of induction of electric current via a time-varying magnetic field (Hallett, 2000). In TMS, a magnetic coil is placed tangential to the subject's scalp over the motor area, and intense time-varying current pulses of about 8 kA run though the coil. The time-varying current in the coil induces a time-varying magnetic field perpendicular to the plane of the coil, and hence the surface of brain tissue, which in turn induces an electric field parallel to the plane of the coil in the brain tissue. The duration of a single pulse TMS is typically within a range of 200 to 600 µs. Unlike TES, the induced magnetic field passes through skin, scalp and skull unimpeded, and as such, TMS is less painful than TES. The maximum magnetic field induced by a magnetic stimulator is about 2.5 Tesla which can induce electric field and tissue current of magnitude 500 volt/m and 15 mA/cm^2, respectively. Furthermore, the strength of the induced magnetic field falls exponentially with increasing distance from the surface. Thus, TMS activates the brain tissue in the outer most 2-2.5 cm.

Due to the horizontal orientation of TMS induced current in the cortex, TMS activates horizontally-oriented interneurons with a higher probability compared to the vertically-oriented pyramidal neurons. Therefore, focal TMS activates pyramidal neurons transynaptically, rather than at the axon of pyramidal tract neurons (Rothwell, 1997). For example, when the handle of the magnetic coil is pointed backward, approximately 45° to the mid-sagittal line, the induced current in the brain is perpendicular to the presumed direction of the central sulcus (Day et al., 1989). The indirect activation of pyramidal neurons by TMS is supported by epidural recordings of descending volleys following application of TMS and TES in patients who have spinal stimulators implanted in the epidural space. The results of epidural recordings have demonstrated that TES produces an early descending volley (referred to as direct wave or D-wave) which at a high intensity of stimulation is followed by indirect multiple waves (I-waves) that peak with a delay period of 1.5 ms from one another. By contrast, focal monophasic TMS results primarily in I-waves, and the number of these I-waves and their amplitude increase with the intensity of stimulation. It is reported that TMS may also generate a D-wave at very high intensities (Di Lazzaro et al., 1999b). D-wave and I-waves were originally observed following electrical stimulation of pyramidal tracts of cats. I-waves have been associated with the synaptic activation of pyramidal neurons through excitatory interneurons while D-waves are associated with a direct activation at the axon of pyramidal neurons (reviewed in (Ziemann & Rothwell, 2000)).

2.2.2 Factors affecting the TMS induced current

Several factors affect the depth and pattern of tissue activation and shape of the TMS induced MEP at the periphery. The geometry of the coil (e.g. circular, figure-8, double-cone, H-coil), the shape of the magnetic pulse generated by the coil (e.g. monophasic or biphasic pulse), and the type of material used to construct the core (e.g. solid-core or air-core) affect the characteristics of the induced current. In regards to the coil geometry, a figure-of-8 coil has a greater focality than a circular coil while the newer generations of deep coils, such as H-coil, have the greatest depth of stimulation. The shape of the induced current also varies between each coil type. For example, the induced electrical field is maximal under the rim of the circular coil, and the strength reduces in the centre, while in the figure-eight coil, the maximum field is in the centre of the coil at the junction of the two circular wings. In addition, biphasic TMS pulses are suggested to be more powerful than monophasic pulses and they generate a more complex pattern of neural activation (Di Lazzaro et al., 2001). Finally, solid-core coil are more efficient than air-core coils in transferring the electrical energy to magnetic field and as a result dissipate less heat. In addition to these parameters, the intensity of the pulse and the positioning of the coil affect the induced current and consequently the activation pattern. Consequently, by changing the intensity and the orientation of the coil different populations of neurons can be activated.

3. TMS combined with electromyography

TMS has been used for both therapeutic and diagnostic purposes (Rossini & Rossi, 2007). In relation to its diagnostic application, TMS-EMG provides a tool to assess the timing of cortical processes, cortico-cortical connectivity, cortical inhibition and facilitation, and the interaction between cortical processes (Anand & Hotson, 2002; Chen, 2004; Daskalakis et al., 2004; Di Lazzaro et al., 2004; Pascual-Leone et al., 2000; Sanger et al., 2001). In this section, several of these TMS paradigms will be discussed in more details, and wherever applicable, evidence supporting their neurophysiological mechanisms will be provided.

3.1 Motor threshold

Motor threshold is often determined by applying single pulse TMS to the motor cortex while the coil is placed at the optimal position for eliciting MEPs from a target muscle. The two muscles which are more easily accessible by TMS stimulation are the abductor pollicis brevis (APB) and the first dorsal interosseous (FDI) muscles. Resting motor threshold (RMT) for a target muscle can be determined through applying single pulse TMS to an area of the motor cortex that generates the largest MEP amplitude for the target muscle, and it is defined as the minimum stimulus intensity that can elicit an MEP of more than 50 μV in at least five out of ten trials in the target muscle (Rossini et al., 1994). It has been demonstrated that NMDA antagonists such as ketamine reduce motor threshold, the block of voltage-gated sodium channels increases motor threshold, and GABA has no influence on motor threshold (for a review refer to (Ziemann, 2004)).

3.2 Short interval cortical inhibition

In short interval cortical inhibition (SICI), a subthreshold conditioning stimulus delivered 1 to 5 ms prior to a suprathreshold test stimulus suppresses the MEP response to the test stimulus compared to the MEP response to a test stimulus delivered alone (Kujirai et al., 1993). It has been suggested that suppression of MEP occurs at the cortical level and is not due to the refractoriness of corticospinal tract (Di Lazzaro et al., 1998; Kujirai et al., 1993). For example, epidural recordings have shown that a preceding subthreshold stimulus that does not produce an I-wave by itself, suppresses the late I-waves of a suprathreshold stimulus that is delivered after 1 to 5 ms (Di Lazzaro et al., 1998). In addition, it was shown that magnetic conditioning stimulus did not suppress the response to an electrical test stimulus which activates the axon of the corticospinal tract (Kujirai et al., 1993). Finally, an electrical conditioning stimulus was less effective in suppressing the response to a magnetic test stimulus suggesting that the inhibition observed in SICI is not due to the refractoriness of corticospinal tract (Kujirai et al., 1993). SICI has been associated with the activity of $GABA_A$ receptor mediated inhibitory neurotransmission, as $GABA_A$ agonists such as lorazepam have been shown to enhance SICI as well as the suppression of the late I-waves (Di Lazzaro et al., 2000).

3.3 Intracortical facilitation

In this paradigm, a subthreshold conditioning stimulus delivered 7 to 20 ms prior to a test stimulus, facilitates the MEP response to the test stimulus (Kujirai et al., 1993). It has been suggested that intracortical facilitation (ICF) is an index of the excitability of the excitatory circuits in motor cortex (Ziemann et al., 1996). Pharmacological studies by Ziemann et al. demonstrated that some NMDA antagonists (such as dextrometorphan) and $GABA_A$ agonists (such as lorazepam) reduce ICF, while $GABA_B$ agonists (such as baclofen) increase ICF (Ziemann, 2004). The reduction of ICF by NMDA antagonist suggests that glutamate may play a role in mediating the cortical response observed in ICF.

3.4 Long interval cortical inhibition

In long interval cortical inhibition (LICI), a suprathreshold conditioning stimulus, delivered within 50 to 200 ms prior to a suprathreshold test stimulus, suppresses the response to the test stimulus compared to the response to the test stimulus delivered alone (Valls-Sole et al., 1992). Epidural recordings suggest that this suppression has a cortical origin at ISI of 100 to 200 ms (Chen et al., 1999; Di Lazzaro et al., 2002a; Nakamura et al., 1997). For example, it was shown that LICI at ISI of 100, 150 and 200 ms resulted in suppression of descending volleys, in particular the late I-waves (Chen et al., 1999; Di Lazzaro et al., 2002a; Nakamura et al., 1997). Several lines of evidence suggest that the LICI induced suppression of MEP responses is related to the activity of $GABA_B$ receptor mediated inhibitory neurotransmission ((McDonnell et al., 2006; Sanger et al., 2001); also reviewed in (Kapogiannis & Wassermann, 2008)). It has been suggested that in LICI, activation of the $GABA_B$ receptors by the conditioning stimulus, inhibits excitation of the motor cortex to the test stimulus that would have otherwise excited the cortex if delivered alone. The $GABA_B$ receptor activation is suggested to peak around 150 to 200 ms post stimulus (McCormick, 1989), and interestingly LICI is optimal when conditioning stimulus precedes the test stimulus by 100 to 150 ms (Sanger et al., 2001).

3.5 Cortical silent period

Cortical silent period (CSP) involves a transient suppression of EMG activity following delivery of a single suprathreshold TMS pulse to the motor cortex during voluntary contraction of the target muscle. Previous studies suggest that early part (i.e. first 50 ms) of CSP is due to spinal mechanism, while the later part is mediated by cortical inhibition (Chen et al., 1999; Inghilleri et al., 1993). Similar to LICI, CSP is also associated with $GABA_B$ receptor mediated inhibitory neurotransmission (Chen et al., 1999; Nakamura et al., 1997; Siebner et al., 1998; Werhahn et al., 1999). For example, Siebner et al. reported a significant prolongation of the CSP duration following a continuous intrathecal administration of baclofen in a patient with generalized dystonia (Siebner et al., 1998). Also, tiagabine, a GABA uptake inhibitor, was shown to enhance LICI and prolong CSP duration (Werhahn et al., 1999). Furthermore, administration of vigabatrin, a selective GABAergic drug that increases the availability of GABA in the brain, has also been shown to enhance LICI and CSP (Pierantozzi et al., 2004). In addition, we have recently shown a significant positive relationship between the suppression of MEP amplitudes in LICI (with an ISI of 100 ms), and the duration of the silent period in the CSP paradigm in healthy subjects (Farzan et al., 2010b).

3.6 Interhemispheric inhibition

Interhemispheric inhibition (IHI), also known as transcallosal inhibition, refers to a phenomenon in which a suprathreshold TMS pulse delivered to one hemisphere can inhibit the MEP response to a suprathreshold TMS pulse that is delivered within 6 to 50 ms to the opposite hemisphere (Ferbert et al., 1992; Gerloff et al., 1998). IHI is conventionally measured at an ISI of 6 to 12 ms, however MEP modulation at an ISI of 40 ms has also been demonstrated but suggested to be mediated by different mechanisms (Chen et al., 2003; Ni et al., 2009). By demonstrating the suppression of the late I-waves, epidural recordings have confirmed that IHI is mediated cortically and most likely through transcallosal pathways (Di Lazzaro et al., 1999a). Furthermore, it was shown that the magnetic conditioning stimulation of contralateral hemisphere did not significantly inhibit the response to an electrical test stimulus (Ferbert et al., 1992). Moreover, triple pulse TMS studies have demonstrated that IHI modulates the MEP response to SICI and LICI which, as previously described, are cortically mediated phenomenon, providing further evidence that IHI itself has a cortical origin (Daskalakis et al., 2002b). Moreover, recently a positive association was found between IHI and the integrity of callosal motor fibers (Wahl et al., 2007). The integrity of callosal motor fiber was examined through diffusion tensor imaging and by measuring the fractional anisotropy, a measure of white matter tract integrity. The results of this study suggest that TMS-EMG combination may also provide useful information about the integrity of the callosal motor fibers.

3.7 Sensory afferent inhibition

Sensory afferent inhibition (SAI) involves the modulation of motor cortex excitability by means of an afferent input produced by the electrical stimulation of digital or medial nerve at the wrist (Tokimura et al., 2000). In SAI, a preceding electrical stimulation of the peripheral nerve suppresses the MEP amplitude elicited by the application of a single pulse TMS to the contralateral motor cortex. There are two forms of SAIs that are suggested to be mediated by slightly different mechanisms: short latency SAI, and long latency SAI. Short SAI, which is investigated more thoroughly, occurs when the peripheral stimulation is delivered about 25 ms prior to the TMS pulse, while long SAI is observed when the sensory input is delivered about 200 ms prior to the TMS pulse. Comparison of TMS and TES and recordings of descending volleys suggest that SAI occurs at the cortical level (Tokimura et al., 2000). The molecular underpinnings of SAI are complex and SAI likely relates to an interaction between several neurotransmitter systems with the possible involvement of the cholinergic neurotransmission (Di Lazzaro et al., 2005; Di Lazzaro et al., 2007; Di Lazzaro et al., 1999c).

3.8 Repetitive TMS

It has been demonstrated that repetitive delivery of TMS pulses (rTMS) as well as repetitive application of TMS pulses paired with electrical peripheral nerve stimulation results in an MEP modulation which would outlast the duration of TMS delivery. Conventionally, rTMS is administered through application of TMS pulses at a frequency of 0.5 Hz (ISI of 2 s) to 50 Hz (ISI of 20 ms). It is thought that the repetitive administration of TMS pulses results in summation of TMS induced alteration of cortical activity, thereby causing an effect which may outlast the stimulation period (Chen et al., 1997; Pascual-Leone et al., 1994). The alteration of cortical activity by rTMS has been typically indexed as a suppression or potentiation of MEP responses to the standard single pulse TMS paradigm before and after an active rTMS session or sometimes by comparing the after effects of active versus sham rTMS. A few studies have also evaluated the effect of rTMS on intracortical inhibition by measuring the changes in CSP and MEP modulation by paired pulse TMS before and after rTMS administration (Daskalakis et al., 2006; Fitzgerald et al., 2004). The results of these studies have demonstrated that on average low frequency rTMS (< 5 Hz) applied to the motor cortex suppresses the MEP amplitudes for about 30 min following the end of the rTMS administration ((Chen et al., 1997); reviewed in (Fitzgerald et al., 2006)). The effect of fast frequency rTMS (> 5 Hz) has been shown to be the facilitation of the MEP amplitudes, however results have been somewhat inconsistent across laboratories (Daskalakis et al.,

2006; Fitzgerald et al., 2006; Maeda et al., 2000), perhaps suggestive of a biphasic effect of fast rTMS with a short period of increased excitability followed by a phase of increased inhibition.

It has been suggested that rTMS combined with EMG may be an effective tool for probing and modifying cortical plasticity. Neural plasticity, a mechanism thought to be critical for learning and memory, represents synaptic strength and the degree of signal transmission between coactive cells which can be weakened (long term depression, LTD) or strengthened (long term potentiation, LTP) in response to the presentation of a strong or weak synchronous synaptic stimulation. The lasting effect of rTMS, reflected through suppression and facilitation of TMS induced MEPs, has been suggestive of the potential value of TMS in probing and inducing LTP and LTD like plasticity in the cortex (reviewed in (Pell et al., 2010)). Owing to this lasting effect, application of rTMS to different brain regions may cause behavioural changes that would outlast the duration of rTMS stimulation (For a review refer to (Ridding & Rothwell, 2007)). This aspect of rTMS has been used to improve and restore functional impairments in several disorders such as stroke, movement disorders, addiction, cognitive as well as psychiatric disorders, with the most promising outcomes observed in the treatment of depression (for a review see (Slotema et al., 2010; Wassermann & Lisanby, 2001)).

Plasticity may also be induced through repeated presentation of a pair of somatosensory afferent stimulation and cortical simulation. This can be achieved through the TMS paradigm paired associative stimulation (PAS) which involves pairing of the peripheral electrical nerve stimulation and single pulse TMS of the contralateral motor cortex repeated at a frequency of 0.1 Hz (Classen et al., 2004; Stefan et al., 2002; Stefan et al., 2000). Choosing an appropriate ISI between peripheral and cortical stimulation (e.g. 25 ms), PAS has been shown to induce a potentiation of MEPs in the target muscle which would last about 40 min following the end of the stimulation (Tsuji & Rothwell, 2002). Moreover, pharmacological studies showed that NMDA antagonists suppressed the PAS induced MEP facilitation, while $GABA_A$ receptor antagonist had no effect (Stefan et al., 2002). Some experimental findings suggest that PAS induced effects have a cortical origin. First, following the PAS intervention and in the presence of facilitated MEPs, the F waves recorded from the median nerve stimulation reflected no change in the excitability of α- motor neurons of the median nerve (Stefan et al., 2002). Second, the MEPs evoked by the electrical stimulation of the brainstem remained unchanged following PAS intervention, while the MEP responses to single pulse TMS were increased compared to the baseline MEP responses (Stefan et al., 2000). These findings along with the transynaptic activation of pyramidal neurons by TMS suggest that PAS-induced MEP potentiation is likely mediated through transynaptic mechanisms in the motor cortex (Stefan et al., 2000), seemingly related to the associative (i.e. Hebbian) LTP of synaptic efficacy (Stefan et al., 2002). According to animal studies and in vitro recordings from neocortical slices, associative LTP occurs at an input to a postsynaptic cell which is conditioned by a synchronous activation of another input to that same cell (Buonomano & Merzenich, 1998). Given that PAS induced MEP potentiation is ISI-dependant, it is inferred that the PAS induced plasticity is likely due to the synchronous arrival of the somatosensory afferent input and the TMS induced activation of horizontally oriented interneurons in the sensorimotor cortex (Classen et al., 2004; Stefan et al., 2002; Stefan et al., 2000).

Recently, it was shown that the delivery of repetitive TMS through a protocol named theta burst stimulation (TBS) may be a more efficient way of altering cortical excitability and probing LTP and LTD like cortical responses (Huang et al., 2005). Theta burst stimulation involves application of 3 bursts of 50 Hz rTMS repeated every 200 ms either continuously for a total of 40 s, or intermittently (every 8 s) for a total of 3 min. The continuous (cTBS) and intermittent delivery of TBS (iTBS) have been shown to result in suppression and facilitation of cortical excitability, respectively, as indexed through suppression and facilitation of MEPs at the periphery (Huang et al., 2005). More importantly, it has been shown that despite the relatively short duration of TBS administration (40 s in cTBS and ~ 3 min in iTBS) compared to the conventional rTMS (~ 25 min), the alteration of cortical excitability by TBS can last for about 70 min which is more than twice as long as the duration of the after effects reported in the conventional rTMS approaches (Di Lazzaro et al., 2011; Thut & Pascual-Leone, 2010).

While the combination of TMS with EMG has been instrumental in assessment of several cortical processes, measuring the effect of cortical stimulation at the periphery has several limitations. First, and foremost and as the motor cortex is concerned, the exact mechanism underlying the generation and modulation of the TMS evoked MEPs remains unclear. While TMS-EMG studies in combination with epidural recordings and electrical stimulation can to some extent confirm the cortical origin of MEP responses, such recordings are invasive and only possible in specific subgroups of patients suffering from neurological disorders. To examine the cortical mechanisms involved in the generation of MEPs in healthy human subjects, therefore, a reliable non-invasive recording from the intact brain is desirable. In the next two sections, we will address how a direct but non-invasive recording of cortical activity would complement the conventional TMS-EMG measures.

4. Recording cortical activity in humans through electroencephalography

Recording electrical activity from the intact surface of mammalian cortex dates back to recordings from the dog's skull in 1870s and to the works of Richard Caton and Vladimir Pravdich-Neminski. Later in 1920s, Hans Berger recorded brain waves from the surface of human scalp and named the technique electroencephalography (EEG) (Buzsáki, 2006; Swartz & Goldensohn, 1998). To date, EEG is still the cheapest and the most widely used neurophysiological technique for measuring cortical local field potentials (Buzsáki, 2006). In EEG, electrical activity of the cerebral cortex is monitored by placing multiple electrodes on the scalp. While TMS induced MEPs, for example, are an outcome of an action potential generated by the activation of pyramidal neurons, cortical potentials recorded from the scalp are not a measure of action potential but they represent the activity of slow and fact acting EPSPs and IPSPs mostly originating from the surface of the cortex (Buzsáki, 2006). Cortical potentials recorded through EEG, therefore, represent the oscillatory activity of the underlying brain tissue. Comparison between monozygotic and dizygotic twins has revealed a high heritability for the temporal structure of amplitude fluctuations in EEG oscillations, implying that EEG may be a reliable neurophysiological technique (Linkenkaer-Hansen et al., 2007).

4.1 Generation and function role of cortical oscillations

While the typical firing rate of a motor unit does not exceed the frequency range of 6-35 Hz, neuronal tissues are capable of oscillating within a wide frequency band ranging from less than 1 Hz to as high as 600 Hz. The results of in vivo and in vitro recordings suggest that the brain generates finite number of discrete frequency bands which are conventionally categorized as delta (1-4 Hz), theta (4-7 Hz), alpha (8-12 Hz), beta (12-28 Hz) and gamma (30-50 Hz) oscillations (Buzsáki, 2006), with some recent experimental findings suggestive of the presence of slower (0.02 Hz to 1 Hz) and faster oscillations (up to 600 Hz) (Buzsáki, 2006). Several factors can affect the frequency of cortical oscillations in humans. In particular, the amplitude and frequency of cortical oscillations have been shown to vary between the mental states of sleep, resting, wakefulness, movement or engagement in complex cognitive functioning. Furthermore, it has been shown that each cortical region may have a specific frequency, with slower alpha oscillations observed more prominently over the posterior and parietal lobes and higher gamma frequencies predominant in the anterior region of the brain (i.e. prefrontal cortex)(Rosanova et al., 2009).

The exact mechanisms underlying the generation of cortical oscillations are not yet fully understood. It is suggested that the presence of various channels in the cell membrane provides neurons with intrinsic properties that allow them to oscillate at various frequencies (Buzsáki, 2006). There are several channels in the cell membrane of neurons through which ions move in and out of the cell. The state of these channels (i.e. open versus close state) is regulated by several mechanisms which are collectively referred to as gating. Four gating mechanisms have been identified: voltage gating, ligand gating, ion-dependent gating, and second-messenger gating. It is suggested that a change in the membrane voltage, release of neurotransmitters, or a change in the concentration of ions can change the state of membrane channels and give rise to an oscillatory activity (Buzsáki, 2006). It is further demonstrated that different population of neurons may selectively respond to inputs of different frequencies (Hutcheon & Yarom, 2000; Pike et al., 2000). For example, in hippocampus of rats, fast spiking GABAergic interneurons respond with highest temporal precision to frequencies in the gamma band, whereas pyramidal cells respond to lower frequency rhythmic inputs (Pike et al., 2000). Furthermore, it has been demonstrated that there may be an inverse relation between the size of the neuronal pool and the frequency of oscillations. That is, low frequency oscillations are generated by a larger population of neurons while higher frequency oscillations may be generated by a smaller number of neurons (Buzsáki, 2006).

The functional role of various cortical oscillations is currently under investigation. The functional role of slow frequency delta oscillations, which in healthy subjects are typically observed during deep sleep, is associated with learning and motivational processes (Knyazev, 2007). The cortical activity within the theta-band has been linked to memory functions, and emotional regulations (Knyazev, 2007). Alpha-band oscillations which are predominant during wakeful resting state are suggested to arise from cortical operations in the absence of sensory inputs, and also may reflect the disengagement of task-irrelevant brain areas (Palva & Palva, 2007). Cortical oscillations within the beta range are shown to be more dominant in the central region of the human cortex, suggestive of their functional role in movement execution and control. It has recently been hypothesized that the functional role of beta oscillations may be related to the maintenance of sensorimotor and cognitive state. That is, oscillations within beta band may be a signal for maintenance of status quo (Engel & Fries, 2010). Consistent with this view, it has been suggested that prolongation of beta oscillations may result in deterioration of flexible behaviour (Engel & Fries, 2010). Finally, the functional role of gamma oscillations has been more closely associated with cognitive control. In this regard, results of several EEG studies have found an association between the oscillataory acitivity in the gamma range and perceptual binding such as the construction of object representations, basic information processing such as sensory processing, and complex cognitive processes such as working memory (Buzsáki, 2006; Engel & Singer, 2001; Fries et al., 2007; Howard et al., 2003; Tallon-Baudry & Bertrand, 1999; Tallon-Baudry et al., 1996; Tallon-Baudry et al., 1998).

Recordings of brain activity through EEG suggest that cortical potentials are a result of summation of different oscillatory activities. Several theories and experimental findings exist to explain why different oscillations may be active at the same time. It has been hypothesized that presence of various oscillations may provide the brain with the ability to function through multiple time scales (Buzsáki, 2006). For example, it has been proposed that different frequencies (e.g. slow versus fast oscillations) may favor different types of computation or different level of connectivity. Based on experimental findings, it was hypothesized that middle-frequency oscillations, such as theta and alpha, may represent top-down processes, while high frequency oscillations, such as gamma, may be related to bottom-up processes (von Stein et al., 2000). Furthermore, the interaction between frequency bands has been proposed to be an essential mechanism for optimal information processing (Roopun et al., 2008). One form of frequency-band interaction is frequency concatenation (Roopun et al., 2008). In this regard, two local networks that are co-activated and oscillate at two different frequency bands may interact and generate a third frequency of oscillations. The period of the new oscillation is the concatenation sum of the original two (Roopun et al., 2008). Another form of frequency-band interaction is nesting. In nesting, phase of a lower frequency band (e.g. theta) may modulate the amplitude of a higher frequency band (e.g. gamma). The theta modulation of gamma oscillations has been observed in the hippocampus ((Bragin et al., 1995); reviewed in (Roopun et al., 2008)). The oscillatory modulation of neuronal responses is suggested to play a key role in information processing perhaps by providing a temporal frame with respect to which neurons may communicate with each other (Fries et al., 2007).

4.2 Cortical oscillations in the motor cortex

The presence of beta oscillations over the precentral region was first reported by Jasper and Andrews EEG recordings from healthy human subjects in 1938 (Jasper and Andrews 1938). It is believed that beta frequency can be further subdivided into narrower frequency bands of low- (12-15 Hz), mid- (15-18 Hz) and high-range (18-30 Hz) beta oscillations, each subserving a distinct functional mechanism. A number of previous studies have attempted to explore the cortical correlate of the EMG signals in order to examine the connectivity between the peripheral muscle and the homologous motor area. This has been typically achieved through computing the coherence between the cortical oscillations measured from the motor cortex through EEG or magnetoencephalography and the EMG recordings from the corresponding peripheral muscle often obtained during voluntary isometric hand contraction (for a review see (Mima & Hallett, 1999)). The findings of these cortico-peripheral coherence studies suggest that beta oscillatory activity in the contralateral motor cortex may underlie the generation of EMG signals in the corresponding body part (Brown et al., 1998). For example, tonic hand muscle contraction has been shown to induce beta oscillations (~15-30 Hz) in the contralateral hemisphere which are coherent with the EMG recordings at the periphery (Brown et al., 1998; Salenius et al., 1997).

The modulation of cortical oscillatory activity before, during and after motor task execution, imagination and observation has been well documented. Several studies have reported on desynchronization of alpha and beta oscillations prior to self-paced hand or finger movement often measured through C3 EEG electrode in the left hemisphere and C4 in the right hemisphere (Pfurtscheller et al., 2000). Following self-paced hand movement, desynchronization of alpha oscillations are observed over the contralateral motor cortex (Pineda, 2005) while beta oscillations (~14-32 Hz) are induced shortly (within one second) after the movement termination (Pfurtscheller et al., 2000). Observation and imagination of motor movement also result in suppression of alpha oscillations in motor areas corresponding to that body part (Pfurtscheller et al., 2000). Furthermore, the peak frequency of the induced beta oscillations may differ between motor areas associated with different body parts. For example, hand movement was shown to induce an oscillatory activity within a frequency range of 16-22 Hz over the hand area, while slightly higher frequency oscillatory activity (19-26 Hz) were recorded in the foot area following foot movement (Neuper & Pfurtscheller, 2001).

The combination of TMS with EMG has offered the possibility to trigger and quantify the magnitude of an involuntary movement, and evoke or slow down activation of a target muscle. As previously described, this is achieved through transynaptic manipulation of corticospinal pathway through application of TMS to the motor area that optimally represents the target muscle on the periphery. However, the specific cortical oscillations that underlie these TMS induced motor responses cannot be clearly identified through only EMG recordings. In the following section, it will be demonstrated that combination of online EEG recording with TMS-EMG would permit examining the functional role of cortical oscillations in each TMS paradigm. The advancement in the EEG amplifier technology that has led to the combination of these modalities will be first briefly described.

5. Combining TMS-EMG with concurrent EEG recording

Simultaneous EEG recording during TMS stimulation was previously unattainable because of the technological shortcomings of EEG amplifiers that would saturate for a long duration due to the large artifact produced by the magnetic stimulation. For example, application of a single monophasic TMS pulse would result in artifact lasting for several seconds after the pulse. Such long lasting artifact blocked the window of time during which neurophysiological processes such as cortical inhibition occur (the first 250 ms following TMS). The newer generation of EEG systems, however, can recover from the TMS artifact within a time window of 10 to 70 ms.

The newer generations of EEG systems offer several strategies to minimize the saturation of amplifiers following TMS. In a majority of TMS-EEG systems, the saturation of EEG amplifiers is avoided by virtue of a sample and hold circuit that pins the amplifier output to a constant level starting from a few milliseconds prior to the TMS application to a few milliseconds after the pulse (Nexstim Ltd., Helsinki, Finland). Some systems are equipped with a magnetic shielding technology in which the EEG electrodes and the amplifiers are shielded from the magnetic artifact (Advanced Neuro Technology, Enschede, Netherland). It is also possible to minimize amplifier saturation and the TMS related artifact through a combination of a wide dynamic range (e.g. recording potentials ranging from -200 to 200 mV in amplitude and with a resolution much lower than 1 μV), high frequency sampling rate (e.g. 20 KHz) and DC filtering (NeuroScan, Compumedics, USA). By employing any of the above strategies, EEG recording can become TMS compatible. Therefore, it is possible to continuously record EEG during TMS stimulation (for a review refer to (Ilmoniemi & Kicic, 2009)).

5.1 Single pulse TMS

Ilmoniemi and colleagues were one of the first research groups that used the interleaved TMS-EEG technique to investigate the effect of TMS on cortical excitability (Ilmoniemi et al., 1997). It was demonstrated that TMS applied to the hand representation area of the human motor cortex elicited a cortical response that spread to the adjacent ipsilateral area as well as to the homologous regions in the opposite hemisphere. It was further shown that the application of TMS to the visual cortex resulted in similar pattern of signal propagation to the contralateral areas, therefore providing evidence that the cortical potentials following motor cortex stimulation were less likely to be a result of peripheral sensory activation. This original experiment resulted in a series of studies that further characterized the EEG substrate of cortical excitability, plasticity and connectivity in healthy subjects (Esser et al., 2006; Kahkonen et al., 2001; Kahkonen et al., 2003; Komssi et al., 2002; Komssi & Kahkonen, 2006; Nikulin et al., 2003; Paus et al., 2001; Thut et al., 2003).

In a number of previous studies it was demonstrated that single pulse TMS applied to the motor cortex generated several EEG peaks within the first 300 ms of TMS stimulation. The EEG components that are commonly replicated across TMS-EEG studies are a negativity at 15 ms (N15), a positivity at 30 ms (P30) followed by N45, P55, N100, P180, and N280 (Komssi & Kahkonen, 2006). Comparing these EEG peaks with the size of MEP responses may permit examining the cortical origin of the TMS induced MEPs. In this regard, it has been shown that TMS induced MEP amplitudes positively correlate with the amplitude of the TMS induced early evoked potential, measured as the peak-to-peak amplitude of the N15-P30 component (Maki & Ilmoniemi, 2010b). In a study by the same group, the relationship between the TMS induced MEPs and the cortical oscillatory activity was explored. It was shown that in the motor cortex, the power of mid-range beta oscillatory activity (12-18 Hz) was weaker before large MEPs as compared to smaller MEPs. Furthermore, the phase of the mid-range beta oscillations recorded over the occipital cortex correlated with the MEP amplitudes (Maki & Ilmoniemi, 2010a). Similarly, Schutter and Hortensius examined the association between cortical oscillatory activity and MEP amplitudes during isometric hand contraction. It was reported that MEP amplitudes could be modeled by the activity of theta (4-7 Hz) and beta (13-30 Hz) cortical oscillations in the right and left primary motor cortex (Schutter & Hortensius, 2011). These authors went a step further and applied this finding to selectively control the therapeutic outcome of transcranial alternative current stimulation (tACS) (for detailed description of tACS readers may refer to (Kanai et al., 2008)). In this experiment, they applied the tACS with two different frequency settings of theta-beta and alpha-alpha configuration which were administered on two separate days. It was shown that the theta-beta tACS significantly increased cortical excitability compared to the alpha-alpha stimulation (Schutter & Hortensius, 2011).

A few studies have also examined the inhibitory components of TMS induced cortical potential. For example, Nikulin et al. demonstrated that following visually triggered hand movement, the N100 component of EEG response was suppressed while the MEP amplitudes were increased (Nikulin et al., 2003). This inverse relationship between the amplitudes of N100 and MEP is thought to reflect the inhibitory nature of N100. Consistent with this finding, the duration of silent period in the CSP paradigm was shown to be positively correlated with the amplitude of the N100 component (Kimiskidis et al., 2008). Interestingly, in a TMS study that investigated the effect of alcohol on TMS evoked cortical potentials, it was shown that following alcohol intake, which is thought to affect the activity

Combination of Transcranial Magnetic Stimulation with Electromyography and Electroencephalography:
Application in Diagnosis of Neuropsychiatric Disorders

77

of GABAergic neurotransmission, the amplitude of N100 response to single pulse TMS was significantly decreased (Kahkonen & Wilenius, 2007). Finally, the effect of age, TMS intensity, sensory attention and response preparation on TMS induced N100 response was investigated in a TMS study conducted in motor cortex of healthy children within an age range of 6-10 years. It was shown that N100 response was attenuated following a task that required a fast response, providing further evidence that N100 was likely related to an inhibitory process (Bender et al., 2005). In addition, N100 response was reported to be larger in children compared to N100 responses of adults in previous studies and a negative correlation was found between N100 response and age in children, suggesting that N100 response may undergo maturation (Bender et al., 2005). Collectively, these findings suggest that GABAergic inhibitory mechanism may underlie the N100 generation. If proved a reliable measure, N100 may be used as a marker for investigating the integrity of the inhibitory responses in healthy and pathological conditions.

5.2 Paired Pulse TMS
5.2.1 Short interval cortical inhibition and intracortical facilitation
One of the first studies evaluating the modulatory effect of paired pulse TMS on cortical evoked potentials is the experiments conducted by Paus et al. (Paus et al., 2001). In this study, SICI and ICF paired pulse paradigms were applied to the left motor cortex of healthy subjects and the amplitude and frequency of EEG responses were compared between single and paired pulse conditions. In this study, three prominent EEG peaks were observed following the singe pulse TMS: N45, P55 and N100. Furthermore, it was shown that single pulse TMS resulted in synchronization of beta oscillations which lasted for several hundred milliseconds after the TMS delivery. Following the ICF paired pulse paradigm, which as discussed before is designed to examine intracortical facilitation, the presence of a subthreshold conditioning stimulus (at an ISI of 12 ms) significantly reduced the amplitude of the EEG N45 component. In addition, the beta oscillatory activity that was recorded following ICF was reported to be smaller as compared to the oscillatory activity following the single pulse condition. By contrast, a conditioning stimulus delivered at an ISI of 3 ms (SICI paradigm) had no effect on either the N45 or beta oscillatory activity.
In a recent study, similar paired pulse experiments were conducted to further confirm and expand the above mentioned findings (Ferreri et al., 2010). In this study, SICI (ISI of 3 ms) and ICF (ISI of 11 ms) paradigms were applied to the left motor cortex of healthy subjects. Several EEG components were observed following single pulse TMS including: N7, P13, N18, P30, N44, P60, N100, P190 and N280. These EEG components were further identified for each stimulation condition and each EEG electrode (19 electrodes). The authors then examined the correlation between the MEP amplitudes and the amplitude of each EEG components in each electrode, after the three TMS conditions of suprathreshold single pulse and the paired pulse conditions of SICI and ICF. It was observed that depending on the stimulation condition (single pulse, SICI or ICF), MEP amplitudes correlated with different EEG components and at a different cortical region. For example, a positive correlation was observed between the MEP amplitude and the P30 component over the non-stimulated motor cortex following the single pulse condition and in the F4 (contralateral prefrontal cortex) following the paired pulse condition. Moreover, N44 peak was attenuated in the contralateral cortex more prominently in the ICF condition, a finding consistent with the earlier report of attenuation of N45 flowing ICF (ISI of 12 ms) as described above (Paus et al., 2001). Furthermore, it was noted that the N100 component was strongest over the

stimulation area (C3 electrode) and its amplitude was larger following the paired pulse conditions as compared to the single pulse condition. Collectively these findings suggest that TMS-EEG offers the possibility to examine not only the MEP-EEG relationship but also the connectivity between cortical regions as it may be evident by comparing the TMS induced EEG activity at the stimulation site with the EEG components recorded in the remaining electrodes.

5.2.2 Long interval cortical inhibition

As briefly described in the introduction, the cortical correlate of LICI has been recently investigated through the combination of TMS-EMG with simultaneous EEG recording. That is, we demonstrated that EMG measures of LICI, measured as the suppression of MEPs in the paired pulse condition compared to the single pulse conditions, were positively correlated with the suppression of the cortical evoked potentials at the site of stimulation (C3 electrode) in the paired pulse condition compared to the single pulse conditions (Daskalakis et al., 2008). In this study, however, instead of examining the peak-to-peak amplitude of EEG components separately, the TMS induced cortical response was identified as the area under the rectified EEG response following the single and paired pulse conditions within the time window of 50 ms (the earliest reliable recording without TMS artifact) to 150 ms (the maximum peak of GABA$_B$ receptor activation). Similarly, the potentiation of MEP response was also examined by comparing the area under the rectified MEP response between the single and paired pulse condition.

Furthermore, in a separate study we found a positive correlation between the duration of the silent period indexed through the CSP paradigm and the extent of EEG and EMG suppression following LICI in a subset of subjects who received both LICI and CSP in their left motor cortex (Farzan et al., 2010b). A key observation was that the silent period seemed to be more strongly correlated with the EEG measures of LICI as compared to the EMG measures of LICI (Farzan et al., 2010b). This observation suggests that EEG measures of LICI maybe a more precise technique for evaluating and comparing the cortical mechanisms that may be common across TMS-EMG paradigms. For instance, it has been suggested that the early (< 50 ms) part of the silent period in the CSP paradigm may originate from spinal mechanism (Chen et al., 1999; Inghilleri et al., 1993). Therefore, by comparing CSP with both EEG and EMG measures of LICI (and other paired pulse paradigms), it may be possible to approximate to what degree each of these paradigms originate from the cortical rather than spinal mechanisms and also to what extent they are mediated by similar processes.

Furthermore, using the above methods, for the first time we examined the modulatory effect of LICI in the DLPFC, a non-motor region of the cortex which is implicated in a number of neurological and psychiatric illnesses (Daskalakis et al., 2008). We were able to show that similar to the motor cortex, LICI applied over the left DLPFC resulted in significant suppression of cortical evoked potentials (30% suppression) in the vicinity of TMS application (i.e. AF3 electrode). However, it was also shown that the extent of EEG suppression following LICI in the DLPFC was not correlated with the EEG or EMG suppression following the application of LICI to the motor cortex (Farzan et al., 2010b), a finding which may further reflect the valuable integration of EEG and paired pulse TMS which allow us to both measure and compare the neurophysiology of motor and non-motor regions of the cortex.

In line with this view, we also examined the effect of LICI on cortical oscillatory activity at the site of TMS stimulation following the LICI application in both the motor cortex and the

Combination of Transcranial Magnetic Stimulation with Electromyography and Electroencephalography:
Application in Diagnosis of Neuropsychiatric Disorders

79

DLPFC (Farzan et al., 2009). Interestingly, it was observed that LICI applied over the motor cortex had a different modulatory effect on the cortical oscillations as compared to the LICI applied to the DLPFC (Farzan et al., 2009). In the motor cortex, delta, theta and alpha oscillations were suppressed without any suppression of beta and gamma oscillations. By contrast, all cortical oscillations were significantly suppressed following the application of LICI to the left DLPFC. The differential effect of LICI on fast cortical oscillations (e.g. gamma oscillations) in the prefrontal and motor cortices provides more insight about the functional roles of these cortical oscillations in each cortical mantel.

5.2.3 Interhemispheric inhibition
Through TMS-EEG it is possible to examine the correlation between functional and structural interhemispheric connectivity in both motor and non-motor regions of the cortex. This is possible through application of suprathreshold single pulse TMS to one hemisphere and examining the propagation of TMS induced cortical evoked activity to the contralateral hemisphere, a cortical process which we suggest may be mediated by similar mechanisms that underlie MEP suppression observed in the conventional IHI paradigm (Voineskos et al., 2010). Using TMS-EEG and diffusion tensor imagining, we investigated the extent of interhemispheric signal propagation from the stimulated site to the contralateral hemisphere as a function of integrity of callosal fibers (Voineskos et al., 2010). We showed that following suprathreshold TMS applied to the left motor cortex, the amount of cortical evoked activity that reached the contralateral hemisphere was inversely correlated with the integrity of callosal motor fibers but not with the integrity of anterior callosal fibers, suggesting an anatomically specific structural-functional relationship. Similarly, we found an anatomically-specific relationship between the extent of interhemispheric propagation of TMS-induced cortical activity from the left DLPFC to the right DLPFC and the fractional anisotropy of anterior callosal fibers (genu) connecting left and right DLPFC, and not with the integrity of callosal motor fibers. That is, in subjects that fractional anisotropy of callosal motor fibers was larger, the propagation of suprathreshold TMS induced activity to the contralateral motor cortex was of smaller magnitude, and in subjects that fractional anisotropy of genu fibers was larger, the extent of propagation of suprathreshold TMS induced activity to the contralateral DLPFC was of a smaller value. These results collectively suggest that in the presence of suprathreshold stimulus, callosal fibers may regulate the cross talk between hemispheres perhaps through similar mechanism that underlie the inhibition of MEPs in the contralateral hand muscle in the conventional IHI paradigm.

5.2.4 Sensory afferent inhibition
The interleaved TMS-EEG was also used to examine the correlation between the cortical and peripheral effects of SAI. In a study conducted by Bikmullina et al., it was demonstrated that the suppression of MEPs following SAI was positively correlated with the attenuation of the amplitude of the EEG N100 component (Bikmullina et al., 2009). This finding supports the findings of earlier studies that suggested a cortical origin for the suppression of MEPs in SAI paradigm. Furthermore, the attenuation of N100 is an interesting observation by itself as it may be a further support for a link between N100 and activity of GABA$_B$ receptor mediated inhibitory mechanism. In this regard, in a triple pulse study, it was demonstrated that SAI had an inhibitory effect on LICI (Udupa et al., 2009). As previously mentioned, suppression of MEPs in LICI has been associated with the activity of slow acting GABA$_B$ receptors.

Therefore, the attenuation of N100 component following SAI is a further support for the inhibitory effect of SAI on GABAergic mechanism and the plausible involvement of GABA$_B$ receptors in generation of N100 component.

Moreover, spectral analysis of EEG response following SAI in rat somatosensory cortex has demonstrated that the extent of SAI varies with the cortical state and the frequency of the underlying cortical oscillations. In particular SAI was enhanced following increases in delta oscillations (Funke & Benali, 2009). The findings of this animal experiment provides further support to reiterate the importance of online EEG recording during TMS-EMG, as some of the inter-subject and inter-laboratory variance that are observed across studies may be explained by the dependence of TMS-EMG measures on cortical states and cortical oscillatory activity immediately before or at the time of TMS stimulation.

5.3 Repetitive TMS

A key advantage of concurrent EEG recording is the ability to directly evaluate the effect of rTMS on cortical excitability. As previously mentioned, slow and fast frequency rTMS applied to the motor cortex may have a differential effect on the cortical excitability. As described earlier, the alteration of cortical excitability by rTMS is conventionally probed through evaluating the changes in MEP responses to single pulse of TMS applied to the motor cortex before and after rTMS session. However, brain is a network of interconnected cortical regions and it is unlikely that rTMS effect would remain solely within the stimulated region. In fact, as described above, the TMS induced cortical evoked activity propagates across cortical mantels and may differentially affect the interconnected local and distant brain regions (Ferreri et al., 2010; Voineskos et al., 2010). Furthermore, evaluation of MEP modulations is limited to investigating the cortical activity of the motor cortex while rTMS treatment is often administered in non-motor regions of the cortex such as the DLPFC in the treatment of depression. Finally, the origin of rTMS mediated modulation of MEP remains a matter of debate. Therefore, recording both cortical and peripheral response before, during and after rTMS would enhance our understanding of the effect of rTMS on both motor and non-motor regions of the cortex and would be critical in examining the exact mechanisms through which rTMS exerts its therapeutic effect. In this vein, research examining the cortico-peripheral effect of rTMS is expanding, some of which will be discussed here.

In one of the earlier studies examining the cortical signature of rTMS induced MEP potentiation, the cortical and peripheral response to single pulse TMS were evaluated before and after 5 Hz rTMS of motor cortex in healthy human subjects (Esser et al., 2006). It was reported that following rTMS, the TMS induced EEG components in response to subthreshold single pulse TMS were selectively potentiated within a time window of 15 to 55 ms. In a similar study, the effect of slow frequency rTMS (0.6 Hz) was assessed by examining the amplitude of EEG N45 response to subthreshold single pulse TMS before and after 15 minutes of rTMS administration (Van Der Werf & Paus, 2006). In this study, it was reported that despite the lack of any rTMS induced MEP modulation, the amplitude of N45 response was reduced. This finding may suggest that EEG response is a more sensitive indicator of rTMS effect as compared to MEP. In another study, the effect of 1 Hz rTMS on cortical oscillations was examined and compared with the suppression of MEPs at the periphery (Brignani et al., 2008). In this study, three 10-min blocks of 1 Hz rTMS was applied to the left primary motor cortex of healthy subjects. Spectral analysis was performed and the power of alpha and beta band oscillations was obtained during each three rTMS blocks. It was shown that the power of cortical oscillations, more prominently alpha oscillations, increased with increase in TMS

Combination of Transcranial Magnetic Stimulation with Electromyography and Electroencephalography: Application in Diagnosis of Neuropsychiatric Disorders

81

duration. The increase in power of cortical oscillations was inversely correlated with the suppression of MEP amplitudes at the periphery. It was suggested that the increase of oscillatory activity may be a representation of altered cortical excitability, possibly related to an increase in the activity of inhibitory mechanism (Brignani et al., 2008). Interestingly, the increase in alpha and beta band cortical oscillations was also documented in a recent study that examined cortical response to 20 Hz rTMS applied to the left primary motor cortex (Veniero et al., 2011). It was demonstrated that synchronization of alpha and beta band cortical oscillations recorded from the C3 electrode was also positively related to the number of delivered stimuli. Furthermore, there was an inverse correlation between the MEP amplitude and synchronization of beta band oscillations, showing that smaller MEP amplitudes were related to higher power of beta oscillations (Veniero et al., 2011).

Theta burst stimulation is a relatively new rTMS approach that has attracted a lot of interest due to its long lasting effect relative to the short administration period. While 25 minutes of 1 Hz rTMS may induce changes lasting for about 30 minutes, only 40 seconds of TBS may result in MEP modulation lasting for more than 60 minutes (Huang et al., 2005). Previous TMS-EMG studies had shown that application of cTBS over the motor cortex results in suppression of MEPs at the periphery. Through combination of TMS-EMG with concurrent EEG recording, it has been demonstrated that the cortico-peripheral effect of cTBS involves a reduction in the cortico-muscular coherence within the cortical beta band oscillations measured thorough EEG C3 electrode in the primary motor cortex (Saglam et al., 2008).

The effect of PAS on cortical evoked potentials has recently been investigated to also examine the cortical origin and EEG substrate of PAS induced LTP in the motor cortex of healthy subjects. In an interesting study by Hubert et al it was shown that the EEG changes following PAS, as opposed to MEP changes, could predict the modification of slow wave (0.5-4.7 Hz) activity during sleep (Huber et al., 2008). In this study, PAS was administered to healthy subjects at two ISIs of 10 ms and 25 ms. Authors then evaluated the cortical evoked potentials in response to single pulse of TMS applied to the motor cortex before and after PAS intervention. Subjects were then allowed to sleep shortly after PAS and their sleep EEG was recorded and analyzed. It was reported that on average PAS at 25 ms resulted in potentiation of TMS-evoked MEPs and PAS at 10 ms resulted in suppression of MEP responses, although the reverse was also observed in a few subjects. The study yielded three interesting findings. First, it was shown that there was a weak but significant correlation between the MEP amplitudes measured through EMG and the cortical evoked potentials measured through EEG. Second, interestingly, the location of maximum cortical activation was over the sensorimotor cortex near the site of stimulation where the effect of afferent and cortical stimulation would most likely overlap, thus further supporting the LTP like mechanisms that underlie PAS-induced MEP potentiation. Finally, in subjects that showed a potentiation of cortical evoked potentials in response to PAS intervention (regardless of the ISI or MEP modulation) the power of slow wave activity was increased during sleep that followed the PAS intervention. By contrast, in subjects that cortical evoked potentials were suppressed following PAS intervention (again, regardless of the ISI or MEP modulation), a relative reduction of slow wave activity was observed. The finding that the modulation of cortical evoked potentials was a better predictor of subsequent changes during sleep is a further support for the significance of probing plasticity and modulation of cortical excitability directly from the cortex.

Furthermore, utilizing the cortical evoked potentials to index PAS induced LTP and LTD like plasticity, a recent study has attempted to examine the PAS induced plasticity in both the motor cortex and DLPFC of healthy subjects. Application of PAS in the DLPFC was achieved by pairing the afferent peripheral stimulation with single pulse TMS applied to the contralateral DLPFC. The preliminary results of this study, currently presented in an abstract form (Rajji TK et al., 2011), shows that in line with findings of Hubert et al. following PAS intervention in the motor cortex, there was a significant correlation between the cortical evoked potentials recorded at the stimulation site and the MEP response at the periphery. It was noted that while all subjects demonstrated potentiation of cortical evoked potentials, MEPs were not potentiated in a subset of subjects. Finally, it was shown that PAS applied to the DLPFC results in significant potentiation of cortical evoked potentials recorded from the DLPFC which is perhaps, if not the first, one of the first studies directly probing LTP like plasticity in the DLPFC of healthy subjects, a cortical region more closely associated with learning and memory.

Similarly, the effect of rTMS on non-motor regions of the cortex can also be evaluated through TMS-EEG. The observation that LICI modulated cortical oscillations differently in the motor compared to the prefrontal cortex (Farzan et al., 2009) suggests that fast versus slow rTMS and cTBS versus iTBS may have differential modulatory effect on cortical oscillations of motor compared to non-motor regions of the cortex such as DLPFC. In fact, in a recent study published by our group it was demonstrated that one session of 20 Hz rTMS applied bilaterally to the left and right DLPFC results in increased power of gamma cortical oscillations during cognitive performance in healthy subjects (Barr et al., 2009) and reduced gamma oscillations in patients with schizophrenia (Barr et al. 2011). Future studies should more systematically investigate the effect of rTMS with different stimulation parameters (e.g. frequency) on motor and non-motor regions of the cortex. Such studies would enhance the efficacy of rTMS therapy.

6. Reproducibility and reliability of TMS-EEG-EMG measures

Research experiments systematically examining the test-retest reliability of TMS induced MEPs are relatively scarce. In this regard, one study has examined the reliability of TMS in identifying the APB muscle motor map between two separate sessions (Corneal et al., 2005). It was also shown that increasing the number of delivered stimuli in TMS paradigms would reduce the intersession variability (Boroojerdi et al., 2000). There are also a few studies that have demonstrated the reliability of TMS induced MEP modulation in the paired pulse paradigms of SICI and ICF (Boroojerdi et al., 2000; Maeda et al., 2002). For example, Maeda et al. reported that SICI was reproducible and correlated between two sessions separated by two weeks (Maeda et al., 2002).

Given the increasing popularity of TMS-EEG-EMG approach as both a therapeutic and diagnostic tool, the number of research experiments examining the reliability and validity of cortical and peripheral indices of TMS is on the rise. The reproducibility of TMS induced cortical responses to single pulse TMS were recently demonstrated in the motor cortex and DLPFC of healthy subjects (Lioumis et al., 2009). Lioumis et al. reported generation of six EEG peaks in the ipsilateral (at latencies 13, 32, 54, 66, 111, 172 ms post TMS) and contralateral (12, 31, 50, 73, 111, 176 ms post TMS) motor cortex following the application of suprathreshold single pulse to the left motor cortex, and six peaks were defined in the ipsilateral DLPFC (first one contaminated by noise, 25, 49, 64, 113, 170 ms post TMS) and contralateral DLPFC (21, 32, 48, 63, 113, and 174 ms post TMS) following suprathreshold TMS to the left DLPFC. It was reported that the amplitudes of TMS evoked cortical

Combination of Transcranial Magnetic Stimulation with Electromyography and Electroencephalography:
Application in Diagnosis of Neuropsychiatric Disorders

83

potentials at various stimulation intensities were highly reliable in both the ipsilateral DLPFC and motor cortex between sessions separated by a one-week interval (test-retest correlation >0.83), while considering the contralateral response, contralateral DLPFC response was more reliable than motor cortex perhaps reflecting the stronger interhemispheric connectivity of the prefrontal cortices (Lioumis et al., 2009).

In a study conducted by our group, we extended the results of previous reports by demonstrating the reliability of cortical and peripheral indices of LICI, as well as the reliability of LICI mediated modulation of each cortical oscillation in both the left motor cortex and left DLPFC (Farzan et al., 2010b). In the motor cortex, we showed that all EEG and EMG measures of LICI were highly reliable, and in the DLPFC all EEG indices of LICI were highly reliable between sessions separated by one-week (Cronbach's alpha ranging from 0.7 to 0.9). Furthermore, we replicated the correlation between EEG measures of LICI and EMG measures of LICI in an extended sample size of 36 subjects. Finally, for the first time we demonstrated a positive correlation between the EEG measures of LICI and the duration of cortical silent period, as indexed through the CSP paradigm. Previous pharmacological studies had linked the cortical silent period and MEP suppression by LICI to the activity of $GABA_B$ receptor mediated inhibitory neurotransmission. Collectively, these findings further confirm the validity and reliability of EEG measures of LICI as indices of GABAergic inhibitory mechanism, and also provide evidence for the cortical origin of MEP modulation and the silent period in the LICI and CSP paradigms, respectively. In the next section, we will discuss how some of these measures can be used to enhance the diagnostic and therapeutic efficacy of TMS.

7. TMS-EEG-EMG in diagnosis and treatment of neuropsychiatric disorders

Since the introduction of TMS in 1985, deficits of TMS induced MEPs have been reported in a number of neurological and psychiatric conditions. Among movement disorders, reduction of SICI (Hanajima et al., 1996; Pierantozzi et al., 2001; Ridding et al., 1995; Strafella et al., 2000), prolongation of silent period, and increases in LICI has been reported in the motor cortex of patients with Parkinson's disease (Berardelli et al., 2008; Berardelli et al., 1996). In another study, impairment of both SICI and ICF was observed in early Parkinson's disease patients not treated with dopamine agonists (Bares et al., 2003). Among neuropsychiatric disorders, reduction of CSP, IHI and SICI was reported in unmedicated patients with schizophrenia, while these measures of cortical inhibition were not significantly impaired in medicated patients with schizophrenia (Daskalakis et al., 2002a). Similarly, the reduction of SICI, IHI and CSP was also demonstrated in the motor cortex of patients with bipolar disorder (Levinson et al., 2007). Application of TMS-EMG in cognitive disorders has shown that patients with Alzheimer's disease have reduced SAI measures (Di Lazzaro et al., 2002b), and it was reported that an oral dose of rivastigmine enhanced SAI in a subgroup of patients (Di Lazzaro et al., 2002b). Reduction of SAI has also been reported in early Alzheimer's disease (Nardone et al., 2008). While these TMS-EMG indices have moved us a step closer to the underlying source of some of these disorders, the exact mechanisms underlying the generation of MEPs and thus the sources of such impairments have remained a matter of debate. Furthermore, the pathophysiology of neuropsychiatric illnesses such as schizophrenia, bipolar disorder and Alzheimer's disease is more closely associated with impairment of non-motor regions of the cortex which are not easily accessible through the conventional TMS-EMG indices of cortical processes.

The combination of TMS-EMG with concurrent EEG recordings permits the assessment of cortical origin of MEP impairments. For example, the cortico-muscular coherence and EEG spectral analysis, discussed in previous sections, can be used to understand the origin of MEP impairments in movement disorders and neurological diseases that have abnormalities of the corticospinal pathway and the cortical oscillatory activity of the motor cortex such as in Parkinson's disease and dystonia (Di Lazzaro et al., 2009; Levy et al.). Furthermore, the combination of TMS with EEG allows for examining cortical processes in neuropsychiatric disorders which are closely associated with impairments of cortical oscillatory activity in the non-motor regions of the cortex. For example, impairments in gamma oscillations have been reported during cognitive performance in the prefrontal cortex in patients with schizophrenia (Basar-Eroglu et al., 2007; Cho et al., 2006). In this regard, we have recently replicated previous studies, such as those by Basar-Eroglu et al. by demonstrating that patients with schizophrenia exhibit excessive power of gamma oscillations during working memory performance (Barr et al., 2010). Given these frontal gamma deficits, we conducted a TMS-EEG-EMG experiment to examine the integrity of LICI induced modulation of gamma oscillations in the DLPFC of patients with schizophrenia compared to healthy subject in whom, as described previously, LICI resulted in a significant inhibition of gamma oscillations following paired pulse stimulation of DLPFC(Farzan et al., 2009). Utilizing these EEG measures of LICI, which were shown to have high test-retest reliability (Farzan et al., 2010b), we have in fact demonstrated that inhibition of gamma oscillations was selectively impaired in the DLPFC of patients with schizophrenia compared to both healthy subjects and patients with bipolar disorder (Farzan et al., 2010a). Interestingly, we observed no deficits in the EEG or EMG measures of LICI in the motor cortex or in modulation of any other frequency bands in the DLPFC. Patients with bipolar disorder were similar to patients with schizophrenia in relation to severity of symptoms, illness duration, and history of psychosis, and about half of them were on antipsychotic medications. In addition, the extent of gamma inhibition did not correlate with the medication dosage, suggesting that the specificity of gamma inhibition deficits to schizophrenia and the DLPFC is less likely to be part of a generalized deficit that is simply related to psychotropic medications and it may represent a candidate endophenotype for schizophrenia. Combining these finding with evidence of impaired gamma modulation during cognitive performance in patients with schizophrenia, it may be hypothesized that the impairments of LICI induced modulation of gamma oscillations in the DLPFC may, at least partly, underlie the excessive power of gamma oscillations that has been reported during working memory performance and perhaps the frontal cognitive deficits in this illness.

In line with these findings, cognitive impairments and the deficits in learning and memory, a process thought to be related to cortical plasticity, constitute one of the core deficits of schizophrenia (Gold & Harvey, 1993). Indeed, in a previous TMS-EMG study, TMS paradigm PAS was used to investigate the integrity of LTP-like plasticity in the motor cortex of patients with schizophrenia (Frantseva et al., 2008). In this study, the effect of PAS in patients with schizophrenia and healthy subjects was evaluated through evaluating the TMS induced MEP response to single pulse of TMS after PAS, and also through examining the effect of PAS on learning a subsequent motor task (rotary pursuit motor task). It was demonstrated that not only patients with schizophrenia had significantly less MEP facilitation in response to PAS, but there was also a correlation between the PAS induced potentiation of MEPs and performance on the motor learning task (Frantseva et al., 2008). That is, patients with schizophrenia who had less MEP potentiation following PAS compared to healthy subjects, also performed poorly on the subsequent motor task

Combination of Transcranial Magnetic Stimulation with Electromyography and Electroencephalography:
Application in Diagnosis of Neuropsychiatric Disorders

85

compared to healthy subjects. Consistent with these finding, both medicated and unmedicated patients with schizophrenia demonstrated a reduced plastic response to 15 min of 1 Hz rTMS applied to the motor cortex compared to healthy subjects (Fitzgerald et al., 2004). It was also shown that the duration of CSP at baseline correlated positively with the rTMS response. That is, patients who had less plastic response to rTMS also had a shorter CSP duration at baseline. The results of these studies would be significantly complemented by examining LTP like plasticity in the DLPFC of patients with schizophrenia through PAS or rTMS combined with EEG. In fact, such experiments are currently underway. Preliminary results of a recent experiment has so far shown that following application of PAS in the DLPFC, patients with schizophrenia demonstrate a deficit in potentiation of cortical evoked potentials recorded from the DLPFC compared to the healthy subjects (Rajji TK et al., 2011).

Furthermore, similar to PAS and LICI, EEG measures of SAI can be used to assess the cortical origin and the cortical oscillatory activity underlying the SAI deficits in Alzheimer's disease. The combination of TMS-EMG with EEG would further permit assessing the effect of afferent sensory stimuli on the prefrontal cortex, which is perhaps more closely associated with the impairment of cognitive disorders. Similar to PAS, this can be conducted through combination of peripheral nerve and single pulse TMS applied to the DLPFC, as opposed to the motor cortex, and examining the amplitude and frequency components of the cortical evoked activity in the DLPFC as well as the spread of the signal to the interconnected cortical regions.

Finally, the neurophysiological measures obtained through TMS-EEG-EMG studies would significantly enhance our understanding of the mechanism through which repetitive TMS exerts its effect, and would further enable us to optimally select stimulation parameters that would benefit individual patients based on their underlying impairment. To this day, the outcomes of repetitive TMS therapy have been inconsistent across studies. There are several reasons for this variability. First, certain stimulation patterns such as intensity, frequency, and number of stimuli delivered can significantly influence the outcome measures. Second, emerging lines of evidence suggest that rTMS effects are highly state dependent (Silvanto et al., 2008a; Silvanto et al., 2008b). That is the level of underlying cortical activity prior to rTMS treatment may influence the rTMS effect and could even be used to predict whether rTMS would suppress or facilitate cortical excitability. However, the classical rTMS treatments, not equipped with any concurrent EEG recordings, have not evaluated or controlled such baseline activities, which explains some of the variability observed in the rTMS studies.

Therefore, online EEG recording during rTMS therapy can improve the efficacy of TMS therapy in several ways. First, proof of concept studies similar to some of the rTMS-EEG experiments described before (Barr et al., 2010; Esser et al., 2006; Saglam et al., 2008; Van Der Werf et al., 2006) should be expanded to more systematically examine the effect of various stimulation parameters (e.g. intensity and frequency) on the cortical evoked potentials that seem to be a better predictor of subtle changes that take place in the cortex, as compared to the conventional MEP responses (Farzan et al., 2010b; Ferreri et al., 2010; Huber et al., 2008; Van Der Werf & Paus, 2006). Second, the results of these studies can then be utilized to custom design rTMS treatment sessions though carefully selecting parameters that would induce a specific response in the cortex (e.g. increased or reduced cortical excitability) similar to the tACS frequency adjustments in a recent study by Schutter and Hortensius (Schutter & Hortensius, 2011). Finally, a major advancement in EEG and TMS technology would hopefully give rise to the design of reliable EEG triggered TMS machines in which continuous online monitoring of underlying cortical potential would trigger the rTMS stimulation whenever the cortical activity reaches a state which would be more prone to be affected by the therapeutic efficacy of a specific rTMS therapy (e.g. low vs. fast frequency) (Rotenberg, 2009). Finally, in an even more advanced design, an EEG-triggered TMS system would be capable of updating the rTMS parameters (e.g. changing the rTMS frequency) during the treatment and based on the online analysis of changes in the cortical activity. Such advances in cortical stimulation technology could revolutionize the TMS field and would be a major step toward making the cortical stimulation a standard treatment approach for several neuropsychiatric disorders.

8. Conclusion

Advances in cortical stimulation and cortical recording techniques over the past few decades have allowed researchers to more systematically and non-invasively investigate the neurophysiological processes from the intact cortex of awake humans. Among such advancements, the concurrent TMS and EMG recordings has been instrumental in identifying and probing cortical processes that underlie generation and modulation of motor evoked potentials. The ability to evaluate cortical processes such as inhibition, excitation and plasticity in healthy subjects has further led to the discovery of pathophysiological processes in various neuropsychiatric disorders. In recent years, the introduction of TMS compatible EEG systems has brought about a significant advancement to the TMS field, enhancing both the diagnostic and therapeutic aspects of TMS. This is achieved through the superior temporal, spatial and spectral precision of TMS-EEG combination in identifying subtle changes of cortical activity before, during and post TMS delivery in both motor and non-motor regions of the cortex. In addition, the integration of EEG data with EMG recordings has provided further confirmation for the cortical origin of the classical TMS-EMG paradigms and has provided new information about the cortical oscillatory activity that underlies the generation and modulation of the peripheral effects. Although today there are only a few number of studies that have systematically investigated the reliability of EEG measures of TMS, the results are promising and suggest that TMS does have a potential for reliably identifying biological markers for several neuropsychiatric disorders. In regards to the future prospect of TMS-EEG-EMG research, it is expected that the integration of online EEG recording during rTMS therapy and advancements of EEG triggered cortical stimulation technology would significantly enhance the therapeutic outcomes of TMS and increase the certainty with which its therapeutic efficacy is predicated for each clinical condition. Such advancement would ultimately assist physicians in selecting patients who would benefit from rTMS therapy.

9. References

Adrian ED, Moruzzi G. (1939). Impulses in the pyramidal tract. *J Physiol*, 97, pp 153-199

Anand S, Hotson J. (2002). Transcranial magnetic stimulation: neurophysiological applications and safety. *Brain Cogn*, 50, pp 366-386

Bares M, Kanovsky P, Klajblova H, Rektor I. (2003). Intracortical inhibition and facilitation are impaired in patients with early Parkinson's disease: a paired TMS study. *Eur J Neurol*, 10, pp 385-389

Barker AT, Jalinous R, Freeston IL. (1985). Non-invasive magnetic stimulation of human motor cortex. *Lancet*, 1, pp 1106-1107

Combination of Transcranial Magnetic Stimulation with Electromyography and Electroencephalography:
Application in Diagnosis of Neuropsychiatric Disorders

87

Barr MS, Farzan F, Arenovich T, Chen R, Fitzgerald PB, Daskalakis ZJ. (2011). The effect of repetitive transcranial magnetic stimulation on gamma oscillatory activity in schizophrenia. *PLoS One,* 6, p e22627

Barr MS, Farzan F, Rusjan PM, Chen R, Fitzgerald PB, Daskalakis ZJ. (2009). Potentiation of gamma oscillatory activity through repetitive transcranial magnetic stimulation of the dorsolateral prefrontal cortex. *Neuropsychopharmacology,* 34, pp 2359-2367

Barr MS, Farzan F, Tran LC, Chen R, Fitzgerald PB, Daskalakis ZJ. (2010). Evidence for excessive frontal evoked gamma oscillatory activity in schizophrenia during working memory. *Schizophr Res,* 121, pp 146-152

Basar-Eroglu C, Brand A, Hildebrandt H, Karolina Kedzior K, Mathes B, Schmiedt C. (2007). Working memory related gamma oscillations in schizophrenia patients. *Int J Psychophysiol,* 64, pp 39-45

Bender S, Basseler K, Sebastian I, Resch F, Kammer T, Oelkers-Ax R, et al. (2005). Electroencephalographic response to transcranial magnetic stimulation in children: Evidence for giant inhibitory potentials. *Ann Neurol,* 58, pp 58-67

Berardelli A, Abbruzzese G, Chen R, Orth M, Ridding MC, Stinear C, et al. (2008). Consensus paper on short-interval intracortical inhibition and other transcranial magnetic stimulation intracortical paradigms in movement disorders. *Brain Stimul,* 1, pp 183-191

Berardelli A, Rona S, Inghilleri M, Manfredi M. (1996). Cortical inhibition in Parkinson's disease. A study with paired magnetic stimulation. *Brain,* 119 (Pt 1), pp 71-77

Bikmullina R, Kicic D, Carlson S, Nikulin VV. (2009). Electrophysiological correlates of short-latency afferent inhibition: a combined EEG and TMS study. *Exp Brain Res,* 194, pp 517-526

Boroojerdi B, Kopylev L, Battaglia F, Facchini S, Ziemann U, Muellbacher W, et al. (2000). Reproducibility of intracortical inhibition and facilitation using the paired-pulse paradigm. *Muscle Nerve,* 23, pp 1594-1597

Bragin A, Jando G, Nadasdy Z, Hetke J, Wise K, Buzsaki G. (1995). Gamma (40-100 Hz) oscillation in the hippocampus of the behaving rat. *J Neurosci,* 15, pp 47-60

Brignani D, Manganotti P, Rossini PM, Miniussi C. (2008). Modulation of cortical oscillatory activity during transcranial magnetic stimulation. *Hum Brain Mapp,* 29, pp 603-612

Brown P, Salenius S, Rothwell JC, Hari R. (1998). Cortical correlate of the Piper rhythm in humans. *J Neurophysiol,* 80, pp 2911-2917

Buonomano DV, Merzenich MM. (1998). Cortical plasticity: from synapses to maps. *Annu Rev Neurosci,* 21, pp 149-186

Buzsáki G (2006). *Rhythms of the Brain,* Oxford University Press, 13 978-0-19-530106-9, New York

Chen R. (2004). Interactions between inhibitory and excitatory circuits in the human motor cortex. *Exp Brain Res,* 154, pp 1-10

Chen R, Classen J, Gerloff C, Celnik P, Wassermann EM, Hallett M, et al. (1997). Depression of motor cortex excitability by low-frequency transcranial magnetic stimulation. *Neurology,* 48, pp 1398-1403

Chen R, Lozano AM, Ashby P. (1999). Mechanism of the silent period following transcranial magnetic stimulation. Evidence from epidural recordings. *Exp Brain Res,* 128, pp 539-542

Chen R, Yung D, Li JY. (2003). Organization of ipsilateral excitatory and inhibitory pathways in the human motor cortex. *J Neurophysiol,* 89, pp 1256-1264

Cho RY, Konecky RO, Carter CS. (2006). Impairments in frontal cortical gamma synchrony and cognitive control in schizophrenia. *Proc Natl Acad Sci U S A,* 103, pp 19878-19883

Classen J, Wolters A, Stefan K, Wycislo M, Sandbrink F, Schmidt A, et al. (2004). Paired associative stimulation. *Suppl Clin Neurophysiol*, 57, pp 563-569

Corneal SF, Butler AJ, Wolf SL. (2005). Intra- and intersubject reliability of abductor pollicis brevis muscle motor map characteristics with transcranial magnetic stimulation. *Arch Phys Med Rehabil*, 86, pp 1670-1675

Daskalakis ZJ, Christensen BK, Chen R, Fitzgerald PB, Zipursky RB, Kapur S. (2002a). Evidence for impaired cortical inhibition in schizophrenia using transcranial magnetic stimulation. *Arch Gen Psychiatry*, 59, pp 347-354

Daskalakis ZJ, Christensen BK, Fitzgerald PB, Roshan L, Chen R. (2002b). The mechanisms of interhemispheric inhibition in the human motor cortex. *J Physiol*, 543, pp 317-326

Daskalakis ZJ, Farzan F, Barr MS, Maller JJ, Chen R, Fitzgerald PB. (2008). Long-interval cortical inhibition from the dorsolateral prefrontal cortex: a TMS-EEG study. *Neuropsychopharmacology*, 33, pp 2860-2869

Daskalakis ZJ, Moller B, Christensen BK, Fitzgerald PB, Gunraj C, Chen R. (2006). The effects of repetitive transcranial magnetic stimulation on cortical inhibition in healthy human subjects. *Exp Brain Res*, 174, pp 403-412

Daskalakis ZJ, Paradiso GO, Christensen BK, Fitzgerald PB, Gunraj C, Chen R. (2004). Exploring the connectivity between the cerebellum and motor cortex in humans. *J Physiol*, 557, pp 689-700

Day BL, Dressler D, Maertens de Noordhout A, Marsden CD, Nakashima K, Rothwell JC, et al. (1989). Electric and magnetic stimulation of human motor cortex: surface EMG and single motor unit responses. *J Physiol*, 412, pp 449-473

Di Lazzaro V, Dileone M, Pilato F, Capone F, Musumeci G, Ranieri F, et al. (2011). Modulation of motor cortex neuronal networks by rTMS: comparison of local and remote effects of six different protocols of stimulation. *J Neurophysiol*, 105, pp 2150-2156

Di Lazzaro V, Oliviero A, Mazzone P, Insola A, Pilato F, Saturno E, et al. (2001). Comparison of descending volleys evoked by monophasic and biphasic magnetic stimulation of the motor cortex in conscious humans. *Exp Brain Res*, 141, pp 121-127

Di Lazzaro V, Oliviero A, Mazzone P, Pilato F, Saturno E, Insola A, et al. (2002a). Direct demonstration of long latency cortico-cortical inhibition in normal subjects and in a patient with vascular parkinsonism. *Clin Neurophysiol*, 113, pp 1673-1679

Di Lazzaro V, Oliviero A, Meglio M, Cioni B, Tamburrini G, Tonali P, et al. (2000). Direct demonstration of the effect of lorazepam on the excitability of the human motor cortex. *Clin Neurophysiol*, 111, pp 794-799

Di Lazzaro V, Oliviero A, Pilato F, Saturno E, Dileone M, Mazzone P, et al. (2004). The physiological basis of transcranial motor cortex stimulation in conscious humans. *Clin Neurophysiol*, 115, pp 255-266

Di Lazzaro V, Oliviero A, Profice P, Dileone M, Pilato F, Insola A, et al. (2009). Reduced cerebral cortex inhibition in dystonia: direct evidence in humans. *Clin Neurophysiol*, 120, pp 834-839

Di Lazzaro V, Oliviero A, Profice P, Insola A, Mazzone P, Tonali P, et al. (1999a). Direct demonstration of interhemispheric inhibition of the human motor cortex produced by transcranial magnetic stimulation. *Exp Brain Res*, 124, pp 520-524

Di Lazzaro V, Oliviero A, Profice P, Insola A, Mazzone P, Tonali P, et al. (1999b). Direct recordings of descending volleys after transcranial magnetic and electric motor cortex stimulation in conscious humans. *Electroencephalogr Clin Neurophysiol Suppl*, 51, pp 120-126

Combination of Transcranial Magnetic Stimulation with Electromyography and Electroencephalography: Application in Diagnosis of Neuropsychiatric Disorders

89

Di Lazzaro V, Oliviero A, Saturno E, Dileone M, Pilato F, Nardone R, et al. (2005). Effects of lorazepam on short latency afferent inhibition and short latency intracortical inhibition in humans. *J Physiol*, 564, pp 661-668

Di Lazzaro V, Oliviero A, Tonali PA, Marra C, Daniele A, Profice P, et al. (2002b). Noninvasive in vivo assessment of cholinergic cortical circuits in AD using transcranial magnetic stimulation. *Neurology*, 59, pp 392-397

Di Lazzaro V, Pilato F, Dileone M, Profice P, Ranieri F, Ricci V, et al. (2007). Segregating two inhibitory circuits in human motor cortex at the level of GABAA receptor subtypes: a TMS study. *Clin Neurophysiol*, 118, pp 2207-2214

Di Lazzaro V, Restuccia D, Oliviero A, Profice P, Ferrara L, Insola A, et al. (1998). Magnetic transcranial stimulation at intensities below active motor threshold activates intracortical inhibitory circuits. *Exp Brain Res*, 119, pp 265-268

Di Lazzaro V, Rothwell JC, Oliviero A, Profice P, Insola A, Mazzone P, et al. (1999c). Intracortical origin of the short latency facilitation produced by pairs of threshold magnetic stimuli applied to human motor cortex. *Exp Brain Res*, 129, pp 494-499

Engel AK, Fries P. (2010). Beta-band oscillations--signalling the status quo? *Curr Opin Neurobiol*, 20, pp 156-165

Engel AK, Singer W. (2001). Temporal binding and the neural correlates of sensory awareness. *Trends Cogn Sci*, 5, pp 16-25

Esser SK, Huber R, Massimini M, Peterson MJ, Ferrarelli F, Tononi G. (2006). A direct demonstration of cortical LTP in humans: A combined TMS/EEG study. *Brain Res Bull*, 69, pp 86-94

Farzan F, Barr MS, Levinson AJ, Chen R, Wong W, Fitzgerald PB, et al. (2010a). Evidence for gamma inhibition deficits in the dorsolateral prefrontal cortex of patients with schizophrenia. *Brain*, 133, pp 1505-1514

Farzan F, Barr MS, Levinson AJ, Chen R, Wong W, Fitzgerald PB, et al. (2010b). Reliability of Long Interval Cortical Inhibition in Healthy Human Subjects: A TMS-EEG Study. *J Neurophysiol,*

Farzan F, Barr MS, Wong W, Chen R, Fitzgerald PB, Daskalakis ZJ. (2009). Suppression of gamma-oscillations in the dorsolateral prefrontal cortex following long interval cortical inhibition: a TMS-EEG study. *Neuropsychopharmacology*, 34, pp 1543-1551

Ferbert A, Priori A, Rothwell JC, Day BL, Colebatch JG, Marsden CD. (1992). Interhemispheric inhibition of the human motor cortex. *J Physiol*, 453, pp 525-546

Ferreri F, Pasqualetti P, Maatta S, Ponzo D, Ferrarelli F, Tononi G, et al. (2010). Human brain connectivity during single and paired pulse transcranial magnetic stimulation. *Neuroimage*, 54, pp 90-102

Fitzgerald PB, Brown TL, Marston NA, Oxley T, De Castella A, Daskalakis ZJ, et al. (2004). Reduced plastic brain responses in schizophrenia: a transcranial magnetic stimulation study. *Schizophr Res*, 71, pp 17-26

Fitzgerald PB, Fountain S, Daskalakis ZJ. (2006). A comprehensive review of the effects of rTMS on motor cortical excitability and inhibition. *Clin Neurophysiol*, 117, pp 2584-2596

Frantseva MV, Fitzgerald PB, Chen R, Moller B, Daigle M, Daskalakis ZJ. (2008). Evidence for impaired long-term potentiation in schizophrenia and its relationship to motor skill learning. *Cereb Cortex*, 18, pp 990-996

Fries P, Nikolic D, Singer W. (2007). The gamma cycle. *Trends Neurosci*, 30, pp 309-316

Funke K, Benali A. (2009). Short-latency afferent inhibition varies with cortical state in rat somatosensory cortex. *Neuroreport*, 20, pp 1313-1318

Gerloff C, Cohen LG, Floeter MK, Chen R, Corwell B, Hallett M. (1998). Inhibitory influence of the ipsilateral motor cortex on responses to stimulation of the human cortex and pyramidal tract. *J Physiol,* 510 (Pt 1), pp 249-259

Gold JM, Harvey PD. (1993). Cognitive deficits in schizophrenia. *Psychiatr Clin North Am,* 16, pp 295-312

Hallett M. (2000). Transcranial magnetic stimulation and the human brain. *Nature,* 406, pp 147-150

Hanajima R, Ugawa Y, Terao Y, Ogata K, Kanazawa I. (1996). Ipsilateral cortico-cortical inhibition of the motor cortex in various neurological disorders. *J Neurol Sci,* 140, pp 109-116

Howard MW, Rizzuto DS, Caplan JB, Madsen JR, Lisman J, Aschenbrenner-Scheibe R, et al. (2003). Gamma oscillations correlate with working memory load in humans. *Cereb Cortex,* 13, pp 1369-1374

Huang YZ, Edwards MJ, Rounis E, Bhatia KP, Rothwell JC. (2005). Theta burst stimulation of the human motor cortex. *Neuron,* 45, pp 201-206

Huber R, Maatta S, Esser SK, Sarasso S, Ferrarelli F, Watson A, et al. (2008). Measures of cortical plasticity after transcranial paired associative stimulation predict changes in electroencephalogram slow-wave activity during subsequent sleep. *J Neurosci,* 28, pp 7911-7918

Hutcheon B, Yarom Y. (2000). Resonance, oscillation and the intrinsic frequency preferences of neurons. *Trends Neurosci,* 23, pp 216-222

Ilmoniemi RJ, Kicic D. (2009). Methodology for combined TMS and EEG. *Brain Topogr,* 22, pp 233-248

Ilmoniemi RJ, Virtanen J, Ruohonen J, Karhu J, Aronen HJ, Naatanen R, et al. (1997). Neuronal responses to magnetic stimulation reveal cortical reactivity and connectivity. *Neuroreport,* 8, pp 3537-3540

Inghilleri M, Berardelli A, Cruccu G, Manfredi M. (1993). Silent period evoked by transcranial stimulation of the human cortex and cervicomedullary junction. *J Physiol,* 466, pp 521-534.

Kahkonen S, Kesaniemi M, Nikouline VV, Karhu J, Ollikainen M, Holi M, et al. (2001). Ethanol modulates cortical activity: direct evidence with combined TMS and EEG. *Neuroimage,* 14, pp 322-328

Kahkonen S, Wilenius J. (2007). Effects of alcohol on TMS-evoked N100 responses. *J Neurosci Methods,* 166, pp 104-108

Kahkonen S, Wilenius J, Nikulin VV, Ollikainen M, Ilmoniemi RJ. (2003). Alcohol reduces prefrontal cortical excitability in humans: a combined TMS and EEG study. *Neuropsychopharmacology,* 28, pp 747-754

Kanai R, Chaieb L, Antal A, Walsh V, Paulus W. (2008). Frequency-dependent electrical stimulation of the visual cortex. *Curr Biol,* 18, pp 1839-1843

Kapogiannis D, Wassermann EM. (2008). Transcranial magnetic stimulation in Clinical Pharmacology. *Cent Nerv Syst Agents Med Chem,* 8, pp 234-240

Kimiskidis VK, Papagiannopoulos S, Kazis DA, Vasiliadis G, Oikonomidi A, Sotirakoglou K, et al. (2008). Silent period (SP) to transcranial magnetic stimulation: the EEG substrate. Brain Stimulation 1. Abstracts from the 3rd international conference on transcranial magnetic simulation and direct current stimulation, pp 315–316

Knyazev GG. (2007). Motivation, emotion, and their inhibitory control mirrored in brain oscillations. *Neurosci Biobehav Rev,* 31, pp 377-395

Combination of Transcranial Magnetic Stimulation with Electromyography and Electroencephalography:
Application in Diagnosis of Neuropsychiatric Disorders

91

Komssi S, Aronen HJ, Huttunen J, Kesaniemi M, Soinne L, Nikouline VV, et al. (2002). Ipsi-
and contralateral EEG reactions to transcranial magnetic stimulation. *Clin
Neurophysiol,* 113, pp 175-184

Komssi S, Kahkonen S. (2006). The novelty value of the combined use of
electroencephalography and transcranial magnetic stimulation for neuroscience
research. *Brain Res Brain Res Rev,* 52, pp 183-192

Krnjevic K, Randic M, Straughan DW. (1964). CORTICAL INHIBITION. *Nature,* 201, pp
1294-1296

Kujirai T, Caramia MD, Rothwell JC, Day BL, Thompson PD, Ferbert A, et al. (1993).
Corticocortical inhibition in human motor cortex. *J Physiol,* 471, pp 501-519

Levinson AJ, Young LT, Fitzgerald PB, Daskalakis ZJ. (2007). Cortical inhibitory dysfunction
in bipolar disorder: a study using transcranial magnetic stimulation. *J Clin
Psychopharmacol,* 27, pp 493-497

Levy R, Lozano AM, Lang AE, Dostrovsky JO. (2010). Event-related desynchronization of
motor cortical oscillations in patients with multiple system atrophy. *Exp Brain Res,*
206, pp 1-13

Linkenkaer-Hansen K, Smit DJ, Barkil A, van Beijsterveldt TE, Brussaard AB, Boomsma DI,
et al. (2007). Genetic contributions to long-range temporal correlations in ongoing
oscillations. *J Neurosci,* 27, pp 13882-13889

Lioumis P, Kicic D, Savolainen P, Makela JP, Kahkonen S. (2009). Reproducibility of TMS-
Evoked EEG responses. *Hum Brain Mapp,* 30, pp 1387-1396

Maeda F, Gangitano M, Thall M, Pascual-Leone A. (2002). Inter- and intra-individual
variability of paired-pulse curves with transcranial magnetic stimulation (TMS).
Clin Neurophysiol, 113, pp 376-382

Maeda F, Keenan JP, Tormos JM, Topka H, Pascual-Leone A. (2000). Interindividual
variability of the modulatory effects of repetitive transcranial magnetic stimulation
on cortical excitability. *Exp Brain Res,* 133, pp 425-430

Maki H, Ilmoniemi RJ. (2010a). EEG oscillations and magnetically evoked motor potentials
reflect motor system excitability in overlapping neuronal populations. *Clin
Neurophysiol,* 121, pp 492-501

Maki H, Ilmoniemi RJ. (2010b). The relationship between peripheral and early cortical
activation induced by transcranial magnetic stimulation. *Neurosci Lett,*

McCormick DA. (1989). GABA as an inhibitory neurotransmitter in human cerebral cortex. *J
Neurophysiol,* 62, pp 1018-1027

McDonnell MN, Orekhov Y, Ziemann U. (2006). The role of GABA(B) receptors in
intracortical inhibition in the human motor cortex. *Exp Brain Res,* 173, pp 86-93

Merton PA, Morton HB. (1980). Stimulation of the cerebral cortex in the intact human
subject. *Nature,* 285, p 227

Mima T, Hallett M. (1999). Electroencephalographic analysis of cortico-muscular coherence:
reference effect, volume conduction and generator mechanism. *Clin Neurophysiol,*
110, pp 1892-1899

Nakamura H, Kitagawa H, Kawaguchi Y, Tsuji H. (1997). Intracortical facilitation and
inhibition after transcranial magnetic stimulation in conscious humans. *J Physiol,*
498 (Pt 3), pp 817-823

Nardone R, Bergmann J, Kronbichler M, Kunz A, Klein S, Caleri F, et al. (2008). Abnormal
short latency afferent inhibition in early Alzheimer's disease: a transcranial
magnetic demonstration. *J Neural Transm,* 115, pp 1557-1562

Neuper C, Pfurtscheller G. (2001). Evidence for distinct beta resonance frequencies in human EEG related to specific sensorimotor cortical areas. *Clin Neurophysiol,* 112, pp 2084-2097

Ni Z, Gunraj C, Nelson AJ, Yeh IJ, Castillo G, Hoque T, et al. (2009). Two phases of interhemispheric inhibition between motor related cortical areas and the primary motor cortex in human. *Cereb Cortex,* 19, pp 1654-1665

Nikulin VV, Kicic D, Kahkonen S, Ilmoniemi RJ. (2003). Modulation of electroencephalographic responses to transcranial magnetic stimulation: evidence for changes in cortical excitability related to movement. *Eur J Neurosci,* 18, pp 1206-1212

Palva S, Palva JM. (2007). New vistas for alpha-frequency band oscillations. *Trends Neurosci,* 30, pp 150-158

Pascual-Leone A, Valls-Sole J, Wassermann EM, Hallett M. (1994). Responses to rapid-rate transcranial magnetic stimulation of the human motor cortex. *Brain,* 117 (Pt 4), pp 847-858

Pascual-Leone A, Walsh V, Rothwell J. (2000). Transcranial magnetic stimulation in cognitive neuroscience--virtual lesion, chronometry, and functional connectivity. *Curr Opin Neurobiol,* 10, pp 232-237

Paus T, Sipila PK, Strafella AP. (2001). Synchronization of neuronal activity in the human primary motor cortex by transcranial magnetic stimulation: an EEG study. *J Neurophysiol,* 86, pp 1983-1990

Pell GS, Roth Y, Zangen A. (2010). Modulation of cortical excitability induced by repetitive transcranial magnetic stimulation: influence of timing and geometrical parameters and underlying mechanisms. *Prog Neurobiol,* 93, pp 59-98

Pfurtscheller G, Neuper C, Pichler-Zalaudek K, Edlinger G, Lopes da Silva FH. (2000). Do brain oscillations of different frequencies indicate interaction between cortical areas in humans? *Neurosci Lett,* 286, pp 66-68

Pierantozzi M, Marciani MG, Palmieri MG, Brusa L, Galati S, Caramia MD, et al. (2004). Effect of Vigabatrin on motor responses to transcranial magnetic stimulation: an effective tool to investigate in vivo GABAergic cortical inhibition in humans. *Brain Res,* 1028, pp 1-8

Pierantozzi M, Palmieri MG, Marciani MG, Bernardi G, Giacomini P, Stanzione P. (2001). Effect of apomorphine on cortical inhibition in Parkinson's disease patients: a transcranial magnetic stimulation study. *Exp Brain Res,* 141, pp 52-62

Pike FG, Goddard RS, Suckling JM, Ganter P, Kasthuri N, Paulsen O. (2000). Distinct frequency preferences of different types of rat hippocampal neurones in response to oscillatory input currents. *J Physiol,* 529 Pt 1, pp 205-213

Pineda JA. (2005). The functional significance of mu rhythms: translating "seeing" and "hearing" into "doing". *Brain Res Brain Res Rev,* 50, pp 57-68

Rajji TK, Sun Y, Farzan F, D'Souza R, Wass C, Mulsant BH, et al. (2011). Assessing plasticity in the dorsolateral prefrontal cortex in patients with schizophrenia. Conference Abstract. The International Congress on Schizophrenia Research, April 2011.

Ridding MC, Rothwell JC. (2007). Is there a future for therapeutic use of transcranial magnetic stimulation? *Nat Rev Neurosci,* 8, pp 559-567

Ridding MC, Sheean G, Rothwell JC, Inzelberg R, Kujirai T. (1995). Changes in the balance between motor cortical excitation and inhibition in focal, task specific dystonia. *J Neurol Neurosurg Psychiatry,* 59, pp 493-498

Roopun AK, Kramer MA, Carracedo LM, Kaiser M, Davies CH, Traub RD, et al. (2008). Temporal Interactions between Cortical Rhythms. *Front Neurosci,* 2, pp 145-154

Rosanova M, Casali A, Bellina V, Resta F, Mariotti M, Massimini M. (2009). Natural frequencies of human corticothalamic circuits. *J Neurosci,* 29, pp 7679-7685

Rossini PM, Barker AT, Berardelli A, Caramia MD, Caruso G, Cracco RQ, et al. (1994). Non-invasive electrical and magnetic stimulation of the brain, spinal cord and roots: basic principles and procedures for routine clinical application. Report of an IFCN committee. *Electroencephalogr Clin Neurophysiol,* 91, pp 79-92

Rossini PM, Rossi S. (2007). Transcranial magnetic stimulation: diagnostic, therapeutic, and research potential. *Neurology,* 68, pp 484-488

Rotenberg A. (2009). Prospects for clinical applications of transcranial magnetic stimulation and real-time EEG in epilepsy. *Brain Topogr,* 22, pp 257-266

Rothwell JC. (1997). Techniques and mechanisms of action of transcranial stimulation of the human motor cortex. *J Neurosci Methods,* 74, pp 113-122

Saglam M, Matsunaga K, Murayama N, Hayashida Y, Huang YZ, Nakanishi R. (2008). Parallel inhibition of cortico-muscular synchronization and cortico-spinal excitability by theta burst TMS in humans. *Clin Neurophysiol,* 119, pp 2829-2838

Salenius S, Portin K, Kajola M, Salmelin R, Hari R. (1997). Cortical control of human motoneuron firing during isometric contraction. *J Neurophysiol,* 77, pp 3401-3405

Sanger TD, Garg RR, Chen R. (2001). Interactions between two different inhibitory systems in the human motor cortex. *J Physiol,* 530, pp 307-317

Schutter DJ, Hortensius R. (2011). Brain oscillations and frequency-dependent modulation of cortical excitability. *Brain Stimul,* 4, pp 97-103

Siebner HR, Dressnandt J, Auer C, Conrad B. (1998). Continuous intrathecal baclofen infusions induced a marked increase of the transcranially evoked silent period in a patient with generalized dystonia. *Muscle Nerve,* 21, pp 1209-1212

Silvanto J, Cattaneo Z, Battelli L, Pascual-Leone A. (2008a). Baseline cortical excitability determines whether TMS disrupts or facilitates behavior. *J Neurophysiol,* 99, pp 2725-2730

Silvanto J, Muggleton N, Walsh V. (2008b). State-dependency in brain stimulation studies of perception and cognition. *Trends Cogn Sci,* 12, pp 447-454

Slotema CW, Blom JD, Hoek HW, Sommer IE. (2010). Should we expand the toolbox of psychiatric treatment methods to include Repetitive Transcranial Magnetic Stimulation (rTMS)? A meta-analysis of the efficacy of rTMS in psychiatric disorders. *J Clin Psychiatry,* 71, pp 873-884

Stefan K, Kunesch E, Benecke R, Cohen LG, Classen J. (2002). Mechanisms of enhancement of human motor cortex excitability induced by interventional paired associative stimulation. *J Physiol,* 543, pp 699-708

Stefan K, Kunesch E, Cohen LG, Benecke R, Classen J. (2000). Induction of plasticity in the human motor cortex by paired associative stimulation. *Brain,* 123 Pt 3, pp 572-584

Strafella AP, Valzania F, Nassetti SA, Tropeani A, Bisulli A, Santangelo M, et al. (2000). Effects of chronic levodopa and pergolide treatment on cortical excitability in patients with Parkinson's disease: a transcranial magnetic stimulation study. *Clin Neurophysiol,* 111, pp 1198-1202

Swartz BE, Goldensohn ES. (1998). Timeline of the history of EEG and associated fields. *Electroencephalogr Clin Neurophysiol,* 106, pp 173-176

Tallon-Baudry C, Bertrand O. (1999). Oscillatory gamma activity in humans and its role in object representation. *Trends Cogn Sci,* 3, pp 151-162

Tallon-Baudry C, Bertrand O, Delpuech C, Pernier J. (1996). Stimulus specificity of phase-locked and non-phase-locked 40 Hz visual responses in human. *J Neurosci,* 16, pp 4240-4249

Tallon-Baudry C, Bertrand O, Peronnet F, Pernier J. (1998). Induced gamma-band activity during the delay of a visual short-term memory task in humans. *J Neurosci*, 18, pp 4244-4254

Thut G, Northoff G, Ives JR, Kamitani Y, Pfennig A, Kampmann F, et al. (2003). Effects of single-pulse transcranial magnetic stimulation (TMS) on functional brain activity: a combined event-related TMS and evoked potential study. *Clin Neurophysiol*, 114, pp 2071-2080

Thut G, Pascual-Leone A. (2010). A review of combined TMS-EEG studies to characterize lasting effects of repetitive TMS and assess their usefulness in cognitive and clinical neuroscience. *Brain Topogr*, 22, pp 219-232

Tokimura H, Di Lazzaro V, Tokimura Y, Oliviero A, Profice P, Insola A, et al. (2000). Short latency inhibition of human hand motor cortex by somatosensory input from the hand. *J Physiol*, 523 Pt 2, pp 503-513

Tsuji T, Rothwell JC. (2002). Long lasting effects of rTMS and associated peripheral sensory input on MEPs, SEPs and transcortical reflex excitability in humans. *J Physiol*, 540, pp 367-376

Udupa K, Ni Z, Gunraj C, Chen R. (2009). Interactions between short latency afferent inhibition and long interval intracortical inhibition. *Exp Brain Res*, 199, pp 177-183

Valls-Sole J, Pascual-Leone A, Wassermann EM, Hallett M. (1992). Human motor evoked responses to paired transcranial magnetic stimuli. *Electroencephalogr Clin Neurophysiol*, 85, pp 355-364

Van Der Werf YD, Paus T. (2006). The neural response to transcranial magnetic stimulation of the human motor cortex. I. Intracortical and cortico-cortical contributions. *Exp Brain Res*, 175, pp 231-245

Van Der Werf YD, Sadikot AF, Strafella AP, Paus T. (2006). The neural response to transcranial magnetic stimulation of the human motor cortex. II. Thalamocortical contributions. *Exp Brain Res*, 175, pp 246-255

Veniero D, Brignani D, Thut G, Miniussi C. (2011). Alpha-generation as basic response-signature to transcranial magnetic stimulation (TMS) targeting the human resting motor cortex: A TMS/EEG co-registration study. *Psychophysiology*,

Voineskos AN, Farzan F, Barr MS, Lobaugh NJ, Mulsant BH, Chen R, et al. (2010). The role of the corpus callosum in transcranial magnetic stimulation induced interhemispheric signal propagation. *Biol Psychiatry*, 68, pp 825-831

von Stein A, Chiang C, Konig P. (2000). Top-down processing mediated by interareal synchronization. *Proc Natl Acad Sci U S A*, 97, pp 14748-14753

Wahl M, Lauterbach-Soon B, Hattingen E, Jung P, Singer O, Volz S, et al. (2007). Human motor corpus callosum: topography, somatotopy, and link between microstructure and function. *J Neurosci*, 27, pp 12132-12138

Wassermann EM, Lisanby SH. (2001). Therapeutic application of repetitive transcranial magnetic stimulation: a review. *Clin Neurophysiol*, 112, pp 1367-1377

Werhahn KJ, Kunesch E, Noachtar S, Benecke R, Classen J. (1999). Differential effects on motorcortical inhibition induced by blockade of GABA uptake in humans. *J Physiol*, 517 (Pt 2), pp 591-597

Ziemann U. (2004). TMS and drugs. *Clin Neurophysiol*, 115, pp 1717-1729

Ziemann U, Rothwell JC. (2000). I-waves in motor cortex. *J Clin Neurophysiol*, 17, pp 397-405

Ziemann U, Rothwell JC, Ridding MC. (1996). Interaction between intracortical inhibition and facilitation in human motor cortex. *J Physiol*, 496 (Pt 3), pp 873-881

Part 5

EMG in Combination with Other Technologies

5

Muscle Force Analysis of Human Foot Based on Wearable Sensors and EMG Method

Enguo Cao, Yoshio Inoue, Tao Liu and Kyoko Shibata
Kochi University of Technology,
Japan

1. Introduction

Sports injuries, traffic accident, childhood diseases and life-style related diseases may cause movement disorder, and especially in aged persons, physical deterioration may leads to high risk of degeneration of motor function and falling in movement problems. Nowadays, in the trend of population aging of many countries, a large proportion of movement disorder patients are difficult to recover completely in the recent medical condition. Therefore, muscle strength and motor function recovery have aroused general concern from the society, musculoskeletal analysis and rehabilitation activities have been greatly progressed in many countries (Yoon et al., 2010), (Vallery et al., 2007), (Peshkin et al., 2005). Furthermore, modern robots are on high speed developing, but multiple-units foot has seldom caught scientists' attention, robot feet are generally treated as a single rigid part which makes gait seems clumsiness (Park et al., 2009), (Ishida et al., 2003). The human walking style is adequate for various situations compared with wheeled mobile robot, and understanding the muscle works of human limb is implemental for medical diagnosis. It is valuable to develop a multiple-units foot for flexible walking robots and rehabilitation training robots. With economical considerations, developing an easy-operating muscle diagnostic system of multiple-units foot is practical for clinical applications.

Muscle force estimation is not easy because some muscles are locating at inner part of limbs and human foot is a complex musculoskeletal system. For direct measurement of muscle forces, electromyography (EMG) method has been frequently applied as a standard clinical tool in identifying activation level of muscles, but in the EMG method the muscle activity result is relative large or small with the unit of % rather than quantitative values with the unit of Newton (Lee et al., 2008), (Merlo et al., 2003). Moreover through surface EMG method only activities of surface muscles could be estimated, but through needle EMG method the invasiveness of needles may cause reluctance of patients (Kizuka et al., 2009). For indirect estimation method, the quantitative muscle forces of human foot could be calculated, but acquirements of motions of limbs, forces applied on limbs, and the construction of musculoskeletal model are essential (Hou et al., 2007).

Up to the present there are various methods to measure human motion and ground reaction force (GRF) for limb dynamics analysis. But many of them are restricted to laboratory environment and sick to adapt to different situations. The commercial motion camera system, which is regarded as the most popular instrument and a standard tool in measuring movement of human limb, could be performed only in laboratory environment and expensive for implements (Ferreira et al., 2009). The force plate, which is the widely used in measuring GRF with high accuracy in various fields, is limited in single stride measurement (Moustakidis et al., 2008). In this situation, wearable sensor systems based on miniature type force sensors, acceleration sensitive units and gyroscopes play more important role in the applicability for continuously walking and climbing stairs or slopes (Liu et al., 2009), (Boonstra et al., 2006). For construction of musculoskeletal dynamic model, the AnyBody Modeling System, which works in a minimum fatigue criterion way, could be introduced in various applications of variable situation. The geometric data of the model could be decided based on measurements of human anatomy model, and through inverse dynamics method quantitative results of muscle forces of human foot could be calculated. Furthermore, the EMG system could be introduced to validate the calculated muscle force results.

In this chapter, muscle forces of human foot were estimated through inverse dynamics method in AnyBody Modeling System based on wearable sensors and EMG method. A wearable sensor system was developed to measure rotational angles, GRF and centres of pressure (COP) of human limbs. Moreover one group of measured GRF and COP data are transferred into two group of GRF on two loading points in the musculoskeletal model. In AnyBody Modeling System a model of multiple-units foot was established to calculate quantitative muscle forces by inverse dynamics analysis. The shank was also built in the model for attaching muscles between foot and shank, and for the angular acceleration of the shank has influence on these muscles in inverse dynamics method. To make the model suit to different individuals, the size factor was indicated based on the length of human foot. To validate our estimation results of muscle forces, a personal surface EMG system was adopted in the experiment and the muscle activation level of Anterior Tibialis (ANT TIB), Peroneus Longus (PL), Gastrocnemius (GAST) and Soleus (SOL) were directly measured. The raw EMG result measured by hard type sensor system was filtered and rectified into integral EMG results, and the integral EMG results were introduced in the validation with the muscle force results of AnyBody Modeling System.

2. Methods

2.1 Wearable sensor system for measuring angular motion, GRF and COP

Angular motions of shank and thigh were measured by two wearable sensors with acceleration sensitive units and gyroscopes. And angular motions, GRF and COP of multiple-units foot were measured by a pair of developed instrument shoes with both force sensors and motion sensors. The measured data were expressed in a general coordinate system which was aligned with the orientation of the shoe, and located on the contacting plane between the shoe and the floor. As shown in Fig. 1, the Z-axis was made vertical, and the Y-axis was chosen to represent the anterior-posterior direction of the shoe on the interface plane contacting with the ground, while the X-axis was chosen such that the global coordinate system would be right-handed (Liu et al., 2008). Accurate location of the sensors is not necessary because the limb segments are regarded as rigid bodies in the study.

In this way the dispersion force on the bottom of shoe was expressed by concentrated GRF and COP, and the measured electrical data of angular motion, GRF and COP of multiple-units foot were transmit into a signal process box, which took the responsibility for wave filtering, data consolidation and transmission, as shown in Fig. 2. The signal process box also played a role of signal synchronization by sending a start pulse to the wearable sensor system combined on the leg, as all the sensors have the same sampling frequency. The

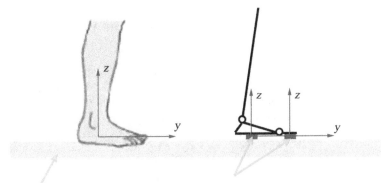

Floor

Fig. 1. Ordinate system of an instrument shoe with multiple sensors to obtain GRF, COP and angular motion of multiple-units foot.

Signal process box

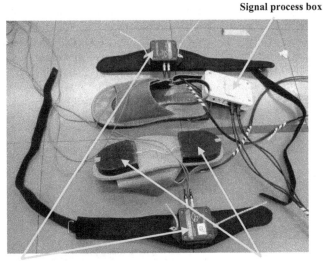

Two wearable motion sensors   **Sensors under a instrument shoe**

Fig. 2. The instrument shoes and two wearable sensors designed to obtain GRF, COP and angular motions of lower limbs during successive walking trial.

motion of shank was measured because muscles joint points in shank have non-separable relationship with the muscles driving the foot, and the process of gait is relied on the co-operation of these muscles. The angular motion of thigh was not involved in the calculation of muscle forces of the foot because there are no muscles connect from thigh to the foot directly, although the motion of thigh was measured in this experiment for the future research. In the wearable motion and GRF sensor system, all the sensors had the sampling frequency of 100 Hz, and the GRF, COP, multiple-units foot and shank rotations had the units of Newton (N), millimeter (mm) and degree (°) respectively. Totally four groups of

GRF, two group of COP and four groups of angular of multiple-units foot were measured by the instrument shoes, moreover one groups of angular of shank and one groups of angular of thigh were measured by the wearable sensors.

2.2 AnyBody modeling system for establishing multiple-units foot model

In human body muscles are activated by the central nervous system (CNS) base on a complicated electro-chemical process. Determining the activation that realizes a desired movement requires an extremely intricate control algorithm. The AnyBody Modeling System is not only a professional musculoskeletal modeling system, but also a kinematics and kinetics analysis system, in which inverse dynamics method is adapted to quantitatively estimate muscle forces. AnyBody imitates the workings of the CNS by computing backwards from the movement and load specified by the user to the necessary muscle forces in a process known as inverse dynamics. Maximum synergism would be the case where all muscles capable of a positive contribution to balancing the external load work together, in such a way that the maximum relative load of any muscle in the system is as small as possible. It means that the body would maximize its endurance and precisely, this criterion might decide survival of the fittest in an environment where organisms are competing with each other for limited resources. So in AnyBody a minimum fatigue criterion way is employed because fatigue is likely to happen first in the muscle working on the maximum relative load, and it makes physiological sense that the body might work that way.

To implement dynamic analysis of human foot, a multiple-units foot and shank model was created in AnyBody Modeling System. As shown in Fig. 3, the coordinates of knee, ankle, and toe joints and muscle joint points were determined by measuring datum of the human lower limb (McMinn et al., 1982). The shank was also built in the model for attaching

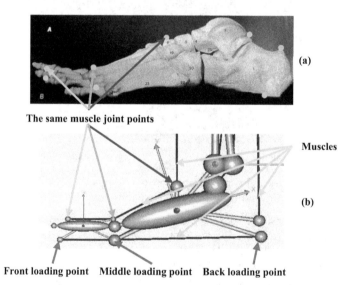

Fig. 3. Method for obtaining coordinates of multiple-units foot model in AnyBody System.
(a) Human anatomy sscannogram for obtaining geometric data of human foot.
(b) Musculoskeletal multiple-units foot model in AnyBody Modeling System.

muscles between foot and shank; furthermore the angular acceleration of the shank has influences on these muscles in the inverse dynamics method. To simulate the true situation of human walking, the GRF were implemented on three loading points locating on the bottom of foot model, and the loads applied on loading points contain both pressure and tangential forces as shown in Fig. 3 (b). The main working muscles involved in the model were ANT TIB, GAST, SOL, PL, Peroneus Brevis (PB), Posterior Tibialis (POST TIB), Extensor Digitorum Longus (EDL) and Flexor Digitorum Longus (FDL), that were built with the maximum strength of 5000 N. Totally seventeen muscle points were created to join muscles, four joints of hip, knee, ankle and toe were created to restrict the activity freedom degree, and three loading points were created to load the GRF and COP. The model worked as an integrated kinetics system after all the units were combined by joints and muscles. The foot model was established based on a rigid barefoot as the instrument shoes nearly have no elasticity, and to make the model suit for different individuals, the model size factor was indicated based on the length of human foot.

2.3 Inverse dynamics method for calculating muscle forces

The GRF, COP and angular motion data measured by the wearable sensor system were imported into the developed multiple-units foot and shank model in AnyBody Modeling System to calculate muscle forces of human foot through an inverse dynamic method. To simulate the true situation of human walking, one group of GRF and COP was transferred into two forces on different locations based on Eq. (1) and Eq. (2), in this way the measured two groups of GRF and COP data were transferred into three groups of force data applied on three loading points on the bottom plane of foot model. In single gait cycle, loads were transferred from posterior foot to the anterior foot continuously and the whole force process was simulated. This transformation can perfectly imitate the GRF variation and COP shifting because the multiple-units foot is regarded as a rigid body system, furthermore real human foot receives GRF mainly on similar three points too. The loads applied on loading points contain both pressure and tangential forces. The pressure force of GRF was expressed on the Z-direction, and the COP_z (x_0, y_0, z_0) on this dirction is defined by Eq. (1), and the tangential force of GRF was expressed on the Y-direction, and the COP_y (x_0, y_0, z_0) on this direction is defined by Eq. (2).

$$x_0 = 0, \quad y_0 = \frac{\sum F_z \bullet y}{\sum F_z}, \quad z_0 = 0 \qquad (1)$$

$$x_0 = 0, \quad y_0 = \frac{\sum F_y \bullet y}{\sum F_y}, \quad z_0 = 0 \qquad (2)$$

F_z — A force on Z-direction.
F_y — A force on Z-direction.
x — X-axis coordinate values of the force.
y — Y-axis coordinate values of the force.
As shown in Fig. 4, the angular motion data of shank, the posterior foot and the anterior foot were measured in general coordinate system as ϕ_{shank}, ϕ_{heel}, ϕ_{toe}. Because all the parts in the model were regarded as rigid bodies, the relative angular motion ($\Delta\phi_{shank}$, $\Delta\phi_{heel}$, $\Delta\phi_{toe}$)

could be calculated by quantitative subtraction. Furthermore in AnyBody Modeling System, the shank, the posterior foot and the anterior foot were driven by $\Delta\phi_{shank}$, $\Delta\phi_{heel}$, $\Delta\phi_{toe}$ respectively as shown in Eq. (3), (4), (5). After all the model units were combined by joints and driven by imported motion data, the AnyBody musculoskeletal model worked as an integrated kinetics system and quantitative muscle forces were calculated out through inverse dynamic process.

$$\Delta\phi_{shank} = \phi_{shank} \tag{3}$$

$$\Delta\phi_{heel} = \phi_{heel} - \phi_{shank} \tag{4}$$

$$\Delta\phi_{toe} = \phi_{toe} - \phi_{heel} \tag{5}$$

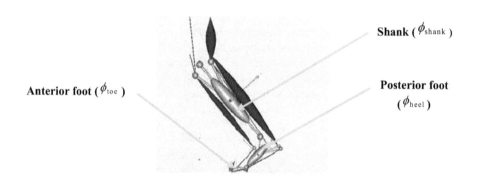

Fig. 4. Angular motion data of shank, the posterior foot and the anterior foot were measured in general coordinate system as ϕ_{shank}, ϕ_{heel}, ϕ_{toe}.

2.4 EMG method for validating muscle force results

The main muscles of human shank and foot were illustrated in Fig. 5, the motions of human limb are motivated by complex teamwork of these muscles, but only several of these muscles were involved in the EMG experiment, that because only the muscles visible in skin surface and offering primary motive power in walking process are possible and worthy for directly analysing. As shown in Fig. 6, the personal-EMG system (P-EMG-0403A01) includes hard type sensor system, filter box and data process system, and based on this system the EMG method was adopted to directly measure muscle activation level of ANT TIB, PL, GAST and SOL. The raw EMG results were filtered and rectified by the filter box and the data process system into integral EMG results that could represent the muscle activation levels. Both the raw EMG and the integral EMG were real time recorded and displayed by the data process system, furthermore the integral EMG results were introduced in the validation with muscle force results calculated by AnyBody Modeling System. Furthermore, one hundred percent standard voluntary contractions (100%SVC) were defined as standard isolation of muscle activity in the respective muscle tests for the normalization of EMG signal (Perry et al., 1986).

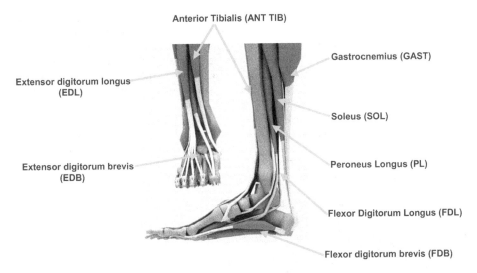

Fig. 5. Illustration of main muscles of human shank and foot.

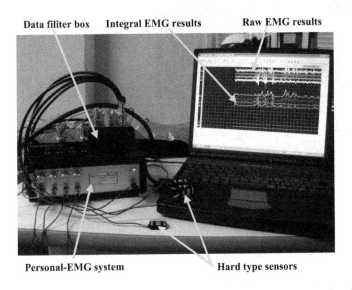

Fig. 6. Personal-EMG system adopted to directly measure muscle activation levels in human lower limb.

3. Experimental study

3.1 Experiment method
The first experiment step is acquisition motion and GRF information of human lower limbs in gait cycle, five adult volunteers (age: 28.5±5 years, weight: 75±6.5 kg.) who had no

musculoskeletal disease history were requireed to performed their normal gait in the experiment. The distance of the performance was four meters, duration time was ten seconds. As shown in Fig. 7, three-dimensional angular motion of thigh, shank, posterior part and anterior part of the multiple-units foot were measured with the unit of degree (°), and three-dimensional GRF and two-dimensional COP were measured by the instrument shoes with the unit of Newton (N) and millimeter (mm) respectively. Because all the limb parts were regarded as rigid segments, precise location of wearable sensors which attached on human limbs was unnecessary, so was the size adjustable of the instrumented shoes for the same reason. The sampling frequency of all sensors were regulated as 100 Hz, signal synchronization was realized by the signal process box which would send a pulse to wearable sensors attached on shank and thigh. To remove noise, low-pass filtering was performed on obtained signals with the cut-off frequency of 10 Hz.

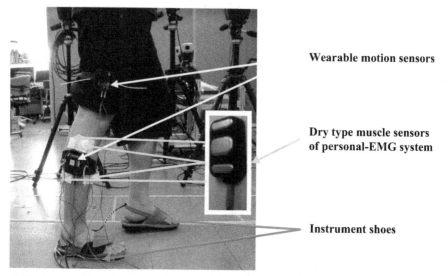

Wearable motion sensors

Dry type muscle sensors of personal-EMG system

Instrument shoes

Fig. 7. Prototype of a volunteer wearing instrument shoes, wearable motion sensors and muscle sensors of personal-EMG in the experiment.

To directly measure muscle activation levels of ANT TIB, PL, GAST and SOL, the personal-EMG system and dry type muscle sensors were adopted in the experiment. The dry type muscle senors, which works on a myoelectricity difference principle, could sensing the muscle activation level while being pasted on the eneurosis zone of muscle surface. Furthermore the measured raw EMG results were real time filtered and rectified into integral EMG results by the personal-EMG application system, and both raw EMG results and integral EMG results were real time displayed for easy checking and adjusting. As shown in Fig. 8, we divided one gait cycle into four steps: contacting step, supporting step, leaving step and swing step. The contacting step starts from the heel contacting the ground and ends in the whole foot bottom plane stamping on the ground, the supporting step represents the process of gravity movement from posterior to anterior while one foot supporting the whole weight, the leaving step stands for the action from the heel leaving the ground to the whole foot leaving the ground, and the swing step means the foot swing forward process without contacting the floor.

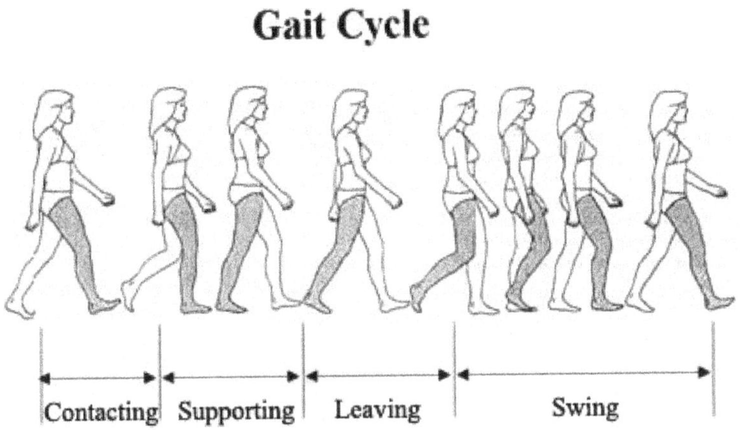

Gait Cycle

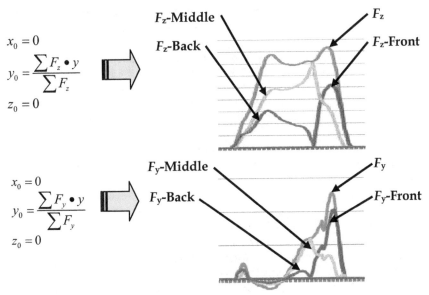

| Contacting | Supporting | Leaving | Swing |

Fig. 8. One gait cycle was divided into contacting step, supporting step, leaving step and swing step.

The second experiment step was calculating the muscle forces in AnyBody Modeling System. For preparation, the measured motion and GRF data of lower limb were transferred into the form that is adequate to the AnyBody system. As a rigid body system, the relative angular motion data ($\Delta\phi_{shank}$, $\Delta\phi_{heel}$, $\Delta\phi_{toe}$) were imported into the model to drive the movement of the shank and the multiple-units foot. The measured GRF data were transformed into three forces on three loading points to imitate GRF variation and COP shifting. As shown in Fig. 9, in Z-axis the entire pressure GRF data measured by sensors was drawn as F_z, and GRF

$$x_0 = 0$$
$$y_0 = \frac{\sum F_z \cdot y}{\sum F_z}$$
$$z_0 = 0$$

F_z-Middle F_z

F_z-Back F_z-Front

$$x_0 = 0$$
$$y_0 = \frac{\sum F_y \cdot y}{\sum F_y}$$
$$z_0 = 0$$

F_y-Middle F_y

F_y-Back F_y-Front

Fig. 9. The GRF were transferred into three forces on three loading points to imitate GRF variation and COP shifting in gait cycle.

transformation data applied on three loading points were drawn as F_z-Front, F_z-Middle and F_z-Back. Futhermore in Y-axis, the entire tangential GRF data were transformed into F_y-Front, F_y-Middle and F_y-Back with the same algorithm. In order to make the foot model suitable for diferent individual, the size factors of foot length were dopted. As shown in Table 1, the size fators of five volunteers were summarized. Finally, the muscle forces and joint moment, while ankle joint muscles collaborating with each other in normal walking, were calculated through the inverse dynamics method in AnyBody Modeling System. This experiment has been approved by the ethics committee of the Department of Intelligent Mechanical System Engineering, Kochi University of Technology.

Subject	Size factor of AnyBody foot model (mm)
1	245
2	240
3	265
4	260
5	235

Table 1. List of size factors of the five subjects in the experiment.

3.2 Experimental results

The muscle force results through indirect AnyBody method and direct EMG method were summarized in this section. In AnyBody Modeling System the complex walking kinematic system requires high collaborations of all units, so the muscle forces of human foot were calculated based on a minimum fatigue criterion way. As shown in Fig. 10, the established AnyBody model, which can demonstrate the walking process and the muscle activation video, made the whole process easier to understand in a visualized way. The muscle activity level could be identified by the muscle bulge level, the value and direction of GRF could be discerned by the length and direction of the arrow in the AnyBody gait process video. The quantitative results of ANT TIB, POST TIB, GAST, SOL, EDL and FDL of five subjects in their normal gait were shown in Fig. 11, in Y-axis the quantitative muscle forces were expressed while in X-axis the time was represented. The muscles connecting shank and foot were classified in foot muscle analysis because these muscles would offer foot driven power, whereas the muscle from thigh to shank were excluded because those muscles could only drive the movement of shank in the gait dynamitic system.

To validate the muscle forces calculated by the musculoskeletal multiple-units foot model, contradistinctive analysis was implemented between AnyBody results and EMG results. Only ANTTIB, PL, SOL and GAST were involved in the analysis becasue these four muscles are powerful muscles for driving the movements of human limbs in normal gait, futhermore these muscles are easy to find in skin surface for surface EMG measurement. As shown in Fig. 12, the AnyBody results were drawn in blue while the EMG results were expressed in shadow, in comparison diagrams the X-axis represented percentage of gait cycle (%GC) while the left Y-axis indicated the muscle force with the unit of Newton, and the right Y-axis indicated the percentage of standard voluntary contraction (%SVC) of muscles. Futhermore for making the discussion clearly, the step division figure of gait cycle was expressed on the top of each diagram.

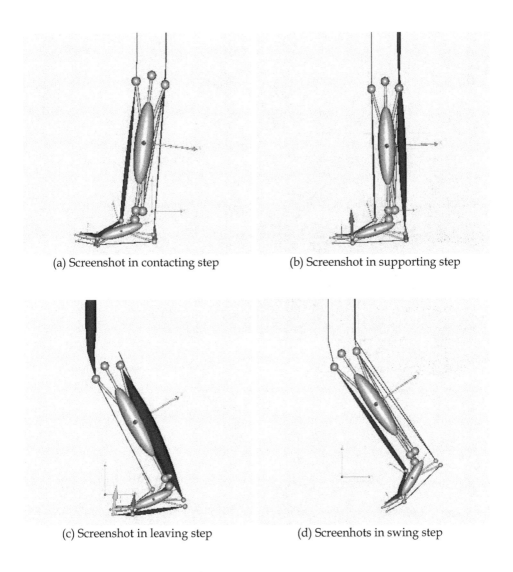

(a) Screenshot in contacting step   (b) Screenshot in supporting step

(c) Screenshot in leaving step   (d) Screenhots in swing step

Fig. 10. Screenshots of gait video in AnyBody Modeling System, four postures in one gait cycle were shown.

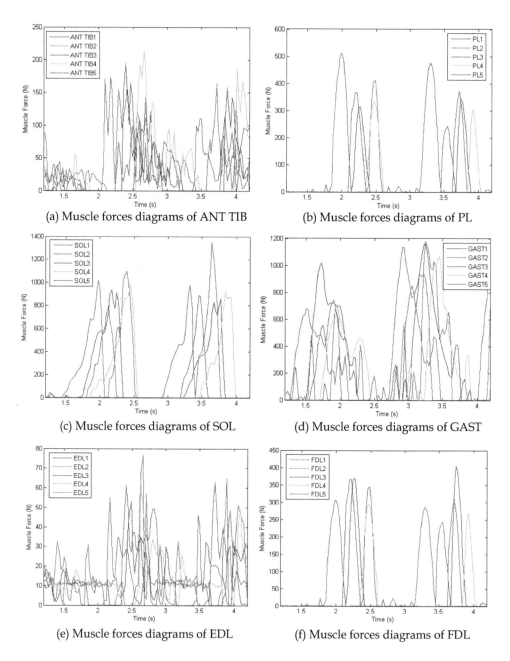

(a) Muscle forces diagrams of ANT TIB

(b) Muscle forces diagrams of PL

(c) Muscle forces diagrams of SOL

(d) Muscle forces diagrams of GAST

(e) Muscle forces diagrams of EDL

(f) Muscle forces diagrams of FDL

Fig. 11. Muscle forces diagrams of ANT TIB, PL, SOL, GAST, FDL and EDL of five subjects obtained in AnyBody Modeling System.

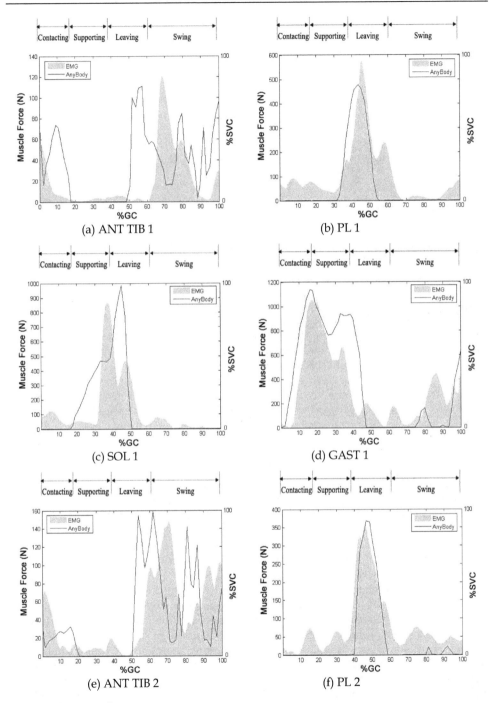

Fig. 12. (Continued)

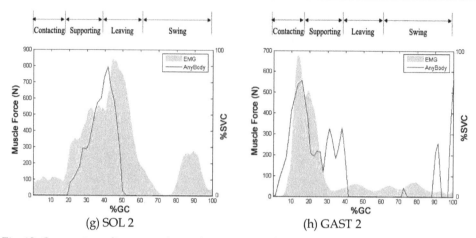

(g) SOL 2　　　　　　　　　　　(h) GAST 2

Fig. 12. Comparison diagrams of muscle activation of ANT TIB, PL, SOL and GAST in one gait cycle. The results of AnyBody Modeling System were drawn in blue while the results of EMG method were expressed in shadow.

4. Discussions

As muscle force results were estimated base on wearable sensor system and AnyBody Modeling system, EMG results had been used to do the comparison as in EMG method the muscle activity result is relatively large or small. As shown in Fig. 11, AnyBody results of five volunteers was exhibited, futhermore reality sense for walking process and similarty could be found among different indivaduals. And in Fig. 12, contradistinctive analysis was implemented between calculated results of AnyBody method and measured results of EMG method, obviously similar comparability could be found although the two results had many differences.

As shown in Fig. 11 (a), (e), the muscle force of ANT TIB and EDL were relatively larger in the first contacting step because the muscles in fronter of shank need to grow up to balance the moment of ankle joint while the heel contacting the floor. And in the last swing step ANT TIB and EDL were larger because they offered forces to drive the limb swing till next gait cycle started. Whereas the values of ANT TIB and EDL were keeping nearly zero in the other steps of gait cycle. As shown in Fig. 12 (a), (e), the value of ANT TIB was relatively high in both AnyBody results and EMG results in the beginning and ending period of one gait cycle, but in the middle steps the AnyBody results were keeping nearly zero while the EMG results were only keeping relatively smaller values.

As shown in Fig. 11 (c), (d), the tensile forces of SOL and GAST increased obviously in the supporting step when the GRF were transfered from posterior foot to anterior foot, moreover the peak value of GAST occurred in this step too. And in the leaving ground step, the SOL continued to increase for pushing human body moving forward and upward till the whole foot separated from the ground and start to swing, moreover the peak value of SOL occurred in this step. The peak Achilles tendon forces occured in the leaving step of our results that ranging from 1.07 kN to 1.66 kN, which were in good agreement with the reported peak Achilles tendon forces of 1430±500 N (Finni et al., 1998). The SOL and GAST were keeping small vaules in the contacting step because the center of gravity were behind the ankle joint. As shown in Fig. 12 (c), (d), (g), (h), the AnyBody results and EMG results were not in high agreement but the variation tendencies were similar.

As shown in Fig. 11 (b), (f), FDL and PL had similar rising period and descending period, and peak values of PL and FDL both occurred in the leaving step, that because the two muscles are both located in the posterior of shank and play a similar role of pushing human body moving forward and upward in the normal human gait. As shown in Fig. 12 (b), (f), in contacting, supporting and swing steps the EMG results of PL showed relatively higher values while the AnyBody results were keeping nearly zero, but in the whole gait cycle obvious comparability could be found between the two results.

5. Conclusions

Muscle forces of human foot were estimated through the inverse dynamics method in AnyBody Modeling System based on wearable sensors and EMG method. The angular motions, GRF and COP of human limb segments could be measured by the developed wearable motion and force sensors with acceleration sensitive units and gyroscopes in various situations. AnyBody Modeling System that professional concerns on musculoskeletal kinematics and kinetics analysis could imported the sensor measured data into a bionic dynamic model. And through invise dynamic method the quantitative muscle forces of human foot could be estimated in AnyBody system. The EMG method was adopted to directly measure muscle activition levels for validation, and the muscle activation results of EMG method have certain comparability with the muscle force results of AnyBody model, futhermore the tendency curves of these muscle forces have reality sense for walking process analysis. This reserch method for human foot appears to be a practical means to determine muscle forces in musculoskeletal analysis and in on-the-spot medical applications. In the future, the muscle force can be made into vector quantity instead of scalar quantity by 3D technology in AnyBody Modeling System as the angular motion and GRF sensors own the capability of 3D measurement.

6. Acknowledgement

The authors wish to acknowledge the support of the volunteer subjects of Robotics and Dynamics Research Lab in Kochi University of Technology.

7. References

Yoon, J.; Novandy, B.; Yoon, C. H. & Park, K. J. (2010). A 6-DOF Gait Rehabilitation Robot With Upper and Lower Limb Connections That Allows Walking Velocity Updates on Various Terrains, *IEEE/ASME Trans. on Mechatronics*, Vol. 15, No. 2, pp. 201–215, ISSN 1083-4435

Vallery, H.; Ekkelenkamp, R.; Buss, M. & Kooij, H. (2007). Complementary Limb Motion Estimation based on Interjoint Coordination: Experimental Evaluation, *Proc. of IEEE 10th Intl. Conf. on Rehabilitation Robotics*, pp. 798–803, ISBN 978-1-4244-1320-1, Noordwijk. Netherlands

Peshkin, M.; Brown, D. A.; Santos-Munné, J. J.; Makhlin, A.; Lewis, E.; Colgate, J. E.; Patton, J. & Schwandt, D. (2005). KineAssist: A Robotic Overground Gait and Balance

Training Device, *Proc. of IEEE 9th Intl. Conf. on Rehabilitation Robotics*, pp. 241–246, ISBN 0-7803-9003-2, Chicago, USA

Park, J.H. & Kim, E.S. (2009). Foot and Body Control of Biped Robots to Walk on Irregularly Protruded Uneven Surfaces, *IEEE Transactions on Systems, Man, and Cybernetics, Part B: Cybernetics*, Vol. 39, No. 1, pp. 289-297, ISSN 1083-4419

Ishida, T.; Kuroki, Y. & Yamaguchi, J. (2003). Mechanical System of a Small Biped Entertainment Robot, *Proceedings of IEEE/RSJ International Conference on Intelligent Robots and Systems*, pp. 1129-1134, ISBN 0-7803-7860-1, Las Vegas, Nevada, USA

Lee, K.S. (2008). EMG-Based Speech Recognition Using Hidden Markov Models With Global Control Variables, *IEEE Transactions on Biomedical Engineering*, Vol. 55, No. 3, pp. 930-940, ISSN 0018-9294

Merlo, A.; Farina, D. & Merletti, R. (2003). A Fast and Reliable Technique for Muscle Activity Detection From Surface EMG Signals, *Transactions On Biomedical Engineering*, Vol. 50, No. 3, pp. 316-323, ISSN 0018-9294

Kizuka T.; Masuda, T.; Kiryu, T. & Sadoyama, T. (2009). *Biomechanism Library Practical Usage of Surface Electromyogram*, Publisher of Tokyo Denki University, ISBN 4-501-32510-0, Tokyo, Japan

Hou, Y.F.; Zurada, J.M.; Karwowski, W.; Marras, W.S. & Davis, K. (2007). Estimation of the Dynamic Spinal Forces Using a Recurrent Fuzzy Neural Network, *IEEE Transactions on Systems, Man, and Cybernetics – Part B: Cybernetics*, Vol. 37, No. 1, pp. 100-109, ISSN 1083-4419

Ferreira, J.P.; Crisostomo, M.M. & Coimbra, A.P. (2009). Human Gait Acquisition and Characterization, *IEEE Transactions on Instrumentation and Measurement*, Vol. 58, No. 9, pp. 2979-2988, ISSN 0018-9456

Moustakidis, S.P.; Theocharis, J.B. & Giakas, G. (2008). Subject Recognition Based on Ground Reaction Force Measurements of Gait Signals, *IEEE Transactions on Systems, Man, and Cybernetics – Part B: Cybernetics*, Vol. 38, No. 6, pp. 1476-1485, ISSN 1083-4419

Liu, K.; Liu, T.; Shibata, K.; Inoue, Y. & Zheng, R.C. (2009). Novel Approach to Ambulatory Assessment of Human Segmental Orientation on A Wearable Sensor System, *Journal of Biomechanics*, Vol. 42, No. 16, pp. 2747-2752, ISSN 0021-9290

Boonstra, M.C.; Slikke, R.M.; Keijsers, N.L.; Lummel, R.C.; Malefijt, M.C. & Verdonschot, N. (2006). The Accuracy of Measuring the Kinematics of Rising from a Chair with Accelerometers and Gyroscopes, *Journal of Biomechanics*, Vol. 39, No. 2, pp. 354-358, ISSN 0021-9290

Liu, T.; Inoue, Y. & Shibata, K. (2008). New Method for Assessment of Gait Variability Based on Wearable Ground Reaction Force Sensor, *30th Annual International IEEE EMBS Conference Vancouver*, pp. 2341-2344, ISSN 1557-170X

McMinn, R.M.H.; Hutchings, R.T. & Logan, B.M. (1982). *Colour Atlas of Foot and Ankle Anatomy*, Year Book Medical Publishers, ISBN 0-815-15829-7, Chicago, USA

Perry, J.; Ireland, M.; Gronley, J. & Hoffer, M. (1986). Predictive Value of Manual Muscle Testing and Gait Analysis in Normal Ankles by Electromyography, *Foot Ankle*, Vol. 6, No. 5, pp. 254-259, ISSN 1071-1007

Finni, T.; Komi, P.V. & Lukkariniemi, J. (1998). Achilles Tendon Loading During Walking: Application of a Novel Optic Fiber Technique, *Eur J Appl Physiol Occup Physiol*, Vol. 77, No. 3, pp. 289-291, ISSN 0301-5548

6

Noninvasive Monitoring of Breathing and Swallowing Interaction

N. Terzi[1,2], D. Orlikowski[2,3], H. Prigent[2,4],
Pierre Denise[6], H. Normand[6] and F. Lofaso[2,4,5]
[1]INSERM, ERI27, Caen; Univ Caen, Caen; CHRU Caen
Service de Réanimation Médicale, Caen
[2]Centre d'Investigation Clinique - Innovations Technologiques, Hôpital Raymond
Poincaré, AP-HP; Université de Versailles-Saint Quentin en Yvelines, Garches
[3]Centre d'Investigation Clinique - Innovations Technologiques 805, Service de
Réanimation et Unité de Ventilation à Domicile, Hôpital Raymond Poincaré, AP-HP
[4]Services de Physiologie - Explorations Fonctionnelles
Hôpital Raymond Poincaré, AP-HP
[5]INSERM, U 955, Créteil
[6]INSERM, ERI27, Caen, Univ Caen; CHRU Caen
Service d'Explorations Fonctionnelles, Caen
France

1. Introduction

The evaluation of swallowing parameters and of interactions between breathing and swallowing is crucial to optimise the management of patients with chronic respiratory failure, as swallowing must occur in precise coordination with breathing. Various techniques have been used to study the physiology and biomechanics of the oral and pharyngeal stages of swallowing. Among them, the two most commonly used, videofluoroscopy and videoendoscopy, provide information on the motion of anatomic structures during swallowing. The determination of muscle activation patterns is best achieved with electromyography (EMG). Most of the initial EMG studies of swallowing used needle electrodes to record intramuscular EMG activity (Doty and Bosma 1956; Perlman, Palmer et al. 1999). Ertekin *et al.* (Ertekin, Pehlivan et al. 1995) were the first to describe an electrophysiological method for investigating swallowing in humans.

Recent advances in the management of respiratory failure have considerably improved the survival of patients with neuromuscular disease (Finder, Birnkrant et al. 2004). For example, the introduction in the 1990s of mechanical ventilation (MV) improved the survival of patients with Duchenne muscular dystrophy (DMD) from about 15 years in the 1960s to more than 30 years now. Quality of life, however, declines over time as the disease progresses. Malnutrition is common: in one study, for instance, 44% of patients had malnutrition (Willig, Bach et al. 1995). The main causes of malnutrition are prolonged swallowing, respiratory failure, and dysphagia, which jeopardize the patient's ability to meet intake needs. Feeding difficulties often develop insidiously, being frequently underestimated by family members and healthcare professionals (Hill, Hughes et al. 2004).

Aspiration is another important consequence of impaired swallowing that becomes increasingly common as the disease progresses (Finder, Birnkrant et al. 2004).
Studies have demonstrated that swallowing dysfunction is closely associated with impaired inspiratory muscle strength (Terzi, Orlikowski et al. 2007; Orlikowski, Terzi et al. 2009) and improve with tracheostomy and mechanical ventilation (Terzi, Prigent et al.; Terzi, Orlikowski et al. 2007). Swallowing and inspiratory muscle strength are being evaluated in patients with acute exacerbations of chronic obstructive pulmonary disease (COPD) requiring noninvasive ventilation.
Noninvasive methods for evaluating swallowing are useful to investigate various disorders and the interactions between breathing and swallowing. Here, after a review of swallowing physiology to explain the EMG evaluation and a discussion of interactions between breathing and swallowing, we describe the most commonly used electrophysiological method, which is noninvasive and easy to perform at the bedside. We do not address methods requiring the connection of measurement devices directly to the airway.

2. Physiology of swallowing

Swallowing is a complex physiological function that was generally investigated using videofluoroscopy, videoendoscopy, manometric methods, or invasive methods providing information on a single pair of muscles involved in swallowing. Swallowing was usually divided into three phases: an initial oral phase; a pharyngeal phase; and an esophageal phase (Dodds 1989). These phases of swallowing involve different in innervation patterns. Thus, the oral phase is usually described as voluntary, the pharyngeal phase as a reflex response, and the esophageal phase as controlled by both the somatic and the autonomic nervous system (Doty and Bosma 1956; Miller 1982).

2.1 Oral phase
The oral phase is mainly voluntary and highly variable in duration depending in humans on taste, environment, hunger, motivation, and consciousness. First, the tongue presses the bolus against the hard palate and initiates displacement of the bolus to the posterior part of the tongue and toward the oropharynx. This stage ends with the triggering of the pharyngeal phase of swallowing.
When the volume swallowed is small (1-2 ml, e.g., saliva), there is no preparatory phase and the oral and pharyngeal phases occur in sequence. In contrast, with large liquid boluses, the oral and pharyngeal phases overlap (Logemann, Kahrilas et al. 1992; Ertekin, Celik et al. 2000). The size of the bolus does not alter the sequence of events during oropharyngeal swallowing but modulates the timing of each phase of the swallow. As volume size increases, pharyngeal transit time increases, as do laryngeal closure and elevation (Ertekin, Aydogdu et al. 1997).
When 20 ml of water is placed in the mouth, normal individuals tend to divide the water into two or more parts, which are swallowed in sequence (Ertekin, Aydogdu et al. 1996). This phenomenon is called piecemeal deglutition.
From this stage to the end of the swallow, breathing is inhibited.

2.2 Pharyngeal phase
The pharyngeal phase is closely related to the oral phase, and the distinction between the two is often unclear. This intimate relationship is expressed by the widespread use of the terms oropharynx and oropharyngeal swallowing.

When the movement of the bolus from the oral cavity to the pharyngeal space triggers the swallowing reflex or response, several closely coordinated events occur in rapid overlapping sequence, transporting the bolus from the oropharynx to the esophagus without allowing aspiration. Coordination of these events may be chiefly under the control of the central pattern generator (CPG) in the brainstem (Miller 1982; Jean 2001). These events are as follows: (i) several reflexes governed by the CPG protect the nasal, laryngeal, and tracheal airways and support laryngeal closure; (ii) the tongue moves backward to push the bolus through the pharynx; (iii) and the upper esophageal sphincter relaxes and opens, allowing the bolus to descend into the esophagus.

Once the pharyngeal phase is initiated, the chain of events is irreversible. The entire oropharyngeal sequence takes only 0.6 to 1.0 second, and this duration is remarkably constant in humans (Ertekin, Pehlivan et al. 1995).

2.3 Esophageal phase
In comparison with the extraordinary complexity and rapidity of the oropharyngeal phase, the esophageal phase of swallowing is simpler and slower. It consists of a peristaltic wave of contraction of the striated and smooth muscles, which propagates to the stomach.

2.4 Neurological control of swallowing
The process of swallowing is an ordered sequence of sensory and motor events. Swallowing is a fundamental motor activity, since it serves two vital functions: by propelling food into the stomach, swallowing subserves the alimentary function; and the swallowing reflex protects the upper respiratory tract, thus preventing aspiration of food particles into the lungs (Miller 1982). Swallowing can occur voluntarily via cerebral cortex activation and/or as a reflex under brainstem control.

The central neural control of swallowing is also divided between the cortex and brainstem. Cortical centers in conjunction with afferent feedback from the musculature initiate and modulate the volitional swallow (Sumi 1969; Car and Roman 1970; Martin and Sessle 1993), whereas the brainstem swallowing CPG generates the sequence of reflex swallowing via the nuclei of the Vth, IXth, and XIIth cranial nerves. Normal swallowing requires coordinated interactions among these outputs. Any disruption in the process of coordination leads to swallowing dysfunction.

The importance of suprabulbar influences in regulating swallowing has been established in animal models in which cortical swallowing regions are disrupted by lesion induction, anesthesia, or cooling (Sumi 1969; Martin and Sessle 1993). In humans, the development of functional magnetic resonance imaging (fMRI) has allowed the identification of the cortical regions involved in voluntary swallowing. The primary motor and sensory areas are consistently active in healthy adults during swallowing. The anterior cingular cortex is also activated during swallowing (Hamdy, Mikulis et al. 1999; Humbert and Robbins 2007).

There is convincing evidence that the sequential and rhythmic patterns of swallowing are formed and organized by a central pattern generator (CPG) located within the medulla oblongata (Jean 2001). The CPG was first described as a swallowing center that can be subdivided into three systems: an afferent system composed of the central and peripheral inputs to the center; an efferent system composed of outputs from the center to various motor neuron pools involved in swallowing; and an organizing system composed of interneuronal networks that program the motor pattern.

Although the central regulation of swallowing is chiefly dependent on the brainstem, which receives sensory input from the oropharynx and esophagus, the initiation of swallowing is a voluntary action that requires the integrity of sensorimotor areas of the cerebral cortex. Therefore, both the brainstem and cortex must be intact to ensure normal swallowing.

3. Interaction between respiration and swallowing

The temporal coordination of pharyngeal and laryngeal swallowing events with breathing is essential to prevent aspiration of oropharyngeal contents into the lungs. Indeed, both breathing and swallowing occur continually, although at different frequencies. As the upper airway is used for both breathing and swallowing, the motor pattern generators for these two activities must work in tight coordination to prevent aspiration and to ensure clearance of lower airway secretions (Feroah, Forster et al. 2002).

The swallowing CPG may play a crucial role in coordinating swallowing and breathing. Within this CPG, some of the premotor and motor neurons can be involved in at least two different tasks, such as swallowing and breathing, swallowing and mastication, and swallowing and phonation (Jean 2001).

During swallowing, mechanisms that protect the airways include adduction of the vocal cords, inversion of the epiglottis, and the upward and forward movement of the larynx away from the flow of the bolus. Respiratory control during swallowing contributes to airway protection.

In 1985, Nishino et al. clarified the effects of swallowing on the pattern of continuous breathing in humans. In adults, approximately 80% of spontaneous or water-induced swallows occurred during the expiratory phase. Furthermore, breathing resumed at the point of the expiratory phase where the interruption had taken place (Nishino, Yonezawa et al. 1985). A striking finding was that most of the water-induced swallows occurred during expiration although the timing of water administration was determined at random. The mechanisms underlying these findings are unclear but may involve reflex-mediated responses, as all the study participants reported being unaware of the breathing phase during which their swallows occurred. One of the main hypotheses is that the timing of swallows is not entirely independent from volitional control. The effects of swallowing on the pattern of continuous breathing were analyzed in detail in this study. Spontaneous (automatic) and volitional (water-induced) swallows occurring during expiration were followed by a small increase in the duration of the interrupted expiration. As the time from expiration onset to swallowing increased, the duration of the expiration increased. Swallows that interrupted the inspiratory phase were followed by short expirations. Thus, swallowing was followed by resetting of the respiratory cycling with a return to the functional residual capacity before the initiation of a new inspiration. This alteration in the breathing pattern may help to clear the airway of secretions and foreign material before the next inspiration, thus contributing to prevent aspiration (Nishino, Yonezawa et al. 1985).

Breathing-swallowing interactions and the underlying mechanisms have been studied in healthy volunteers by measuring a variety of parameters including the duration of deglutition apnea (Nishino, Yonezawa et al. 1985; Selley, Flack et al. 1989; Martin, Logemann et al. 1994; Klahn and Perlman 1999) and the timing of breathing events relative to swallows (Perlman, Schultz et al. 1993; Martin, Logemann et al. 1994; Paydarfar, Gilbert et al. 1995; Klahn and Perlman 1999). Several factors that influence breathing-swallowing interactions were identified. Interestingly, many studies showed that breathing-swallowing coordination was influenced by neurological disorders affecting the brain, spinal cord, or peripheral nerves.

Studies in unconscious patients demonstrated that several mechanisms integrating breathing and swallowing remained operative, leading to changes in the breathing pattern during repeated swallows. These findings are consistent with a role for brainstem control (Nishino and Hiraga 1991), especially as both the respiratory center and the swallowing CPG are located in the same area of the brainstem. In contrast, other studies demonstrated that the cortex influences breathing-swallowing interactions in unconscious patients (Hadjikoutis, Pickersgill et al. 2000).

In the other direction, alterations in breathing patterns and ventilation may influence the coordination of swallowing and breathing. This effect is of particular importance in patients with chronic respiratory failure, in whom close breathing-swallowing coordination is essential to maintain adequate ventilation despite the limited ventilatory capacity. Alterations in breathing-swallowing coordination have been reported in patients with chronic obstructive pulmonary disease (COPD) (Shaker, Li et al. 1992) and in awake healthy volunteers subjected to added respiratory loads (Kijima, Isono et al. 1999). Tachypnea and lung volume have also been demonstrated to influence breathing-swallowing coordination.

Alterations in breathing-swallowing coordination chiefly affect temporal coordination. When temporal coordination is disrupted, most swallows are followed by an inspiration, which significantly increases the risk of aspiration.

4. Breathing-swallowing interaction in neuromuscular patients

Elucidation of breathing-swallowing interactions in patients with specific neuromuscular diseases is of considerable interest. Patients with neuromuscular disease have achieved substantial survival gains in recent years as a result of advances in the management of respiratory failure (Finder, Birnkrant et al. 2004). The introduction of mechanical ventilation (MV) in the 1990s improved survival in patients with Duchenne muscular dystrophy (DMD) from about 15 years in the 1960s to more than 30 years now. Quality of life, however, declines over time as the disease progresses. Malnutrition is common: in one study, for instance, 44% of patients had malnutrition (Willig, Bach et al. 1995; Finder, Birnkrant et al. 2004). The main causes of malnutrition are prolonged swallowing, respiratory failure, and dysphagia, which jeopardize the patient's ability to meet intake needs. Feeding difficulties often develop insidiously, being frequently underestimated by family members and healthcare professionals (Hill, Hughes et al. 2004). Aspiration is another important consequence of impaired swallowing that becomes increasingly common as the disease progresses (Finder, Birnkrant et al. 2004).

To the best of our knowledge, breathing-swallowing interactions initially received little research attention (Hadjikoutis, Pickersgill et al. 2000). Moreover, improvements in the management of chronic respiratory failure translate into differences in breathing conditions across patients and over time, and this variability is likely to complicate the evaluation of breathing-swallowing interactions. These breathing conditions are now well defined and include spontaneous breathing (SB), (Raphael, Chevret et al. 1994), noninvasive mechanical ventilation (NIV) (Bach, Alba et al. 1993; 1999; Mehta and Hill 2001; Annane, Orlikowski et al. 2007), tracheostomy with SB (Bach and Alba 1990; Chadda, Louis et al. 2002), and tracheostomy with MV (Bach and Alba 1990; Bach 1993; Simonds 2003).

In contrast to spontaneously breathing patients, tracheostomized patients receiving assist-control MV cannot prolong their expiratory phase. Consequently, the ventilator determines whether expiration or inspiration occurs after swallowing. Under normal breathing conditions, swallows are nearly always followed by expiration (Nishino, Yonezawa et al. 1985; Smith, Wolkove et al. 1989; Paydarfar, Gilbert et al. 1995), which may contribute to prevent aspiration.

In studies of breathing-swallowing interactions in neuromuscular patients with chronic respiratory failure, we found that SB was associated with piecemeal deglutition leading to an increase in the time needed to swallow a water bolus, as well as with inspiration after nearly half the swallows. These abnormalities may contribute to feeding difficulties. They correlated with the reduction in respiratory muscle performance, suggesting a relationship between breathing-muscle performance and swallowing-muscle performance. Accordingly, tongue strength and indices of global and respiratory strength varied in parallel throughout the course of Guillain-Barré syndrome (Orlikowski, Terzi et al. 2009). Tongue strength can be considered representative of the strength of the various muscles involved in swallowing. Another hypothesis is that respiratory failure alone may alter breathing-swallowing coordination. In keeping with this possibility, breathing-swallowing abnormalities were documented in COPD patients with respiratory failure but no upper-airway muscle-strength abnormalities. These findings indicated a need for evaluating the positive impact of MV on breathing-swallowing interactions in patients with respiratory failure.

First, in tracheostomized NM patients who were able to breathe spontaneously, we demonstrated that MV decreased both piecemeal deglutition and swallowing time per bolus (Terzi, Orlikowski et al. 2007).

Second, we evaluated the impact of tracheostomy with MV on swallowing performance in patients with DMD. To this end, we assessed swallowing performance and breathing-swallowing coordination before and after tracheostomy in the same patients. Piecemeal deglutition over several breathing cycles occurred in all patients. Before tracheostomy, half the swallows were followed by inspirations. Tracheostomy was associated with significant decreases in total bolus swallowing time and number of swallows per bolus, compared to the values before tracheostomy. These findings indicated that invasive ventilation via a tracheostomy improved swallowing. Several hypotheses can be put forward to explain this effect. Breathing and swallowing use the same initial pathway and, therefore, competition occurs between these two functions. Under physiological conditions, this competition is well controlled via close coordination of breathing and swallowing. Respiratory failure exacerbates the competition, giving preference to breathing over swallowing and altering the coordination between these two activities. Our results suggest that, by reversing the respiratory failure and separating the breathing and swallowing pathways, invasive MV may have a positive impact on swallowing in patients with respiratory failure.

The question is now whether treating the respiratory failure without separating the breathing and swallowing pathways, e.g., by using NIV, improves swallowing performance in patients with respiratory failure. We are currently studying the impact of NIV on swallowing in patients with chronic obstructive pulmonary disease (COPD) admitted to the intensive care unit for acute respiratory failure. The first results strongly support a beneficial effect of NIV on swallowing performance.

All these studies underline the clinical usefulness of noninvasive dynamic evaluations of breathing-swallowing interactions in order to detect patients at risk for swallowing dysfunction due to respiratory failure. All our studies were done using a previously described noninvasive method (see below).

5. From bench to the bedside

EMG can be used to demonstrate the sequential and orderly activity of the muscles involved in swallowing and breathing. The anatomical components of the swallowing apparatus include the bony and cartilaginous support structures, striated and smooth muscles, and neural elements.

The muscles involved in swallowing have been studied in experimental animals and, to some extent, in humans. In dogs, the pattern of EMG activity was studied in the oral and pharyngeal muscles during swallowing elicited reflexively by electrical and mechanical stimuli (Doty and Bosma 1956). Needle electrodes were used to record intramuscular EMG activity during swallowing from a large complex of oral, pharyngeal, and laryngeal muscles in anesthetized animals. Descriptive studies based on this technique consistently found that the nonvolitional component of swallowing was controlled by a CPG (Miller 1972; Suzuki, Tokuriki et al. 1977; Kobara-Mates, Logemann et al. 1995). In humans, most of the intramuscular EMG studies of the pharyngeal phase of swallowing focused on a single muscle or muscle pair (Basmajian and Dutta 1961; Perlman, Luschei et al. 1989). Such studies can shed valuable light on the properties of the muscle of interest. However, they provide no information on the dynamics of swallowing.

To evaluate the dynamics of swallowing, researchers used quantitative surface EMG of the submental complex (SM) composed of submandibular/suprahyoid muscles including the mylohyoid, genohyoid, and anterior digastric muscles. All the muscles in this complex contract simultaneously to initiate a swallow and function as laryngeal elevators (Miller 1982). Consequently, submental surface EMG activity provides considerable information about the onset and duration of the oropharyngeal swallowing phase, as contraction of the SM complex pulls the hyoid bone into an anterosuperior position, thereby elevating the larynx and initiating the other reflexive changes that constitute the pharyngeal phase of swallowing (Donner, Bosma et al. 1985; Dodds, Logemann et al. 1990; Ertekin, Pehlivan et al. 1995). However, pharyngeal and laryngeal EMG recording during swallowing was difficult to perform noninvasively and usually required the insertion of a needle electrode. However, laryngeal motion can be detected fairly easily using a mechanical sensor.

To evaluate swallowing, we used a method previously described by Ertekin et al. (Ertekin, Aydogdu et al. 1998). Skin-surface electrodes are placed on the chin to record submental muscle activity and a piezo-electric sensor is placed between the cricoid and thyroid cartilages on the midline to detect laryngeal motion (Figure 1) (Terzi, Orlikowski et al. 2007). Breathing-swallowing coordination is assessed by using respiratory inductive plethysmography to record thoracic and abdominal movements. All signals are digitized and recorded on a personal computer equipped with an MP 150 data acquisition system (Biopac Systems, Goleta, CA, USA). The system software (AcqKnowledge) is configured to display the EMG signals, laryngeal movements, thoracic and abdominal movements simultaneously on separate channels.

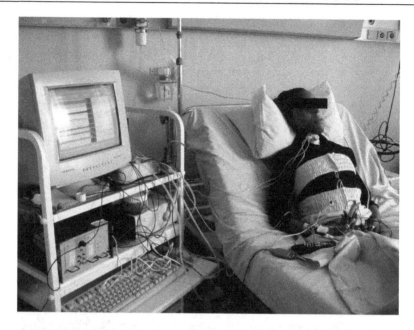

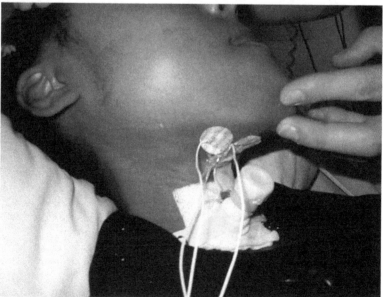

Fig. 1. Noninvasive monitoring. Extracted from Terzi et al. (Terzi, Orlikowski et al. 2007)

First, using this method we have demonstrated that the breathing-swallowing interaction was associated with piecemeal deglutition in neuromuscular patients, contrary to healthy subjects (Figure 2).

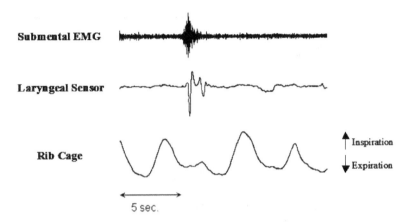

Healthy subjects

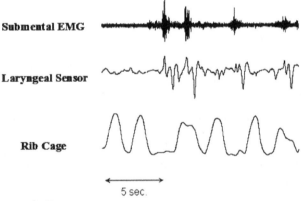

Patient with Neuromuscular disease

Fig. 2. Example of recordings in healthy subjects, and in patient with neuromuscular disorder. Extracted from Terzi et al. (Terzi, Orlikowski et al. 2007).

Piecemeal deglutition and breathing-swallowing anormalities was also demonstrated when neuromuscular patients were tracheostomized, however swallowing performance improved with mechanical ventilation (Figure 3).

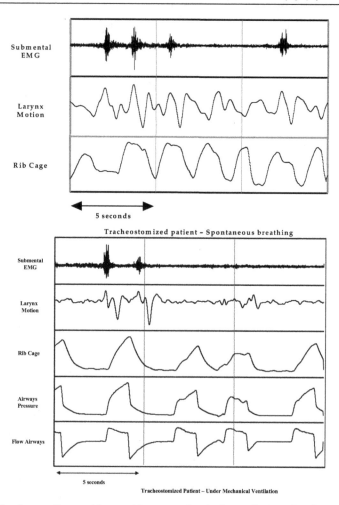

Fig. 3. Example of recordings with or without mechanical ventilation. Swallowing performance was improved by mechanical ventilation.

6. References

(1999). "Clinical indications for noninvasive positive pressure ventilation in chronic respiratory failure due to restrictive lung disease, COPD, and nocturnal hypoventilation--a consensus conference report." Chest 116(2): 521-534.

Annane, D., D. Orlikowski, et al. (2007). "Nocturnal mechanical ventilation for chronic hypoventilation in patients with neuromuscular and chest wall disorders." Cochrane Database Syst Rev(4): CD001941.

Bach, J. R. (1993). "A comparison of long-term ventilatory support alternatives from the perspective of the patient and care giver." Chest 104(6): 1702-1706.

Bach, J. R. and A. S. Alba (1990). "Tracheostomy ventilation. A study of efficacy with deflated cuffs and cuffless tubes." Chest 97(3): 679-683.

Bach, J. R., A. S. Alba, et al. (1993). "Intermittent positive pressure ventilation via the mouth as an alternative to tracheostomy for 257 ventilator users." Chest 103(1): 174-182.

Basmajian, J. V. and C. R. Dutta (1961). "Electromyography of the pharyngeal constrictors and levator palati in man." Anat Rec 139: 561-563.

Car, A. and C. Roman (1970). "[Deglutitions and oesophageal reflex contractions induced by electrical stimulation of the medulla oblongata]." Exp Brain Res 11(1): 75-92.

Chadda, K., B. Louis, et al. (2002). "Physiological effects of decannulation in tracheostomized patients." Intensive Care Med 28(12): 1761-1767.

Dodds, W. J. (1989). "Physiology of swallowing." Dysphagia 3(4): 171-178.

Dodds, W. J., J. A. Logemann, et al. (1990). "Radiologic assessment of abnormal oral and pharyngeal phases of swallowing." AJR Am J Roentgenol 154(5): 965-974.

Donner, M. W., J. F. Bosma, et al. (1985). "Anatomy and physiology of the pharynx." Gastrointest Radiol 10(3): 196-212.

Doty, R. W. and J. F. Bosma (1956). "An electromyographic analysis of reflex deglutition." J Neurophysiol 19(1): 44-60.

Ertekin, C., I. Aydogdu, et al. (1996). "Piecemeal deglutition and dysphagia limit in normal subjects and in patients with swallowing disorders." J Neurol Neurosurg Psychiatry 61(5): 491-496.

Ertekin, C., I. Aydogdu, et al. (1997). "Effects of bolus volume on oropharyngeal swallowing: an electrophysiologic study in man." Am J Gastroenterol 92(11): 2049-2053.

Ertekin, C., I. Aydogdu, et al. (1998). "Electrodiagnostic methods for neurogenic dysphagia." Electroencephalogr Clin Neurophysiol 109(4): 331-340.

Ertekin, C., M. Celik, et al. (2000). "The electromyographic behavior of the thyroarytenoid muscle during swallowing." J Clin Gastroenterol 30(3): 274-280.

Ertekin, C., M. Pehlivan, et al. (1995). "An electrophysiological investigation of deglutition in man." Muscle Nerve 18(10): 1177-1186.

Feroah, T. R., H. V. Forster, et al. (2002). "Effects of spontaneous swallows on breathing in awake goats." J Appl Physiol 92(5): 1923-1935.

Finder, J. D., D. Birnkrant, et al. (2004). "Respiratory care of the patient with Duchenne muscular dystrophy: ATS consensus statement." Am J Respir Crit Care Med 170(4): 456-465.

Hadjikoutis, S., T. P. Pickersgill, et al. (2000). "Abnormal patterns of breathing during swallowing in neurological disorders." Brain 123 (Pt 9): 1863-1873.

Hamdy, S., D. J. Mikulis, et al. (1999). "Cortical activation during human volitional swallowing: an event-related fMRI study." Am J Physiol 277(1 Pt 1): G219-225.

Hill, M., T. Hughes, et al. (2004). "Treatment for swallowing difficulties (dysphagia) in chronic muscle disease." Cochrane Database Syst Rev(2): CD004303.

Humbert, I. A. and J. Robbins (2007). "Normal swallowing and functional magnetic resonance imaging: a systematic review." Dysphagia 22(3): 266-275.

Jean, A. (2001). "Brain stem control of swallowing: neuronal network and cellular mechanisms." Physiol Rev 81(2): 929-969.

Kijima, M., S. Isono, et al. (1999). "Coordination of swallowing and phases of respiration during added respiratory loads in awake subjects." Am J Respir Crit Care Med 159(6): 1898-1902.

Klahn, M. S. and A. L. Perlman (1999). "Temporal and durational patterns associating respiration and swallowing." Dysphagia 14(3): 131-138.

Kobara-Mates, M., J. A. Logemann, et al. (1995). "Physiology of oropharyngeal swallow in the cat: a videofluoroscopic and electromyographic study." Am J Physiol 268(2 Pt 1): G232-241.

Logemann, J. A., P. J. Kahrilas, et al. (1992). "Closure mechanisms of laryngeal vestibule during swallow." Am J Physiol 262(2 Pt 1): G338-344.

Martin, B. J., J. A. Logemann, et al. (1994). "Coordination between respiration and swallowing: respiratory phase relationships and temporal integration." J Appl Physiol 76(2): 714-723.

Martin, R. E. and B. J. Sessle (1993). "The role of the cerebral cortex in swallowing." Dysphagia 8(3): 195-202.

Mehta, S. and N. S. Hill (2001). "Noninvasive ventilation." Am J Respir Crit Care Med 163(2): 540-577.

Miller, A. J. (1972). "Significance of sensory inflow to the swallowing reflex." Brain Res 43(1): 147-159.

Miller, A. J. (1982). "Deglutition." Physiol Rev 62(1): 129-184.

Nishino, T. and K. Hiraga (1991). "Coordination of swallowing and respiration in unconscious subjects." J Appl Physiol 70(3): 988-993.

Nishino, T., T. Yonezawa, et al. (1985). "Effects of swallowing on the pattern of continuous respiration in human adults." Am Rev Respir Dis 132(6): 1219-1222.

Orlikowski, D., N. Terzi, et al. (2009). "Tongue weakness is associated with respiratory failure in patients with severe Guillain-Barre syndrome." Acta Neurol Scand 119(6): 364-370.

Paydarfar, D., R. J. Gilbert, et al. (1995). "Respiratory phase resetting and airflow changes induced by swallowing in humans." J Physiol 483 (Pt 1): 273-288.

Perlman, A. L., E. S. Luschei, et al. (1989). "Electrical activity from the superior pharyngeal constrictor during reflexive and nonreflexive tasks." J Speech Hear Res 32(4): 749-754.

Perlman, A. L., P. M. Palmer, et al. (1999). "Electromyographic activity from human laryngeal, pharyngeal, and submental muscles during swallowing." J Appl Physiol 86(5): 1663-1669.

Perlman, A. L., J. G. Schultz, et al. (1993). "Effects of age, gender, bolus volume, and bolus viscosity on oropharyngeal pressure during swallowing." J Appl Physiol 75(1): 33-37.

Raphael, J. C., S. Chevret, et al. (1994). "Randomised trial of preventive nasal ventilation in Duchenne muscular dystrophy. French Multicentre Cooperative Group on Home Mechanical Ventilation Assistance in Duchenne de Boulogne Muscular Dystrophy." Lancet 343(8913): 1600-1604.

Selley, W. G., F. C. Flack, et al. (1989). "Respiratory patterns associated with swallowing: Part 1. The normal adult pattern and changes with age." Age Ageing 18(3): 168-172.

Shaker, R., Q. Li, et al. (1992). "Coordination of deglutition and phases of respiration: effect of aging, tachypnea, bolus volume, and chronic obstructive pulmonary disease." Am J Physiol 263(5 Pt 1): G750-755.

Simonds, A. K. (2003). "Home ventilation." Eur Respir J Suppl 47: 38s-46s.

Smith, J., N. Wolkove, et al. (1989). "Coordination of eating, drinking and breathing in adults." Chest 96(3): 578-582.

Sumi, T. (1969). "Some properties of cortically-evoked swallowing and chewing in rabbits." Brain Res 15(1): 107-120.

Suzuki, M., M. Tokuriki, et al. (1977). "Electromyographic studies on the deglutition movement in the goat." Nippon Juigaku Zasshi 39(3): 243-253.

Terzi, N., D. Orlikowski, et al. (2007). "Breathing-swallowing interaction in neuromuscular patients: a physiological evaluation." Am J Respir Crit Care Med 175(3): 269-276.

Terzi, N., H. Prigent, et al. "Impact of tracheostomy on swallowing performance in Duchenne muscular dystrophy." Neuromuscul Disord 20(8): 493-498.

Willig, T. N., J. R. Bach, et al. (1995). "Nutritional rehabilitation in neuromuscular disorders." Semin Neurol 15(1): 18-23.

7

Affective Processing of Loved Familiar Faces: Contributions from Electromyography

Pedro Guerra, Alicia Sánchez-Adam, Lourdes Anllo-Vento and Jaime Vila
University of Granada,
Spain

1. Introduction

Human faces stand among the most unique stimuli in social and emotional communication. By looking at faces we can access a broad range of significant information about the other, such as personal identity, emotional state (facial expression), sex, age, race, attractiveness, attitudes (whether they are friendly or hostile), intentions, and thoughts (Dekowska et al., 2008; Adolphs, 2009). Because of its relevance in everyday interactions, the face has been the target of much study throughout the past decades. Most studies on the psychology of face perception and recognition have focused on emotional facial expressions, following the pioneering work of Tomkins (1962), Izard (1971, 1977, 1994), and Ekman (1984, 1992) (see Russell, 1994; Dimberg, 1997; Whalen et al., 1998; Öhman et al., 2001; Adolphs, 2002; Eimer & Holmes, 2007; Vuilleumier & Pourtois, 2007; Li et al., 2010), based on the evolutionary perspective outlined by Darwin in his book *The expression of emotions in man and animals* (1872). More recently, a large body of research has been devoted to delineate the brain mechanisms involved in face perception and identity recognition (see Adolphs, 2002; Faihall & Isahi, 2006; Dekowska et al., 2008; Li et al., 2010). In this context, studies using central electrophysiological techniques, such as electroencephalography (EEG), event-related potentials (ERPs), or magnetoencephalography (MEG), and metabolic techniques, such as positron emission tomography (PET) or functional magnetic resonance imaging (fMRI), have proven particularly useful in describing the chain of events taking place in the processing of facial information and the neural circuitry responsible for face recognition, respectively. Thus, several event-related components such as P1, N170, N250r, P300, and N400, have been used to determine the temporal sequence that goes from pictorial/structural encoding to retrieval of biographical/emotional information (Bentin et al., 1996; Bruce & Young, 1986; Eimer, 2000a; Herrmann et al., 2005; Schweinberger, 2011). Imaging techniques, on their part, have helped identify the specific brain areas involved in face perception and recognition, including recognition of emotional expression and personal identity (Adolphs, 2002; Gobbini & Haxby, 2007; Zeki, 2007, Haxby & Gobbini, 2011). These brain areas constitute a distributed network with a core system responsible for the analysis of visual appearance (posterior superior temporal sulcus, inferior occipital and fusiform gyri), and an extended system that underlies the retrieval of person knowledge (medial prefrontal cortex, temporo-parietal junction, anterior temporal cortex, precuneus, and posterior cingulate), action understanding (inferior temporal and frontal operculum, and intraparietal sulcus), and emotion (amygdala, insula, and striatum/reward system).

In the context of this broad literature, a subset of studies has looked into the emotional processing associated with recognition of familiar loved faces (i.e., relatives, friends, own children, or romantic partner) by using electrophysiological or fMRI indices of brain activity (Aron et al., 2005; Baçar et al., 2008; Bartels & Zeki, 2000, 2004; Bobes et al., 2007; Fisher et al., 2005; Grasso et al., 2009; Grasso & Simons, 2011; Herzmann et al., 2004; Langeslag et al., 2007; Xu et al., 2011). A major shortcoming in this literature, besides the need to integrate it with research on the neural mechanisms of social and cultural cognition (Tomasello et al., 2005; Amodio & Frith, 2006; Herrmann et al., 2007), is the lack of evidence regarding the elicitation of a genuine positive emotional response to loved familiar faces. This is in part due to the presence of two significant confounding factors in most experimental studies: emotional arousal and familiarity.

Emotional arousal refers to the intensity of an emotion, regardless of its affective valence (positive or negative). Arousal-related ERP modulation is a robust phenomenon that primarily affects long-latency components (Oloffson et al., 2008). Those studies focusing on the modulation of brain responses (ERPs) associated with processing of loved familiar faces have consistently found enhanced P300 and Late Positive Potential (LPP) amplitudes when comparing loved familiar faces to control familiar (newly-learned) and neutral faces. However, similar amplitude increases have been reported in response to highly unpleasant stimuli such as mutilated faces or attacking animals, thus casting doubt on whether the larger late positivity evoked by loved faces reflects activation of positive emotional mechanisms or plain emotional arousal (Palomba et al., 1997; Cuthbert et al., 2000; Schupp et al., 2000, 2004; Sabatinelli et al., 2007; Bradley, 2009).

On its part, familiarity has been defined as a form of explicit or declarative memory (Gobbini & Haxby, 2007; Voss & Paller, 2006, 2007) that is affected by factors such as length of time spent with an individual, number of previous encounters, duration of the relationship, or information accumulated about that individual. Attempts to control for familiarity effects include viewing faces of acquaintances, famous people, or newly learned faces. However, familiarity of loved faces will always exceed that of control faces because of the amount of time spent with them (Grasso et al., 2009). Studies on ERP modulation associated with familiarity have consistently found increases in late positivities at posterior locations (Eimer, 2000a, b; Voss and Paller, 2006; Yovel and Paller, 2004). Interestingly, these same effects have been reported in studies of loved familiar faces (Bobes et al., 2007; Grasso et al., 2009; Herzmann et al., 2004; Langeslag et al., 2007).

Here we propose that studies on the processing of loved familiar faces would benefit from the use of those tools developed in the context of emotional processing research, with special emphasis on the potential contribution of electromyographic recordings.

The picture-viewing paradigm used by Lang and colleagues (Bradley & Lang, 2007; Codispoti, Bradley, & Lang, 2001; Lang, 1995; Lang & Davis, 2006; Lang, Davis, & Öhman, 2000) allows us to disentangle those effects attributable to picture valence (either positive or negative) from those elicited by emotional arousal (intensity of emotion, regardless of its affective valence). In this paradigm, a broad set of central and peripheral measures are simultaneously recorded while participants view pleasant, neutral, and unpleasant pictures taken from the International Affective Picture System (IAPS; Lang, Bradley, & Cuthbert, 2008), an instrument that provides normative ratings of valence, arousal, and dominance for each picture. Research conducted within this framework has consistently shown that highly pleasant pictures are associated with (a) a pattern of accelerative changes in the heart rate, (b) reduced eye-blink startle responses, (c) increases in zygomatic muscle activity, and (d) decreases in corrugator supercilii muscle activity. The inverse pattern is observed with highly arousing unpleasant pictures. Moreover, highly arousing pleasant and unpleasant pictures, when compared to neutral ones, provoke (a) increases in skin conductance, and (b) larger amplitudes for both P3 and LPP components obtained at central-parietal locations (Bradley et al., 2001; Lang & Bradley, 2010). Therefore, two different sets of measures can be identified: one that consistently responds to affective valence, and a second one that is most sensitive to variations in emotional arousal.

Both eye-blink startle and facial EMG have been extensively investigated in the context of emotional processing (see Bradley & Lang, 2007, for a review), and their ability to differentiate affective states has been repeatedly established. The startle reflex consists of a chain of extensor-flexor movements that spread throughout the body (Landis & Hunt, 1939) in response to intense and abrupt stimulation (i.e., an intense white noise). Rapid closing of the eyes constitutes one of the most stable components of this reflex in humans and it can be easily measured by placing electrodes over the orbicularis muscle under the eye. In studies of emotional modulation of the startle reflex using the picture-viewing paradigm, startle eye-blink is consistently potentiated when viewing highly arousing unpleasant pictures, and inhibited when facing highly arousing pleasant pictures, compared to neutral ones (Bradley & Lang, 2007). This valence-mediated effect has been interpreted in terms of the *motivational priming hypothesis* (Lang et al., 1997). According to this model, perceptual stimuli that engage the aversive motivational system potentiate the reflex, whereas those stimuli that engage the appetitive motivational system provoke startle inhibition. The same linear relationship between startle amplitude and affective valence is observed in a large variety of perceptual settings: using pictures (Bradley et al., 2001), films (Jansen & Fridja, 1994), sounds (Bradley & Lang, 2000), and odors (Miltner, 1994).

Facial EMG also provides reliable indices of affective engagement. Special attention has been given to the activation of the corrugator supercilii and zygomatic major muscles in different induction contexts, such as perception, anticipation, and imagery (Bradley & Lang, 2007). The corrugator supercilii muscles are located above and between the eyes and are responsible for drawing down the eyebrows. The zygomatic major muscles originate in the cheeks bones and exert their action by lifting the corner of the mouth obliquely and upwards. Activity in these two sets of muscles is associated with frowning and smiling, respectively.

Since the pioneering work of Schwartz and colleagues (Brown & Schwartz, 1980; Schwartz et al., 1976a, b) and until recently, corrugator supercilii and zygomatic major EMG have been often used to study emotional processing. Processing of unpleasant material elicits larger corrugator activity than neutral or pleasant stimuli (Bradley et al., 2001; Cacioppo et al., 1986; Lang et al., 1993; Larsen et al., 2003). Lang and colleagues (1993) found a linear relationship between activity of the corrugator muscle and the hedonic valence of the pictures, with unpleasant slides eliciting the largest contraction, and pleasant pictures causing inhibition of the corrugator muscles. This same linear gradation was obtained by Larsen, Norris, and Cacioppo (2003) in a study that measured facial EMG in response to three different kinds of stimuli: pictures, sounds, and words. When looking at corrugator activity as a function of emotional picture contents (Bradley et al., 2001), slides depicting mutilations and contamination-related scenes elicit the largest activity in this muscle compared to other unpleasant material.

The relationship between zygomatic activity and affective valence is somewhat more complex. Lang and colleagues (1993) obtained a quadratic relationship between emotional valence and zygomatic activity, with highly pleasant pictures eliciting the largest responses, when compared to either neutral or unpleasant material. However, significant zygomatic activation was also found for unpleasant pictures, compared to neutral stimuli. Larsen and colleagues (2003) confirmed this finding for emotional pictures and sounds, but not for affective words. Because the zygomatic major is involved in smiling and smiling has an unquestionable communicative function in humans, it has been argued that its activity is malleable according to rules of social display. Ekman, Davidson, and Friesen (1990), however, noted that a true smile (the so-called Duchenne smile) is accompanied by simultaneous activation of the zygomatic and orbicularis muscles, while social smiles devoid of positive emotion involve only zygomatic activity.

In this chapter, we summarize the results of three studies aimed at unraveling the mechanisms underlying the processing of loved familiar faces, while distinguishing the relative effects of affective valence, undifferentiated emotional arousal, and familiarity, with special emphasis on zygomatic and orbicularis activity. All three studies combine the following elements: (a) an experimental paradigm that allows differentiation of valence versus arousal effects, (b) simultaneous recording of a broad set of psychophysiological measures, and (c) different sets of stimuli that differ in valence, arousal, and familiarity ratings.

2. Methodology

2.1 Experiment 1

Experiment 1 was aimed at investigating the neurophysiological mechanisms associated with the affective processing of loved familiar faces by combining peripheral and central electrophysiological measures while separating the relative contributions of valence (i.e., positive vs. negative affect), arousal (i.e., more vs. less activation), and familiarity (i.e., known vs. unknown faces). Event-related potentials, skin conductance, heart rate, and electromyography of the *zygomatic major* muscle were obtained along with subjective ratings of valence, arousal, and dominance for each picture. Because of the scope of the present chapter, we will focus on the activity of the zygomatic muscle.

2.1.1 Participants

Thirty female undergraduate students, ranging between 20 and 27 years of age, took part in the study. Subjects were required to have a current romantic relationship (between 6 months and 6 years in duration) and to live in close proximity to five loved ones, including the partner, so as to be able to take their photographs. None of the participants reported current physical or psychological problems and none were under pharmacological treatment. All were right-handed and had normal or corrected to normal vision. All subjects signed informed consent forms and received course credit for their participation.

2.1.2 Materials and design

Participants viewed faces belonging to one of five categories in two separate blocks that differed in picture presentation rate and were administered in counterbalanced order. The slow block, whose results are presented here, consisted of an initial 5-min baseline period, followed by 50 trials with the following structure per trial: 4-sec baseline, 4-sec picture presentation, and 4-sec post-picture period. Inter-trial intervals (ITI) varied randomly between 8 and 12 seconds. The study included 5 photographs of faces in each of 5 categories: loved ones, neutral, unknown, famous, and baby faces. In addition to the partner, faces of loved ones could include parents, siblings, second-degree relatives, and friends. Neutral faces were selected from Ekman and Friesen's (1978) "Facial Action Coding System". Unknown faces were selected among the photographs of loved ones provided by some other participant, after ensuring that those pictures did not depict anyone known to that participant. Famous faces were selected by each participant prior to the experimental session, from a set of 9 photographs portraying people that frequented Spanish media. Participants were asked to identify famous people as such, and were expected not to feel strong attraction or rejection towards them. Finally, faces of babies were selected from the IAPS (Lang et al., 2008) among those with valence scores over 7 (rating scale ranging from 1 to 9) according to Spanish norms (Moltó et al., 1999; Vila et al., 2001). Pictures of loved ones were provided by each participant a few days before the experiment and after they had followed full detailed instructions on how to take the photographs (i.e., loved ones had to look straight at the camera with neutral expression in front of a light background). All pictures were edited using Corel-Draw Photopaint software (version 7). Photographs were matched in size, color, and background. All were cropped down to 650 x 650 pixels, transformed into gray scale (8 bits), and surrounded by a black background.

Each picture was presented twice following a double Latin Square design. The first Latin Square included a 5x5 matrix, where each row and each column contained only one picture belonging to the same category. The second Latin Square was an inverted mirror of the first one. Participants, in groups of 5, were randomly assigned to 5 different sequences (each of those starting with a different picture category) to ensure that all categories were equally distributed within the complete sample. In addition, 15 participants had the slow presentation block followed by the fast presentation block, while the other 15 participants had the inverse order.

Subjects were instructed to simply look at the pictures for the entire time they were on the screen, while trying to withhold from blinking or, if necessary, blinking during the ITI. After the second block, participants evaluated the valence, arousal, and dominance of each single picture according to the Self-Assessment Manikin (Bradley & Lang, 1994).

2.1.3 Apparatus

A Coulbourn polygraph, model V-Link, was used for the recording of zygomatic activity. Stimulus control and peripheral physiological data acquisition were accomplished using an IBM-compatible computer running VPM data acquisition and reduction software (Cook III, 1997). E-Prime software (Psychological Tools, Pittsburgh) controlled the actual presentation of the pictures using a second Pentium 4 computer connected to the master computer through the serial port. Finally, a digital camera, model Kodak Easy Share DX6490, was used to obtain the photographs of loved ones.

2.1.4 Zygomatic EMG recording

Zygomatic EMG activity was recorded using miniature In Vivo Metrics silver/silver chloride electrodes. The raw EMG was amplified by 5000 and band-pass filtered (90-1000 Hz) by means of a Coulbourn V75-04 bioamplifier. The signal was subsequently rectified and integrated using a Coulbourn V75-23A integrator. Time constant for zygomatic activity was 500 ms. The integrated EMG was sampled at 100 Hz and averaged every one half-second for the length of the trial. Each value was expressed in terms of differential scores with respect to the averaged EMG activity during the 4 sec preceding stimulus onset.

2.1.5 Statistical analysis

Zygomatic EMG data were averaged across trials within the same face category and order of block presentation, and analyzed by means of repeated measures ANOVA, using a 5 x 16 design, with the first factor being Face Category (Loved, Neutral, Unknown, Famous, and Babies faces), and the second factor being Time, expressed in 16 one half-second bins following stimulus onset. The Greenhouse-Geisser epsilon correction was applied to correct for sphericity. Analysis of significant interactions was performed identifying the levels of the interacting factors explaining the significant effects, followed by post-hoc pairwise comparisons using Bonferroni test.

2.1.6 Results

Figure 1 shows changes in zygomatic activity during face presentation when the slow block was presented in first and second place, respectively. Regardless of task order, only loved familiar faces evoked a clear response, starting right after stimulus onset and continuing until the end of the 8-sec recording period. Although less pronounced, a response can also be observed for baby faces. The ANOVA revealed significant effects of Face Category $(F(4,116)=9.74, p<0.002, \eta p^2=0.251)$, Time $(F(15, 435)=3.56, p<0.04, \eta p^2=0.109)$, and Face Category x Time $(F(60, 1740)=3.59, p<0.007, \eta p^2=0.110)$.

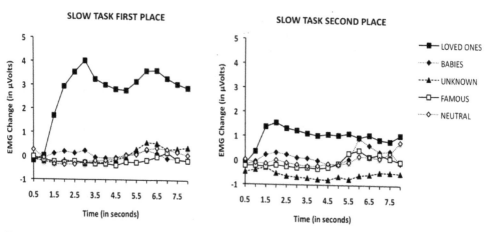

Fig. 1. Zygomatic activity across categories in the slow task as a function of task order.

Analysis of the Face Category x Time interaction yielded significant Face Category effects for all Time points from second 1.5 to second 8 (all p-values < 0.02). Except for seconds 6 and 6.5, loved familiar faces prompted a larger response than all other categories (all p-values < 0.04). Significant differences were also found between babies and neutral faces in seconds 2.5 and 3 (both p-values < 0.05). No differences were found between famous and unknown faces.

Figure 2 displays the average zygomatic response across the four subcategories of loved faces. Separate ANOVAs for each pair of subcategories yielded significant differences between partner and friend $(F(1, 18)=4.015, p<0.05, \eta p^2=0.157)$, though only in the first trial. Differences between partner and parent $(F(1, 21)=3.75, p<0.07, \eta p^2=0.160)$, and partner and sibling ($F(1,19)=3.346$, $p<0.08$, $\eta p^2=0.165$), also during the first trial, were marginally significant. No other significant differences were found.

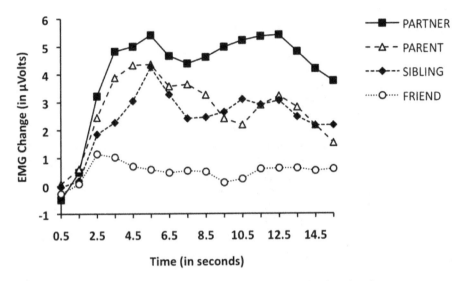

Fig. 2. Zygomatic activity as a function of subcategory of loved familiar faces.

2.2 Experiment 2

In Experiment 1, familiarity of the faces was indirectly controlled by comparing loved faces with famous faces and, additionally, by examining the responses to loved faces differing in their familiarity (partner, parents, friends, and siblings) among themselves. The findings of the experiment above suggest that familiarity is not a major determinant of the substantial zygomatic activity differences obtained in that study. However,, two problems affect the familiarity issue in Experiment 1: on the one hand, the degree of familiarity of loved faces and famous faces is not comparable, since the former will always exceed any other category; on the other hand, the first experiment did not equate subcategories of loved faces in number or order of presentation. In fact, of the 30 participants, 15 included both parents among the 5 loved faces; 6 included only the father, and 8 did not include any parent. Similarly uneven numbers were associated with the rest of loved familiar faces (siblings, second-degree relatives, and friends) freely chosen by participants.

In this second experiment, we examined psychophysiological responses in a design that controlled for familiarity differences among pictures and that included five different face categories: boyfriend, father, control-boyfriend, control-father, and baby faces.

2.2.1 Participants

Thirty-five female undergraduate students, ranging in age between 20-29 years, took part in this study. Inclusion criteria were the same as in Experiment 1. None of the participants reported current physical or psychological problems and none were under pharmacological treatment. All were right-handed and had normal or corrected-to-normal vision. All subjects signed informed consent forms and were given course credit for their participation.

2.2.2 Materials and design

Subjects viewed faces belonging to one of five categories in a passive picture viewing paradigm: boyfriend, father, control-boyfriend, control-father and baby. A few days before the experimental session, participants provided photographs of their boyfriend and their father according to detailed instructions provided by the experimenters (i.e., neutral expression, face looking straight at the camera, and subject standing in front of a light background). Control-boyfriend and control-father pictures were selected among the boyfriend and father photographs provided by other participants, once the experimenter ensured that the pictures did not depict someone known to the participant. The baby picture was selected from the IAPS (Lang et al., 2008) and had a valence score over 7 (rating scale from 1 to 9) according to the Spanish norms (Moltó et al., 1999; Vila et al, 2001). Pictures provided by participants were taken using a Nikon D-60 camera. All pictures were edited using Corel-Draw Photopaint software (version 7). All of them were matched in size, color, and background. All photographs had 650 x 650 pixels, were transformed to a gray scale (8 bits), and inserted into a circle surrounded by a black background. Pictures were presented by using Presentation software (Neurobehavioral Systems, CA) on a 19-in flat monitor located approximately 0.6 m from the participant.

Each picture was presented 20 times following a quadruple Latin Square design. The first Latin Square consisted of a 5x5 matrix that included one picture category in each row and each column. The rest of the Latin Squares were inverted mirrors of the first one. Five different sequences of pictures were created, each one starting with a different category, so as to be equally distributed within the 35 participants. Participants, in groups of five, were randomly assigned to one of the five sequences. After a 5-min baseline period, 100 picture trials were presented with the following structure per trial: 4-sec baseline, 4-sec picture presentation, and 4-sec additional recording period. The inter-trial interval varied randomly from 1 to 3 seconds (with an average of 2 sec). No recording was obtained during that period.

Participants were instructed to simply look at the pictures for the entire time they were projected on the screen.

2.2.3 Physiological measures

Zygomatic major EMG activity was obtained using miniature In Vivo Metrics silver/silver chloride electrodes. EMG activity was sampled at 100 Hz. The raw EMG signals were amplified by 5000 and band-pass filtered (13-1000 Hz) with a Coulbourn V75-04 bioamplifier. They were subsequently rectified and integrated using a Coulbourn V75-23A integrator. Time constant for zygomatic activity was 500 ms. Activity in the orbicularis muscle was recorded by placing two miniature In Vivo Metrics silver/silver chloride electrodes under the left eye. The raw EMG signal was amplified by 5000 and band-pass filtered (28-500 Hz) with a Coulburn V75-04 bioamplifier and a V75-48 High Performance Filter. Orbicularis EMG was subsequently integrated by a V75-23A integrator with a time-constant of 20 ms. Integrated EMG was recorded with a sampling rate of 100 Hz and averaged every one half-second during the period of face presentation. Subsequently, each value was expressed in terms of differential scores with respect to the averaged EMG during the 4 sec preceding stimulus onset.

Stimulus control and peripheral physiological data acquisition were accomplished using an IBM-compatible computer running VPM data acquisition and reduction software (Cook III, 1997).

2.2.4 Data reduction and analysis
Both zygomatic and orbicularis EMG data were averaged across trials within the same face category. Zygomatic activity was analyzed by repeated measures ANOVA using a 5x16 design, with the first factor being Category (boyfriend, father, control-boyfriend, control-father, and baby), and the second factor being Time (the 16 one half-second bins following picture onset). Post-hoc pairwise comparisons were performed using the same procedure than in the previous study. For correlation analysis between zygomatic and orbicularis EMG, the maximum amplitude values during the whole period of picture presentation were obtained across categories and the Pearson bivariate correlation calculated.

2.2.5 Results
Figure 3 shows changes in zygomatic activity for each of the 5 face categories. Only boyfriend and father pictures prompted visible responses starting right after stimulus onset. In addition, the face of the romantic partner elicited a larger response compared to the face of the father.

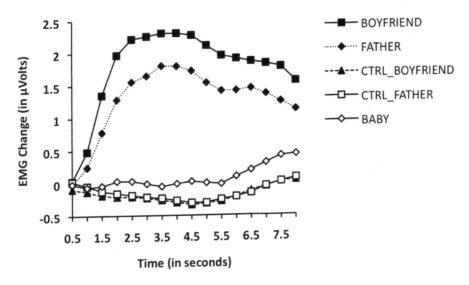

Fig. 3. Zygomatic activity across categories in study 2.

The ANOVA results yielded significant effects for Category ($F_{(4,136)}$ = 12.825, $p < 0.0001$, ηp^2 = 0.274), Time (15,510) = 4.889, $p < 0.017$, ηp^2 = 0.126), and Category x Time ($F_{(60,2040)}$ = 7.307, $p < 0.001$, ηp^2 = 0.177). Planned comparisons revealed the following results: (a) loved faces produced a significantly larger EMG response than control ($p < 0.001$) and baby ($p < 0.001$) faces, and (b) the face of the boyfriend produced a significantly larger EMG response than the different of the father ($p < 0.02$).
Significant positive correlations were found between the zygomatic and orbicularis muscle activity evoked by loved familiar faces, but not by unknown or baby faces (see Figure 4), thus suggesting that the Duchenne smile effect was present in these data.

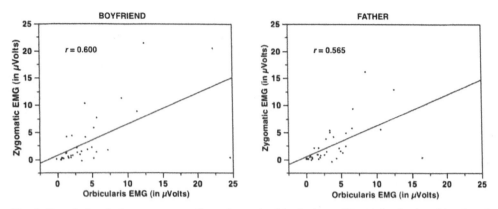

Fig. 4. Correlation between zygomatic major and orbicularis oculii activity for boyfriend and father faces.

2.3 Experiment 3

Experiments 1 and 2 have shown that processing of loved familiar faces elicits a pattern of responses that are indicative of a positive emotional state. Further evidence supporting the view that loved familiar faces engage the appetitive motivational system would be available if the same loved familiar faces proved to be efficient inhibitors of some defensive response (e.g., the startle reflex). Consequently, this third experiment was conducted to explore whether faces perceived as highly positive (i.e., loved familiar faces) were able to inhibit the startle reflex when compared to either neutral (i.e., unknown) or unpleasant (i.e., mutilated) faces. Additionally, Experiment 3 was designed so as to replicate previous findings regarding central and peripheral physiological reactions to loved familiar faces

2.3.1 Participants

Forty-two undergraduate students (12 males) participated in this experiment. Inclusion criteria were the same as in Experiments 1 and 2. None of the participants reported current physical or psychological problems and none were under pharmacological treatment. All were right-handed and had normal or corrected-to-normal vision. All subjects signed informed consent forms and received course credit for their participation

2.3.2 Materials and design

Participants viewed faces in a passive picture viewing paradigm, which belonged to three face categories: loved familiar faces (partner, father, mother, and best-friend), neutral faces (control-boyfriend, control-father, control-mother, and control-best-friend), and unpleasant faces[1]: This latter category included pictures from the IAPS (Lang, Bradley, & Cuthbert, 2008) that were present in the Spanish normative ratings (Moltó et al., 1999; Vila et al., 2001). The participants provided photographs of loved familiar persons a few days before the experiment and according to full detailed instructions on how to take the photographs (i.e.,

---

[1] International codes for unpleasant pictures were: 3000, 3051, 3060, and 3080)

pictures could not be taken by the participant him/herself, and people in the pictures should look straight at the camera with a neutral expression in front of a light background). Neutral pictures were selected among the loved familiar pictures provided by other participants after ensuring those pictures did not depict anyone known to that participant. Photographs of loved familiar persons were taken using a Nikon D-3000 camera. All pictures were edited using Corel Draw Photopaint (version 7). They were matched in size, color, and background. All photographs were cropped to 650 x 650 pixels, transformed to a gray scale (8 bits), and inserted into a circle surrounded by a black background. Pictures were presented using Presentation Software (Neurobehavioral Systems, CA) on a 19-in flat monitor located at approximately 60 cm from the participant.

Participants were randomly assigned to 6 different picture-presentation sequences that were created following a set of eight 3x3 Latin Squares. In each of those 3x3 matrices, one out of the four pictures included in each category was discarded so that, in total, each picture was presented 6 times during the whole task. To control for order effects, each sequence started with a different category.

The task started with a 5-min baseline period, followed by 72 trials with the following structure per trial: 4-sec baseline, 6-sec picture presentation, and 4-sec post-picture interval. Two-thirds of the pictures (48) were presented together with a startle probe (a burst of white noise at 105dBs, 50-ms duration and nearly instantaneous rise time) at 4, 4.5, 5, or 5.5 sec after picture onset. The same number of startle probes was assigned to each picture (n=4). In addition, 8 startle probes were delivered during the inter-trial interval in order to minimize noise predictability. The inter-trial interval varied randomly between 2 and 4 sec (with an average of 3 sec). Throughout the whole task a fixation point was presented in the centre of the screen to minimize eye movements. Participants were instructed to simply look at the pictures for the entire time they were on the screen.

2.3.2 Physiological measures

Zygomatic and orbicularis EMG activity were both measured using miniature silver chloride electrodes, and acquired using two Coulbourn V75-04 bioamplifiers. Band-pass filter settings for zygomatic and orbicularis raw signals were 13-1000 Hz, and 28-500 Hz, respectively. Both signals were amplified by 5000 and then rectified and integrated using a Coulbourn V76-24 integrator. Time constants for zygomatic and orbicularis muscles were 500 and 20 ms, respectively. Both raw signals were acquired at a sampling rate of 100 Hz during baseline with an increase in sampling rate for orbicularis muscle activity to 1000 Hz from 500 ms before the onset of the startle probe up to 500 ms after probe onset.

2.3.3 Data reduction and analysis

Zygomatic EMG activity was determined by subtracting the activity in the 3 sec before picture onset from that occurring at each half-second after picture presentation. Amplitude of the startle reflex was defined as the difference in microvolts between the peak and the onset of the orbicularis muscle response in a time window between 20 and 120 ms after stimulus onset, computed following the algorithm described by Balaban et al. (1986). To control for between-subject variability, startle magnitudes for each subject were converted to t scores.

Zygomatic activity was analyzed by repeated measures ANOVA using a 3x12 design with the first factor being Category (loved familiar faces, unknown faces, and unpleasant faces) and the second factor being Time (the 12 half-second² increments following stimulus onset). Startle reflex magnitude was analyzed using repeated measures ANOVA with Face Category as single factor.

Finally, correlational analysis between zygomatic and orbicularis muscle activity was conducted as in the previous study, except that the maximum amplitude values were obtained during the first 4 seconds of picture presentation in order to avoid orbicularis EMG contamination by the startle probe.

2.3.4 Results

As can be observed in Figure 5, loved familiar faces prompted a clear zygomatic response, starting right after picture presentation and continuing until the end of the picture-presentation interval. No activation of the zygomatic muscle was observed for all other picture categories.

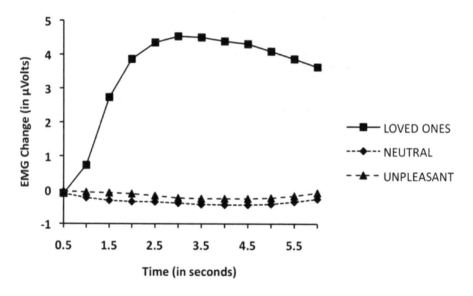

Fig. 5. Zygomatic activity response across face category.

The ANOVA yielded significant effects for Face Category ($F_{(2,82)}$ = 16.629, p <0.001, ηp^2 = 0.289), Time ($F_{(11,451)}$ = 13.065, p <0.001, ηp^2 = 0.242), and Face Category x Time ($F_{(22,902)}$ = 15.594, p <0.001, ηp^2 = 0.276).

Analysis of the Face Category x Time interaction revealed significant Face Category effects for all Time points from the second 1.5 to the end of the picture presentation. At all these Time points, loved familiar faces differed significantly from all others (all p-values <0.007). No significant effects were found between neutral and unpleasant faces at any Time point.

The correlational analysis revealed a significant positive covariation between zygomatic and orbicularis EMG only for loved familiar faces, as can be seen in Figure 6.

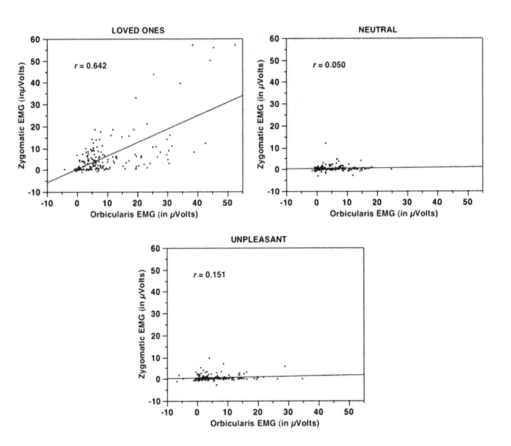

Fig. 6. Correlation between zygomatic major and orbicularis oculii across face category.

Finally, a clear modulation of the startle response was observed: loved familiar faces inhibited the startle response whereas mutilated faces potentiated the startle response, compared to neutral (unknown) faces, as can be seen in Figure 7. The ANOVA results yielded a significant main effect of Face Category ($F(2,82) = 25.135$, p <0.0001, $\eta p^2 = 0.380$). Planned comparisons revealed significant differences (a) between loved familiar and neutral faces ((p<0.01)), (b) between neutral and unpleasant faces (p<0.002), and (c) between loved familiar and unpleasant faces (p<0.0001).

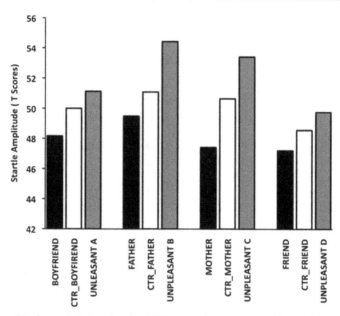

Fig. 7. Startle eyblink modulation for the different subcategories of loved familiar faces.

3. Discussion

The results of the three studies highlight the relevance of including electromyographic measures to advance knowledge on the psychological and physiological mechanisms underlying the affective processing of faces associated with identity recognition. The three studies were highly consistent in showing a large zygomatic major response to faces of loved ones, a response that starts around one second after picture onset and lasts for several seconds after picture offset. This response was totally absent or greatly diminished to all other categories of faces used as control in our three studies: unknown, famous, baby, neutral, and unpleasant faces. In all cases, the faces were photographs in black and white and with no emotional expression. Moreover, in the three studies, loved and unknown faces were physically identical since they were interchangeable across participants, guaranteeing that the observed differences among faces in physiology and subjective ratings were due to identity recognition and not to differences in emotional expression or physical features of the faces.

The sequence of the three studies was also highly consistent in confirming that the processing of loved familiar faces involves activation of an intense positive emotional response that cannot be explained by undifferentiated emotional arousal or familiarity. In the first study, the arousal effect was controlled by simultaneously recording heart rate and skin conductance. In the context of Lang's picture-viewing paradigm (Bradley & Lang, 2007), heart rate is an unambiguous index of emotional valence (positive versus negative emotion), whereas skin conductance is an index of emotional arousal (the intensity of the emotion, regardless of its positive or negative valence). Both indices confirmed that the zygomatic response to the loved faces was reflecting the presence of an intense positive emotional response. In this study, the familiarity effect was indirectly controlled by comparing famous versus unknown faces, as well as loved faces with different levels of familiarity among themselves. No differences were found between famous and unknown faces, and the few differences found among loved faces were contrary to the familiarity explanation: larger responses to the less familiar (partner) than to the more familiar (parent and siblings) faces.

In the second and third study, the confounding arousal and familiarity effects were further controlled by including a second electromyographic measure (the orbicularis muscle activity) and by using an experimental design that better controlled for familiarity. The simultaneous recording of the zygomatic and orbicularis muscles provides two additional specific indices of emotional valence: the Duchenne smile and the eye-blink startle response. As mentioned in the introduction, the Duchenne or true smile is characterized by simultaneous activation of the zygomatic and orbicularis muscles, whereas social smile devoid of positive emotion involves only zygomatic activation (Ekman et al., 1980). The significant correlation found between zygomatic and orbicularis muscle activity only for loved faces in our second and third study is another piece of evidence supporting the conclusion that viewing faces of loved ones induces a feeling of genuine positive affect that cannot be explained in terms of arousal or familiarity.

On the other hand, the eye-blink startle response is perhaps the most robust physiological response showing emotional modulation by affective valence. Numerous studies (see Bradley & Lang, 2007, for a review) have consistently demonstrated that viewing highly pleasant pictures (e.g., erotica or sport images) reduces the magnitude of the eye-blink startle response, whereas viewing highly unpleasant pictures (e.g., mutilation or threatening images) increases its magnitude, compared to neutral pictures (e.g., household objects or non-emotional faces). In these studies, however, the startle magnitude while viewing neutral pictures not always occupies an intermediate position with significant differences with respect to both pleasant and unpleasant images. The results of our third study, showing significant differences between our three categories of faces (loved, neutral, and unpleasant), are not only an independent confirmation of Lang's *motivational priming hypothesis* (startle inhibition during activation of the appetitive motivational system by pleasant pictures and startle potentiation during activation of the aversive motivational system by unpleasant pictures, compared to neutral ones). They are also an unambiguous demonstration that viewing loved familiar faces induces an intense positive emotion capable of inhibiting defensive reflexes.

The electromyographic results of our second and third study also contribute to disentangle the confounding effects of familiarity in the processing of loved familiar faces. The control of familiarity has always been a major methodological problem in this type of studies. Although difficult to separate, emotional valence and familiarity are not inevitably confounded. In studies using the picture-viewing paradigm with pleasant, neutral, and unpleasant pictures from the IAPS, the enhanced zygomatic response while viewing pleasant pictures has been interpreted in terms of positive affect, rather than familiarity, since all pictures are new and there is no explicit memory involvement. But in studies on loved familiar faces, familiarity is necessarily confounded with emotion, since both memory and emotion are involved in their processing. Our second and third study controlled for familiarity by comparing the face of the romantic partner (with less than 6 years relationship) with the face of the parent of same sex (with more than 18 years relationship). Therefore, two categories of loved familiar faces, differing in amount of familiarity, were compared. Both studies (although the details of the third one are not reported here) replicated the results of the first study revealing larger zygomatic responses to the less familiar face (i.e., the romantic partner) than to the more familiar face (i.e., the parent), thus disconfirming the familiarity hypothesis.

It should be noted, however, that the three studies reported here not only recorded EMG responses. A broad set of autonomic (heart rate and skin conductance), electromyographic (zygomatic and orbicularis muscle activity), and brain (N100, P200, P3, and LPP) responses was recorded, in addition to subjective indices of valence, arousal, and dominance, the three general dimensions of emotional reactions (see Osgood, Suci & Tannenbaum, 1957; Mehrabian & Russel, 1974; Bradley & Lang, 2007). The results of the three studies revealed a very consistent pattern of physiological and subjective responses to loved familiar faces: (a) increases in heart rate, skin conductance, zygomatic activity, and the event-related potentials P3, and LPP; (b) decreases in eye-blink startle magnitude and the event-related potential N200; and (c) higher ratings of positive valence and arousal, but lower ratings of dominance. This set of physiological and subjective responses suggests that the processing of loved familiar faces involves a complex pattern of psychophysiological mechanisms that single physiological measures, whether central or peripheral, would fail to capture accurately. The use of both central and peripheral measures to investigate the affective processing of familiar faces contrasts with the dominant trend in current cognitive and affective neuroscience, almost limited to central physiological measures (EEG, ERP, MEG, PET, or fMRI). In the context of studies on emotional processing, the neglect of peripheral physiological measures, such as facial EMG or heart rate, has the shortcoming of not providing unambiguous evidence of the type of response being elicited, confounding emotional valence, undifferentiated emotional arousal, and familiarity.

But the shortcoming of a neuroscience approach that ignores peripheral physiological measures has much wider implications. It assumes a model of brain function apparently unrelated to efferent motor components. As Robert Sperry emphasized in 1952, the human brain primarily evolved not to contemplate and understand the world but to facilitate behavioral adaptation: *The primary function of the brain is essentially the transformation of sensory patterns into patterns of motor coordination* (Sperry, 1952, p. 297)... *Cerebration, essentially, serves to bring into motor behavior additional refinement, increased direction toward distant, future goals, and greater over-all adaptiveness and survival value. The evolutionary increase in man's capacity for perception, feeling, ideation, imagination, and the like, may be regarded, not so much as an end in itself, but as something that has enabled us to behave, to act, more wisely and efficiently* (Sperry, 1952, p. 299). Sperry's neuroscience approach implies that mental and motor processes are intimately associated and that research on brain mechanisms of psychological processes should integrate both central and peripheral physiological measures.

This approach not only has distinguished roots in early behaviorism and motor theory of thought and emotion (Watson, 1913; Washburn, 1928; Jacobson, 1929). It also has relevant defendants among more recent psychophysiologists and cognitive neuroscientists. McGuigan published in 1978 a book entitled *Cognitive Psychophysiology: Principles of covert behavior* gathering together a bulk of experimental studies showing the close covariation between electromyographical measures at different muscle locations and numerous cognitive processes. Based on these data, he suggested that all brain circuits are basically neuromuscular circuits, a proposal not too different from Sperry's ideas on mind-body interactions. More recent developments within cognitive and affective neuroscience are also beginning to suggest the need to integrate brain and bodily responses in order to fully comprehend the brain mechanisms underlying psychological processes. The embodied cognition (Lenggenhager et al., 2006; De Vega, Glenberg & Graesser, 2008; Niedenthal et al., 2009) and social cognition (Tomasello et al., 2005; Amodio & Frith, 2006; Herrmann et al., 2007; Losin et al., 2010) groups are perhaps the most relevant cognitive movements of this new approach within neuroscience research. The basic idea of both movements is that bodily responses and affective social interactions are integral part of our cognitive representations in the brain and that both, central and peripheral responses, play a crucial role in successful behavioral adaptation and survival.

In summary, the present chapter summarizes a set of three studies aimed at investigating the affective processing of loved familiar faces using a set of central and peripheral physiological measures, including electromyographic recordings of the zygomatic major and orbicularis oculii muscle, in the context of Lang's picture-viewing paradigm. The results of the three studies support the conclusion that viewing the faces of familiar loved ones elicits an intense positive emotional reaction that cannot be explained either by familiarity or arousal alone. The three studies highlight the relevance of integrating central and peripheral measures to advance knowledge on the brain mechanisms underlying affective processing.

4. Ackowledgements

This research was supported by a grant from the Junta de Andalucía (Project P07-SEJ-02964).

5. References

Adolphs, R. (2009). The social brain: neural basis of social knowledge. *Annual Review of Psychology*, Vol. 60, (September 2008), pp. 693–716, ISSN: 0066-4308.

Adolphs, R. (2002). Neural systems for recognizing emotion. *Current Opinion in Neurobiology*, Vol. 12, No. 2, (April 2002), pp. 169-177, ISSN: 0959-4388

Amodio, D.M., & Frith, C.D. (2006). Meeting minds: The medial frontal cortex and social cognition. Nature Reviews/Neuroscience, Vol. 7, (April 2006), pp. 268-277, ISSN: 1471-003X.

Aron, A., Fisher, H., Mashek, D.J., Strong, G., Li, H., & Brown, L.L. (2005). Reward, motivation, and emotion systems associated with early-stage intense romantic love. *Journal of Neurophysiology*, Vol. 94, No. 1, (March 2005), pp. 327-337, ISSN: 0022-3077.

Baçar, E., Schmiedt-Fehr, C., Örniz, A., & Baçar-Eroglu, C. (2008). Brain oscillations evoked by face of a loved person. *Brain Research*, Vol. 1214, (June 2008), pp. 105-115, ISSN: 00068993.

Balaban, M.T., Losito, B.D., Simons, R.F., & Graham, F.K. (1986). Off-line latency and amplitude scoring of the human reflex eye blink with Fortran IV. Psychophysiology, 23, 612.

Bartels, A. & Zeki, S. (2000). The neural basis of romantic love. *NeuroReport,* Vol. 11, No. 17, (November 2000), pp. 3829-2834, ISSN: 0959-4965.

Bartels, A. & Zeki, S. (2004). The neural correlates of maternal and romantic love. *NeuroImage*, Vol. 21, No. 3, (March 2004), pp. 1155-1166, ISSN: 10538119.

Bentin, S., Allison, T., Puce, A., Perez, E., McCarthy, G., 1996. Electrophysiological studies of face perception in humans. *Journal of Cognitive Neuroscience*, Vol. 8, No. 6, (November 1996), pp. 551–565, ISSN: 0898-929X.

Bobes, M.A., Quiñonez, I., Perez, J., Leon, I., & Valdés-Sosa, M. (2007). Brain potentials reflect access to visual and emotional memories for faces. *Biological Psychology*, Vol. 75, No. 2, (May 2007), pp. 146-153, ISSN: 0301-0511.

Bradley, M.M., & Lang, P.J. (2007). Emotion and Motivation. In: *Handbook of Psychophysiology, Third Edition*, John T. Cacioppo, Louis G. Tassinary, & Gary Berntson, pp. 581-607.

Bradley, M.M. (2009). Natural selective attention: orienting and emotion. *Psychophysiology*, Vol. 46, No. 1, (January 2009), pp. 1–11, ISSN: 0048-5772.

Bradley, M.M., Codispoti, M., Cuthbert, B.N., Lang, P.J. (2001). Emotion and motivation I: defensive and appetitive reactions in picture processing. *Emotion*, Vol 1, No. 3, (September 2001), pp. 276–298, ISSN: 1528-3542.

Bradley, M.M., Lang, P.J. (2000.) Measuring emotion. behavior, feeling, and physiology. In: Lane, R.D., Nadel, L. (Eds.), *Cognitive Neuroscience of Emotion*. Oxford University Press, New York, pp. 242– 276.

Brown, S. L., & Schwartz, G. E. (1980). Relationships between facial electromyography and subjective experience during affective imagery. *Biological Psychology*, Vol. 11, No. 1, (August 1980), pp. 49–62, ISSN: 0301-0511.

Bruce, V., & Young, A. (1986). Understanding face recognition. *British Journal of Psychology*, Vol. 77, No. 3, (August, 1986), pp. 305-327, ISSN: 2044-8295.

Cacioppo, J. T., Petty, R. E., Losch, M. E., & Kim, H. S. (1986). Electromyographic activity over facial muscle regions can differentiate the valence and intensity of affective reactions. *Journal of Personality and Social Psychology*, Vol. 50, No. 2, (February 1986), pp. 260–268, ISSN: 0022-3514.

Codispoti, M., Bradley, M.M., Lang, P.J., 2001. Affective reactions to briefly presented pictures. *Psychophysiology*, Vol. 38, No. 3, (April 2001), pp. 474–478, ISSN: 0048-5772.

Cook III, E.W. (1997). VPM Reference Manual [Computer Software]. Author, Birmingham, Alabama.

Cuthbert, B. N., Schupp, H. T., Bradley, M. M., Birbaumer, N., & Lang, P. J. (2000). Brain potentials in affective picture processing: Covariation with autonomic arousal and affective report. *Biological Psychology*, Vol. 52, No. 2, (March 2000),pp. 95-111, ISSN: 0301-0511.

Dekowska, M., Kuniecki, M., & Jaskowski, P. (2008). Facing facts: Neuronal mechanisms of face perception. *Acta Neurobiologiae Experimentalis*, Vol. 68, No. 2, pp. 229-252.

De Vega, M., Glenberg, A.M., & Graesser, A.C. (2008). *Symbols and embodiment: debates on meaning and cognition*. Oxford University Press: New York.

Dimberg, U. (1997). Psychophysiological reactions to facial expressions. In U. Segerstrale and P. Molnar (Eds.), *Nonverbal communication: Where nature meets culture* (pp.27-60). Mahwah, NJ: Erlbaum.

Eimer, H., & Holmes, A. (2007). Event-related potential correlates of emotional face processing. *Neuropsychologia*, Vol. 45, No. 1, pp. 15-31, ISSN: 0028-3932.

Eimer, M. (2000a). Event-related brain potentials distinguish processing stages involved in face perception and recognition. *Clinical Neurophysiology*, Vol. 111, No. 4, (April 2000), pp. 694–705, ISSN: 1388-2457.

Eimer, M. (2000b). Effects of face inversion on the structural encoding and recognition of faces: evidence from event-related brain potentials. *Cognitive Brain Research*, Vol. 10, No. 1-2, (September 2000), pp. 145–158, ISSN: 0926-6410.

Ekman, P. (1980). Face of man: Universal expression in a New Guinea village. New York: Garland.

Ekman, P. (1992). Facial expression and emotion. *American Psychologist*, Vol. 48, No. 4, (April 1992), pp. 376-379, ISSN: 0003-066X.

Ekman, P., Davidson, R. J., Friesen, W. V. (1990). The Duchenne smile: Emotional expression and brain physiology II. *Journal of Personality & Social Psychology*, Vol. 58, No. 2, (February 1990), pp. 342-353, ISSN: 0022-3514.

Fairhall, S.L., & Ishai, A.(2007). Effective connectivity within the distributed cortical network for face perception. Cerebral Cortex, Vol. 17, No. 10, (December 2006), pp. 2400-2406, ISSN: 1047-3211.

Fisher, H., Aron, A., & Brown, L.L. (2005). Romantic love: An fMRI study of a neural mechanism for mate choice. *The Journal of Comparative Neurology*, Vol. 493, No. 1, (December 2005), pp. 58-62, ISSN: 1096-9861.

Gobbini, M.I., & Haxby, J.V. (2007). Neural systems for recognition of familiar faces. *Neuropsychologia*, Vol. 45, No. 1, 32-41, ISSN: 0028-3932.

Grasso, D.J., & Simons, R.F. (2011). Perceived parental support predicts enhanced late positive event-related brain potentials to parent faces. *Biological Psychology*, Vol. 86, No. 1, (January 2011), pp. 26-30, ISSN: 0301-0511.

Grasso, D.J., Moser, J.S., Dozier, M., & Simons, R. (2009). ERP correlates of attention allocation in mothers processing faces of their children. *Biological Psychology*, Vol. 81, No. 2, (May 2009), pp. 95-102, ISSN: 0301-0511.

Haxby, J.V., & Gobbini, M.I. (2011). Distributed Neural Systems for Face Perception. In: *The Oxford Handbook of Face Perception*, Andrew J. Calder, Gillian Rhodes, Mark H. Johnson, & James Haxby, pp. 93-110, Oxford University Press, New York.

Herrmann, E., Call, J., Hernández_Lloreda, M.V., Hare, B., & Tomasello, M. (2007). Humans have evolved specialized skills of social cognition: The cultural intelligence hypothesis. *Science*, Vol. 317, No. 5843, (September 2007), pp. 1360-1366, ISSN: 0036-8075.

Herrmann, M.J., Ehlis, A.C., Ellgrin, H., & Fallgatter, A.J. (2005). Early stages (P100) of face perception as measured with event-related potentials (ERPs). *Journal of Neural Transmission*, Vol. 112, No. 8, (December 2004), pp. 1073-1081, ISSN: 0300-9564.

Herzmann, G.H., Schweinberger, S.R., Sommer, W., & Jentzsch, I. (2004). What's special about personally familiar faces? A multimodal approach. *Psychophysiology*, Vol. 41, No. 5, (September 2004), pp. 688-701, ISSN: 0048-5772.

Izard, C. (1971). *The face or emotion*. New York: Appleton-Century-Crofts.

Izard, C. (1977). *Human emotions*. New York: Plenum Press.

Izard, C. (1994). Innate and universal facial expressions: Evidence from developmental and cross-cultural research. *Psychological Bulletin*, Vol. 115, No. 2, (March 1994), pp. 288-299, ISSN: 0033-2909.

Jacobson, E. (1929). *Progressive Relaxation*. Oxford, England: University of Chicago Press.

Jansen, D.M., Fridja, N.H. (1994). Modulation of the acoustic startle response by film-induced fear and sexual arousal. *Psychophysiology*, Vol. 31, No. 6, (November 1994), pp. 565- 571, ISSN: 0048-5772.

Lang, P. J., Greenwald, M. K., Bradley, M. M., & Hamm, A. O. (1993). Looking at pictures: Affective, facial, visceral, and behavioral reactions. *Psychophysiology*, Vol. 30, No. 3, (May 1993), pp. 261-273, ISSN: 0048-5772.

Lang, P.J. (1995): The emotion probe: Studies of motivation and attention. *American Psychologist*, Vol. 50, No. 5, (May 1995), pp. 372-385, ISSN: 0003-066X.

Lang, P.J., & Bradley, M.M. (2010). Emotion and the motivational brain. *Biological Psychology*, Vol. 84, No. 3, (July 2010), pp. 437-450, ISSN: 0301-0511.

Lang, P.J., Bradley, M.M., & Cuthbert, B.N. (2008). *International affective picture system (IAPS): Affective ratings of pictures and instruction manual. Technical Report A-8*. University of Florida, Gainesville, FL.

Lang, P.J., Davis, M., 2006. Emotion, motivation, and the brain: reflex foundations in animal and human research. *Progress in Brain Research*, Vol. 156, pp. 3–29.

Lang, P.J., Davis, M., Öhman, A., 2000. Fear and anxiety. Animal models and human cognitive psychophysiology. *Journal of Affective Disorders*, Vol. 61, No. 3, (December 2000), pp. 137–159, ISSN: 0165-0327.

Lang, P.J.,Bradley,M.M.,&Cuthbert,B.N.(1997).Motivated attention: Affect, activation and action. In P.J.Lang, R.F.Simons, & M.T.Balaban (Eds.), Attention and orienting: Sensory and motivational processes. Hillsdale, NJ: Lawrence Erlbaum Associates, Inc.

Langeslag, S.J.E., Hansma, B.M., Franken, I.H.A. & Strien, J.W.V. (2007). Event-related potential responses to love-related facial stimuli. *Biological Psychology*, Vol. 76, No. 1-2, (September 2007), pp. 109-115, ISSN: 0301-0511.

Larsen, J.T., Norris, C.J., & Cacioppo, J.T. (2003). Effects of positive and negative affect on electromyographic activity over zygomaticus major and corrugator supercilii. *Psychophsysiology*, Vol. 40, No. 5, (September 2003), pp. 776-785, ISSN: 0048-5772.

Lenggenhager, B., Smith, S.T., & Blanke, O. (2006). Functional and Neural Mechanisms of Embodiment: Importance of the Vestibular System and the Temporal Parietal Junction. *Reviews in Neurosciences*, Vol. 17, No. 6, pp. 643-657, ISSN: 0306-4522.

Li, H., Chan, R.C.K., McAlonan, G.M., & Gong, Q. (2010). Facial emotion processing in schizophrenia: A meta-analysis of functional neuroimaging data. *Schizophrenia Bulletin*, Vol. 36, No. 5, pp. 1029-1039, ISSN: 745-1701.

Mehrabian, A., & Russell, J.A. (1974). *An approach to environmental psychology*. Cambridge, MA: M.I.T. Press.

Losin, E.A., Dapretto, M., & Iacobini, M. (2010). Culture and neuroscience: additive or synergistic? *Social Cognitive & Affective Neuroscience*, Vol. 5, No. 2-3, (January 2010), pp. 148-158, ISSN: 1749-5016.

McGuigan, F.J. (1978).*Cognitive psychophysiology: Principles of covert behavior*. Englewood Cliffs. NJ: Prentice-Hall.

Miltner, W. (1994). Emotional qualities of odors and their influence on the startle reflex in humans. *Psychophysiology*, Vol. 31, No. 1, (January 1994), 107– 110, ISSN: 0048-5772.

Niedenthal, P. M., Winkielman, P., Mondillon, L., Vermeulen, N. (2009). Embodiment of emotion concepts. *Journal of Personality and Social Psychology*, Vol 96, No. 6, (Jun 2009), pp. 1120-1136, ISSN: 0022-3514.

Öhman, A., Lundqvist, D., & Esteves, F. (2001). The face in the crowd: A threat advantage with schematic stimuli. *Journal of Personality and Social Psychology*, Vol. 80, No. 3, (March 2001), pp. 381-396, ISSN: 0022-3514.

Oloffson, J.K., Nordin, S., Sequeira, H., & Polich, J. (2008). Affective picture processing: An integrative review of ERP findings. *Biological Psychology*, Vol. 77, No. 3, (March 2008), pp. 247-265, ISSN: 0301-0511.

Osgood, C.E., Suci, G., & Tannenbaum, P. (1957) *The measurement of meaning.* Urbana, IL: University of Illinois Press.

Palomba, D., Angrilli, A., & Mini, A. (1997). Visual evoked potentials, heart rate responses and memory for emotional pictorial stimuli. *International Journal of Psychophysiology,* Vol. 27, No. 1, (July 1997), pp. 55-67, ISSN: 0167-8760.

Russell, J.A. (1994). Is there universal recognition of emotion from facial expression? A review of the cross-cultural studies. *Psychological Bulletin,* Vol. 115, No. 1, (January 1994), pp. 102-141, ISSN: 0033-2909.

Sabatinelli, D., Lang, P.J., Keil, A., & Bradley, M.M. (2007). Emotional perception: correlation of functional MRI and event related potentials. *Cerebral Cortex,* Vol. 17, No. 5, pp. 1085-1091, ISSN: 1047-3211.

Schupp, H.T., Cuthbert, B.N., Bradley, M.M., Cacioppo, J.T., Ito, T., & Lang, P.J. (2000). Affective picture processing: The late positive potential is modulated by motivational relevance. *Psychophysiology,* Vol. 37, No. 2, (March 2000), pp. 257-261, ISSN: 0048-5772.

Schupp, H.T., Junghöfer, M., Weike, A.I., & Hamm, A.O. (2004). The selective processing of briefly presented affective pictures: An ERP analysis. *Psychophysiology,* Vol. 41, No. 3, (May 2004), pp. 441-449, ISSN: 0048-5772.

Schwartz, G. E., Fair, P. L., Salt, P., Mandel, M. R., & Klerman, G. L. (1976a). Facial muscle patterning to affective imagery in depressed and nondepressed subjects. *Science,* Vol. 192, No. 4238, (April 1976), pp. 489–491, ISSN: 0036-8075.

Schwartz, G. E., Fair, P. L., Salt, P., Mandel, M. R., & Klerman, G. L. (1976b). Facial expression and imagery in depression: An electromyographic study. *Psychosomatic Medicine,* Vol. 38, No. 5, (September 1976), pp. 337-347, ISSN: 0033-3174.

Schweinberger, S.R. (2011). Neurophysiological correlates of Face Recognition. In: *The Oxford Handbook of Face Perception,* Andrew J. Calder, Gillian Rhodes, Mark H. Johnson, & James Haxby, pp. 345-366, Oxford University Press, New York.

Sperry, R.W. (1952). Neurology and the mind-brain problem. *American Scientist,* 40, No. 2, (April 1952), pp. 291-312, ISSN: 0003-0996.

Tomasello, M., Carpenter, M., Call, J., Behne, T., & Moll, H. (2005). Understanding and sharing intentions: The origins of cultural cognition. *Behavioral and Brain Sciences,* Vol. 28, No. 5, pp. 675-735, ISSN: 0140-525X.

Tomkins, S.S. (1962). *Affect, imagery and consciousness: Vol. I. The positive affects.* New York: Springer.

Voss, J.L., & Paller, K.A. (2006). Fluent conceptual processisng and explicit memory for faces are electrophysiologically distinct. *The Journal of Neuroscience,* Vol. 26, No. 3, (January 2008), pp. 926-933, ISSN: 1529-2401.

Voss, J.L., & Paller, K.A. (2007). Neural correlates of conceptual implicit memory and their contamination of putative neural correlates of explicit memory. *Learning and Motivation,* Vol. 14, pp. 259-267, ISSN: 1072-0502.

Vuilleumier, P. & Pourtois, G. (2007). Distributed and interactive brain mechanisms during emotion face perception: Evidence from functional neuroimaging. *Neuropsychologia,* Vol. 45, No. 1, pp. 174-194, ISSN: 0028-3932.

Washburn, M.F. (1928). Emotion and Thought: A Motor Theory of Their Relations. In: Martin L. Reymert (Ed.), *Feelings and Emotions: The Wittenberg Symposium.* Worcester, MA: Clark University: 104-115.

Watson, J.B. (1913). Psychology as the Behaviorist views it. *Psychological Review*, Vol. 20, No. 2, (March 1913), pp. 158-177, ISSN: 0033-295X.

Whalen, P.J., Rauch, S.L., Etcoff, N.L., McInerney, S.C., Lee, M.B., & Jenike, M.A. (1998). Masked presentations of emotional facial expressions modulate amygdala activity without explicit knowledge. *The Journal of Neuroscience*, Vol. 18, No. 1, (January 1998), pp. 411-418, ISSN: 0270-6474.

Xu, X., Aron, A., Brown, L., Cao, G., Feng, T., & Weng, X. (2011). Reward and motivation systems: A brain mapping study of early-stage romantic love in Chinese participants. *Human Brain Mapping*, Vol. 32, No. 2, (February 2011), pp. 249-257, ISSN: 1097-0193.

Yovel, G., & Paller, K.A. (2004). The neural basis of the butcher-on-the-bus phenomenon. When a face seems familiar but is not remembered. *NeuroImage*, Vol. 21, No. 2, (February 2004), pp. 789-800, ISSN: 10538119.

Zeki, S. (2007). The neurobiology of love. *FEBS Letters*, Vol. 581 No. 14, (June 2007), pp. 2575-2579, ISSN: 0014-5793.

Part 3

EMG New Frontiers in Research and Technology

8

Water Surface Electromyography

David Pánek, Dagmar Pavlů and Jitka Čemusová
Department of Physiotherapy, Faculty of Physical Education and Sport,
Charles University
Czech Republic

1. Introduction

Registration of electrical muscle activity with the use of surface electromyography (SEMG) is today already a routine neuro-physiological method. Over the course of a few decades it has moved from the field of the purely experimental to the area of rehabilitation medicine, kinesiology, and sports issues. Together with this trend, interest has begun to deepen in the study of all types of movement patterns stereotypes conducted in a water environment and in a dry environment. This has also opened a new area of electromyographic diagnostics that represents a modification of the basic methodology of surface EMG in a water environment, so-called Water Surface Electromyography -WaS-EMG (Pánek et al., 2010).

Although current modern technology allows a huge number of computer post-processing of an acquired native recording, a key phase of the actual recording of electrical activity remains in the hands of the experimenter. For these reasons significant attention is paid to the methodology and issue of correct placement and fixing of electrodes in all neuro-physiological methods. In general approach, recording an EMG signal in a water environment is no different from the common methodology of surface EMG, but there are certain specifics in that case. Currently, great attention is paid in the literature to the issue of the different effect of water and dry environments on the nature of the EMG recording itself (Kelly et al., 2000; Masumoto et al., 2004, 2008; Rainoldi et al., 2004; Veneziano et al., 2006), and thus on the course of a defined movement stereotype (Kelly et al., 2000; Masumoto et al., 2004, 2005, 2008; Pavlů & Panek, 2008; Holländerova, 2011; Sladká, 2011).

In this work we take up the issue of Water Surface Electromyography (WaS-EMG), both in terms of research and the practical, including a summary of the results of several of our experiments.

2. WaS-EMG methodology

In our workplace we use a telemetric EMG instrument, the TelemyoMini 16, which is made by the Neurodata company. We evaluate and process the acquired data with the help of MyoResearch XP Master Edition software for concurrent video monitoring. However, the following items are also needed to complement the equipment for recording an EMG signal in a water environment (Fig. 1):

1. Water-resistant sac for the EMG amplifier and transmitter.
2. Special bipolar electrodes with a set of two-sided adhesive patches that are necessary for solidly affixing the electrodes to the skin.

3. Covering, waterproof patches for the electrodes, which prevent moistening and the subsequent release of electrodes into the water.
4. An abrasive and conductive paste.
5. Alcohol benzine.
6. Electrode conductive cream (from GE Medical System).
7. Universal Silicone.

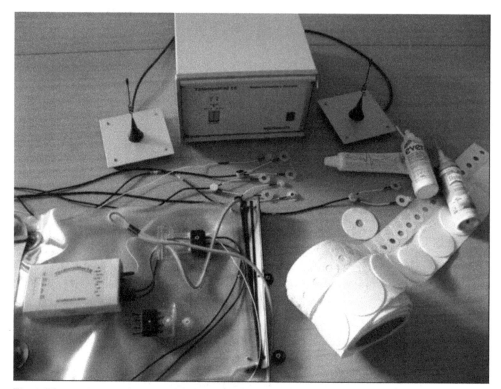

Fig. 1. The equipment for recording EMG singnal in a water environment (Pánek et al., 2010).

2.1 Preparatory phase of measurement

Significant attention must be paid to placing the EMG transmitter in the water-resistant sac. Unless we ensure proper sealing of the sac, the damage will reach large financial sums. Closing the main opening of the sac poses no problems, but sealing the openings for the bipolar electrode cables is more complicated. Because this involves relatively complex and precise work, we recommend immediately preparing all the cables that we have at our disposal. If we do not use all the cables in the measurement, we can secure the remaining cables with water-resistant adhesive tape right to the sac. We place the cables in grooves already prepared in the sealing rubber, which is divided into two halves and secured with a screw. Nevertheless, it is still necessary to assure that it is water-resistant by sealing the cables in the grooves with common Universal Silicone. This method makes it possible to later free up the cables and clean the grooves in the sealing rubber without problems. Before closing the main opening of the sac it is good to place the transmitter on a polystyrene board, which will allow the transmitter to float. In this way we can avoid loss of the EMG signal at the moment when the proband is moving actively in the water, which can lead to the EMG transmitter being submerged below water level (Pánek et al., 2010).

2.2 Application of electrodes on the skin

For recording an EMG signal in a water environment we use special bipolar electrodes (Fig.2). This involves Ag/AgCl disk electrodes that are 5 mm in diameter, which are embedded in plastic periphery so that only the central part, which is placed against the skin, remains free.

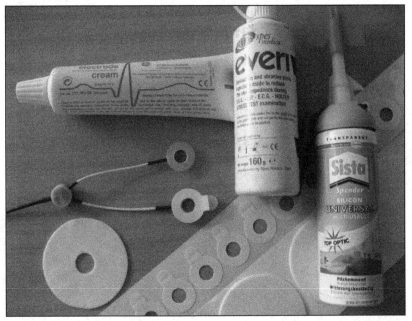

Fig. 2. WaS- EMG electrodes intended for water environments with accessories (Pánek et al., 2010).

Here, too, the basic rule applies that the electrodes are affixed to thoroughly cleaned and degreased skin. In our case, we used an abrasive tape and alcohol benzine. We stick two-sided adhesive tape, which copies the round shape of the electrode and is supplied together with the electrodes, to the plastic disk of the electrode, which is placed against the skin. Only then do we apply the conductive gel to the electrode. In our experience this phase is very important, because too much gel markedly increases the risk of the electrode coming loose during the course of the experiment. Of course a small amount does not ensure proper adherence of the electrode to the skin, it increases the impedance between the electrodes and the skin, and there is a weakening and disruption of the electrical signal. Each subsequent correction of the attachment to the skin is, due to the wet environment, significantly complicated. After sticking the electrode to the skin, we cover it with a special round sealing patch with a central opening, which we place precisely over the electrode. We also paste over the electrode cable; passing the cable through the central opening has not worked, as in water the electrode itself always came unstuck. Maintaining the recommended distance between electrodes at 1cm (DeLuca, 2002) is impossible for use of this methodology, as any decrease in the diameter of the covering patch leads to the electrode becoming unstuck. However, it follows from our experience that covering the individual patches by about 1/3 of their diameter is stable, and the electrodes do not fall off in water.

2.3 Affixing the water-resistent sac to the body, and entering the pool

After applying all the electrodes on the skin we can proceed to affixing the water-resistant sac to the body. It seemed to us that the best option is to pull the sac's blue hanger (Fig. 3) over the head and loosen it sufficiently so that during movement in water it will slip into the C-Th area and not cause an unpleasant feeling of pulling in the area of the neck. We adjust the sac's strap in the area of the torso in such a way that during movements the sac can be above water surface level.

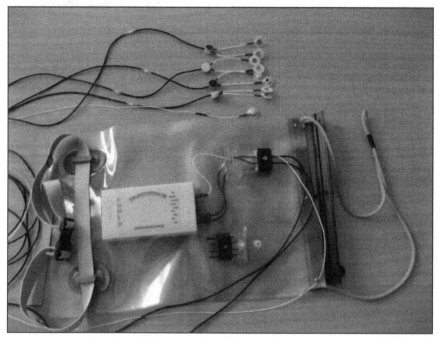

Fig. 3. Water-resistant sac with EMG transmitter and electrodes (Pánek et al., 2010).

It is necessary to affix the loose cables from the bipolar electrodes placed on the skin to the proband's body, because they can both obstruct movement and lead to detachment of the electrode from the preamplifier placed for the electrode itself, and their free movement can also affect the EMG signal (Rainoldi et al., 2004). It is possible to use water-resistant straps that are used in various water sports for affixing loose cables, but there is the possible risk of allergic contact reactions. One variant appears to be to cut patches for the electrodes that do not come unstuck in water or cause allergic reactions.

Because we are working in a wet environment, we must protect the EMG instrument itself and the notebook against damage. We select a place that is relatively well protected against direct contact with water. For this reason, most of the affixing of electrodes and the overall preparation of the proband proceed further from optimal entry into the water.

In Figure 4 we see how the proband climbs over the side area of the pool only with the help of an assistant who holds the sac and the loose cables. We consider this method of entering the pool to be simply unsuitable, because its result can be only yanking or unsticking an electrode.

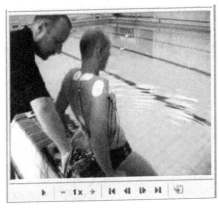

Fig. 4. Unsuitable entry into swimming pool

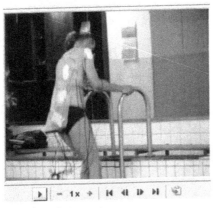

Fig. 5. Recommended entry into pool.

For this reason we recommend that the proband enter the pool in a freely accessible place, in our case by the steps, and on the side of the pool, where it is possible to comfortably stand on the bottom (Fig. 5). In this way the proband can't demage the loose cables and the water-resistant sac, which remains on the water surface behind the proband. When using the telemetric EMG instrument it is necessary to ensure that the water-resistant sac remains above the water level during the course of the experiment. We achieved this by placing lightening floats right in the sac (Fig. 6), or we used an assistant who always kept the sac above water level, thereby limiting increased movement of loose cables during the course of the probands' motor activity (Sladká, 2011).

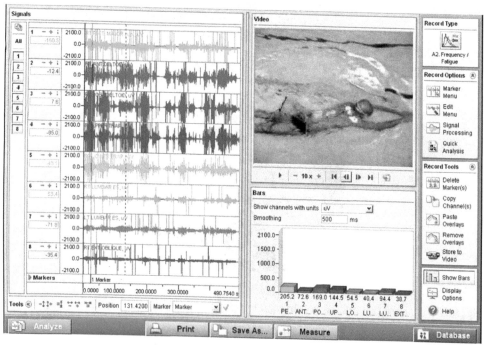

Fig. 6. WaS-EMG: Recording of swimming (Pánek et al, 2010).

The issue of the difference between telemetric measurement and direct connection of the EMG instrument and the electrodes by cables has already been dealt with in the study by Clarys et al. (Clarys et al., 1985). When using both methods for registering an EMG signal no difference was found. And for this reason, due to the more advantageous manipulation with the telemetric system, this method is primarily recommended for recording electrical activity of muscles.

Other technical parameters of registration are also taken up by Masumoto and Mercer (Masumoto & Mercer, 2008), who evaluated whether it is better to use a water-resistant suit or to affix each electrode covered by water-resistant tape with a foam cushion. Although a water-resistant suit appears to be better, there are also many disadvantages. The suit must both fit every individual, thereby increasing the price of the measurement, and the cables must leave through holes in the suit, resulting in potential places for leaks. And, last but not least, it is not entirely clear whether the suit limits the proband's dynamic movement. For these reasons, according to Masumoto and Mercer it is better to apply each electrode separately, with covers of waterproof tape.

3. Effect of water environment on the amplitude and spectral characteristics of an EMG signal

During electromyographic studies in a water environment, and especially when comparing the motor behaviour of an individual in water and on a dry land, the relevant question arises as to how the water environment affects the native EMG signal, and what the specific changes are in muscle activity caused by the change in gravitation and by the resistance of the water environment.

The original studies by Clarys et al. (Clarys et al., 1985) and Pöyhönem et al. (Pöyhömen et al. 1999) pointed to decreased amplitude of the EMG signal in the course of maximal voluntary contraction (MVC) in water compared to EMG activity on a dry land. But it was not clear whether this result was affected by methodological limitations or physiological changes caused by the water environment. That is to say, in both cases the authors did not use waterproof attachment of electrodes or attachment of electrode by means of adhesive tape (Sulkova, 2011).

A significant contribution to the solution of this problem is the study by Rainoldi et al. (Rainoldi et al., 2004). The authors monitored the EMG activity of the brachial biceps muscle during maximal voluntary contraction on a dry land, in standing water, and in a flowing water at 25° C. In all cases they compared the individual parameters of the EMG signal (average rectified value, root mean square, mean frequency, median frequency) during isometric contraction with and without attachment of electrodes by means of water-resistant adhesive tape and with attachment of free electrode cables. The results of the study indicated that without the covering tape over the electrodes, the amplitude of the signal is recorded in standing and flowing water as lower (by 6.7%) than during contractions on a dry land. A dramatic change appeared during isometric contractions in flowing water without the covering tape, when there was a significant increase of the frequency component in the low frequency band of 0-20Hz, which affected all of the monitored parameters. The incidence of this artefact was caused by the movement of free cables, and after they were affixed and the electrodes were glued on it disappeared. The conclusion of this study was to recommend the use, when registering EMG activity in water, water-resistant adhesive tape, whereby we can rule out the occurrence of marked artefacts and ensure constant conditions during the course of the entire experiment.

Da Silva Carvalhoa et al. (Da Silva Carvalhoa et al., 2010) present many studies that stress the importance of water-resistant tape when measuring EMG in a water environment, but also several practices that cast this fact in doubt. They conducted an experiment that should have clarified the inconsistency. We can see the following from the results: during isometric contractions in water without taping, there was a EMG amplitude decreased in to 50%. When comparing isometric contractions in a water environment with the use of covering tape, the results were in accord with those that were measured on a dry land with and without tape. So according to them, the covering tape used on a dry surface does not affect the EMG amplitude, yet it had a marked effect on the EMG recording in a water environment.

Similarly, Veneziana et al. (Veneziano et al., 2006) also recommend the use of covering tape in a water environment and on dry land, because among other things, the covering tape also develops a certain mechanical pressure on the skin and the muscle tissue under the electrode.

Many authors thus agree on the necessity of attaching the electrodes with water-resistant tape, which eliminates the artificially lowered amplitude of the EMG recording and the spectral changes in water. We thus ensure that the EMG signals acquired on a dry land and in water can be correctly reproduced and compared. When adhering to the correct methodology for attaching the electrodes the water environment does not affect the registered electrical activity of the muscle or the maximum muscle contraction.

Another discussed question is whether we should normalise the EMG data to the maximal voluntary contraction (MVC) in water or on a dry land. Masumoto and Mercer (Masumoto

& Mercer, 2008) recommend that it all be normalised to MVC on a dry land, because most prior studies were conducted in precisely by this way. Silvers and Dolny (Silvers & Dolny, 2001) tested maximal voluntary contraction on a dry land and in water on 12 probands. From the results they conclude that no marked difference was found between individual MVC values on a dry land and under water. So they also recommend normalisation to MVC values registered on a dry surface.

4. Effect of water temperature on the native EMG signal

The heat conductivity of water is 23 times higher than the conductivity of air. Dewhurst et al. (Dewhurst et al., 2005) documents that the temperature of a muscle is, under ordinary conditions, always higher than the temperature on the surface of the body. In a water environment there is a faster exchange of heat between the water and tissues, and therefore the organism cools earlier than on the air.

Proximal muscles are warmer at rest, by an average of 4.1° C, than distal muscles. Muscle temperature changes the most in the first 5 minutes after being submerged in water, and in 15 minutes their temperature equals the temperature of ambient water (Petrofsky J, 2005).

Petrofsky and Laymon (Petrofsky & Laymon, 2005) tracked the effect on an EMG signal in connection with water temperature on 7 probands. They registered EMG activity from the upper and lower extremities (m. biceps brachii, m. brachioradialis, m. quadriceps femoris, m. gastrocnemius) after 20 minutes of submersion in water at temperatures of 24°, 27°, 34° a 37° C. For all four examined muscles there was no statistically significant difference between the MVC values and the median frequency among the three highest water temperature. Nevertheless, after submersion in the coolest water (24° C), all of the monitored muscles showed a significant MVC decrease (by up to 44.8%), a shift of the median frequency by 32 Hz in the direction of lower values, and a slower speed of action potential conduction in the muscle fibre by 2m/s in comparison with the value achieved in the warmest water.

A similar issue was taken up in the diploma thesis by Stejskalová (Stejskalová, 2011), where she evaluated the amplitude changes in isometric contraction after 5 minutes in water at temperatures of 15° C, 24° C, 35° C for 30%, 50%, and 70% of the maximum output muscle strength measured by pressing a hand dynamometer. She registered EMG activity from finger flexors and the wrist of the right upper extremity, which was submerged in a water bath at the level of half the forearm. The results of the study, as opposed to the work of Petrofsky and Laymon (Petrofsky & Laymon, 2005), did not show any effect of water temperature on the EMG recording. This finding explains the shorter period of the extremity's submersion in water, when for the first time after 15 minutes the temperature between the ambient water and the muscle stabilize which subsequently appears in cool water as changes of electromyographic activity.

The water temperature and duration of submersion are significant factors that affect the EMG record. For these reasons, the stimulation of the water temperature must be stated and considered. According to Jandová (Jandová, 2009), after an isothermic bath the water bath temperature was designated as 34-35° C. But this involved baths in their entirety for which no physical activity was assumed. At a temperature of 25-32° C, the bath was cooling, hypothermal. At a temperature of 25° C there was already a decline in body temperature of 1° C after 7 minutes (Jandová, 2009). Most electromyographic studies in a water environment work at temperatures between 27 and 34° C (Miyoshi et al., 2004; Masumoto et al., 2004, 2009; Veneziano et al., 2006; Shono et al., 2007; Kaneda et al., 2008; Pavlů & Pánek, 2008).

5. Comparison of movement in a water environment and on a dry land

The growing popularity of all sorts of rehabilitation and fitness procedures in water has led to many studies that deal with dynamic regimens of muscle activity and their comparison when done on dry land or in water. The specificity of the water environment leads, in comparison with dry surfaces, to different muscle timing through a change in the proportional representation of activity agonistic-antagonistic muscles, and through a different compensation mechanism that follows from a certain postural "instability" in movements in water. Most published works deal with the issue of normal or modified gait or the monitoring of activity of muscles of the lower extremities in variously defined movements. Less attention is paid to the activity of muscles of the upper extremities, mostly with a focus on the shoulder girdle.

5.1 WaS-EMG analysis of walking in water

Movements in a water environment are affected by the viscosity of the water, which is eight hundred times as great as that of air. Bodies submerged in water are lighter than in air thanks to the buoying force. This buoying force of water decreases the vertical burden in a water environment against to walking on a dry land. This result was objectivised on the basis of treading on a Kistler pressure-sensitive surface in a water environment (Miyoshi et al., 2004).

Masumoto et al. (Masumoto et al., 2004) monitored muscle activity during walking on a treadmill in a water environment with the use of an water counterflow and without, and they compared it with walking on a dry land. They monitored muscles in the lower extremities (m.gluteus medius, m.rectus femoris, m.vastus medialis, m.biceps femoris, m.gastrocnemius lateralis, m.tibialis anterior) and bilaterally on the trunk (mm.paravertebrales in the area of the fourth lumbar vertebra and the m.rectus abdominis). The gait speed in a water environment (30 m/min, 40 m/min, 50 m/min) was half that of the gait speed on a dry surface. The depth of the water in the pool reached the level of the processus xiphoideus. Significantly lower electrical activity values were found in the monitored muscles when walking in a water environment with a counterflow and without a counterflow in comparison with identical movement on a dry land, the difference amounting to 10-20%. These results corresponded to previous studies, which also describe decreased EMG activity in a water environment compared with identical movement on a dry land (Clarys et.al., 1985; Fujisawa et al., 1998; Pöyhömen et al., 1999; Kelly et al., 2000). The following year Masumoto et al. (Masumoto et al., 2005) published a further study. In which, while keeping the previous conditions, they again monitored the activity of muscles of the lower extremity and trunk musculature while walking on a treadmill backwards on a dry land and in a water environment (with and without a water counterflow). They arrived at similar reasults. The sole exception was heightened activity of paravertebral muscles in the area of the fourth lumbar vertebra. They explained the increase in their activity in water by citing the greater resistance of the water environment, greater demands on balance, and backwards walking.

In the work of Shono et al. (Shono et al., 2007), electrodes were placed on muscles of the right lower extremity: m.tibialis anterior, m.gastrocnemius medialis, m.vastus medialis, m.rectus femoris, m.biceps femoris. Gait was measured among sixty years old women at speeds of 20 m/min., 30 m/min, and 40 m/min in a water environment, and then at twice these speeds on a dry land. The gait cadence was lower (by nearly one-half) and the stride length was longer in a water environment, if the same gait speeds in both environments were compared. However, when comparing the same intensity of movement, i.e., approximately 30 m/min in a water environment against 60 m/min on a dry land, the stride length was not significantly different. At a corresponding intensity of movement, nearly identical activity for the m. tibialis anterior, m. vastus medialis, and m. biceps femoris was recorded, but the m. gastrocnemius medialis and m. rectus femoris showed lower activity in a water environment. When comparing the results of the same speeds, activity of the tibialis anterior, vastus medialis, and biceps femoris was higher in a water environment, while activity of the gastrocnemius medialis and the rectus femoris was the same.

Pöyhönen (Pöyhönen T, 2001) evaluated the muscle activity of the m. quadriceps femoris and the m. biceps femoris during flexing and extension of the knee on a dry land and in a water environment. In the water environment the test was run with and without the use of a "Hydro Boot." Eighteen persons without any physical problems took part in the study. The underwater EMG results showed a decline in time in the concentric activity of the agonist muscles with concurrent activity of the antagonist muscles without the "Hydro Boot." When measuring activity in a water environment with and without the resistance boot the probands were seated on a chair so that they are submerged up to the mid-sternum level. In the results, the EMG amplitudes were similar in both cases. The authors are of the opinion that with and without the use of the boot the size of the EMG amplitude was similar, especially thanks to the "power-speed" relationship of the muscle contraction. But it was pointed out that if a muscle acts as an agonist it is active in roughly the first 50-60% of the extent of the movement. If it is acting as an antagonist it is active in roughly the last 50-60% of the extent of the movement, while on a dry surface an agonist is active throughout the entire period of movement and an antagonist shows only a little activity.

5.2 WaS-EMG analysis of muscle timing during cycling on dry land and in a water environment

In the work of Sladká (Sladká, 2011), with the help of surface EMG, was compared the timing of muscles of four probands aged 23-24, while riding a bicycle on a dry land and in a water environment. In the experiment she used two identical Sapilo water bicycles (Fig. 7). She placed WaS-EMG electrodes on the right and left paravertebrales muscles and the m. biceps femoris, m. gastrocnemius lateralis, m. vastus medialis, and m. tibialis anterior of the left, non-dominant extremity.

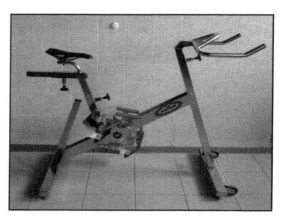

Fig. 7. Sapilo water bicycle.

The temperature of the water in the pool was 32° C (±0.5° C), and the temperature of the air was 28° C (±0.5° C). The depth of the water was up to 125 cm. The measurement itself of the EMG recording was made while riding on the water bicycle, first on a dry surface and then in the water. The pedalling speed was 60 revolutions per minute. The pedalling time on the dry land and in the water was one minute.

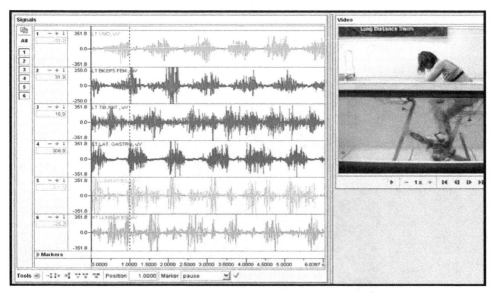

Fig. 8. EMG recording with a synchronized video recording. The interrupted vertical line captures the left lower extremity at the beginning of the pedal revolution (Sladká, 2011).

The results of the study did not show changes in the timing of the monitored muscles of the lower extremity when riding a bicycle on dry land and in a water environment. Due to greater demands related to stabilizing the pelvis in the water environment, there was co-contraction of both paravertebral muscles. On dry land this tendency was not recorded. At the same time, it was found that in the water environment pedalling was more regular than pedalling on dry land.

5.3 Analysis of muscles of the pectoral girdle with the help of WaS-EMG

The already outlined general trend towards decreasing electromyographical activity for identical movements in water versus dry land has also been described by many authors studying muscle activity in the area of the pectoral girdle (Rouard & Clarys, 1995; Fujisawa et al., 1998; Pavlů & Pánek, 2008).

Kelly et al. (Kelly et al., 2000) broadened their question to include the issue of the speed of abduction in the shoulder joint with a concurrent comparison of the activity of muscles of the rotator cuff and the synergies of the shoulder during exercise on dry land and in water. Six probands took part in the research. In the water environment, the probands were submerged up to neck level. In both environments they caused abduction in their shoulder joints at speeds of 30°/s, 45°/s, and 90°/s. The results showed that when the selected speed corresponded to 30°/s and 45°/s, the activity of the muscles (supraspinatus, infraspinatus, subscapularis, and the front, middle and back parts of the deltoideus) was smaller than on dry land. At 90°/s, the muscle activity especially of the m. subscapularis, increased markedly.

Holländerová (Holländerová, 2011), during the course of her study, which was conducted in our workplace, evaluated the timing and size of activation of muscles during abduction in the shoulder joint as opposed to the resistance of a flexible pull on dry land and in water. The flexible resistance was provided with the help of Thera-Band yellow dye. Four probands took part in the study. EMG activity was registered from the m. trapezius pars superior et inferior and the m. deltoideus pars medialis muscles (Fig. 9).

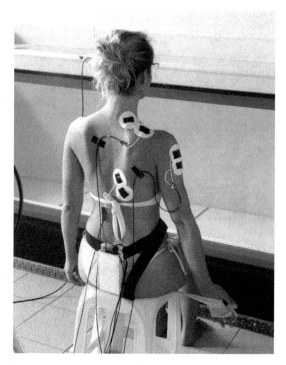

Fig. 9. Localization of WaS-EMG electrodes during study of muscle activity against flexible resistance with the help of Thera-Band yellow dye (Holländerová, 2011).

The water temperature was 32° C. The probands caused abduction in the shoulder joint at a speed of 30°/s to the horizontal position of the brachium, first on a dry surface and then in water, which reached the level of the procesus spinosus vertebra C5. They continually repeated abduction of the brachium 10 times, and 7 stable cycles were evaluated (Fig. 10). The results of the study indicated a decrease in monitored muscle activity in the water environment; the most marked change was captured in the m. trapezius pars superior muscle - 47-57% - in the other two muscles the change ranged between 19 and 29%. She also found different muscle timing, coinciding with an earlier study (Pavlů & Pánek, 2008), between movement in water and on dry land, but this was individual and there was no common trend.

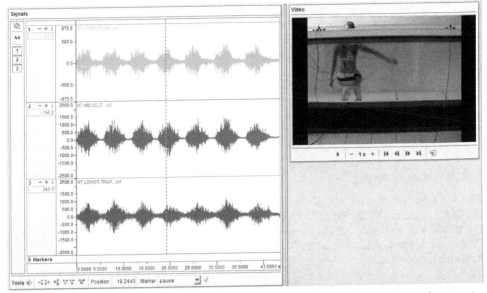

Fig. 10. EMG activity in the course of 7 cycles of brachial abduction in a water environment (Holländerová, 2011).

6. Conclusion

WaS-EMG is a relatively modern method for studying electrical muscle activity in an environment that was formerly rather inaccessible for neuro-physiological methods. Nevertheless, there are many studies that make it possible to follow up on acquired knowledge relating primarily to methodological measurement and the effect of a captured biological signal. In summary, here are the most basic of them:

1. For registering electrical activity it is best to use separate electrodes. Water resistant suits and garments are mainly more expensive, they place greater limitation on the probands' activity, and they are more likely to leak water onto the electrodes.

2. Electrodes should be attached with water-resistant tape, which should also affix loose cables. This limits the occurrence of artefacts from cable movements that appear in the 0-20 Hz frequency band.

3. Pasted on electrodes should be used for measurements on dry land as well, because this does not change the character of the EMG signal between the water environment and on a dry land.

4. For measurement of the maximal voluntary contraction (MVC) should be used movements on a dry land. This is a simple method, and furthermore, is also in standard use in prior publications.

5. In dynamic modes it is good to engage in a defined movement activity in water at half the speed of that on dry land. The greater viscosity of water as against air can lead, especially during faster movements, to the change in the native EMG recording.

6. The optimal water temperature is between 27 and 34° C. Cooler water leads to lower electrical muscle activity. Higher temperatures are uncomfortable for the performance

of movement activities. Stable temperatures of muscles and the ambient water are reached in approximately 15 minutes.

7. When making an identical movement in water and in a dry environment, in the water environment there is decreased muscle activity versus the identical movement on a dry land.

8. The change on the size of muscle activity in a water environment depends on the speed of the movement on a dry land, and primarily for fast movements, when greater effect of water's viscosity is emphasized.

9. If we study movements that are more demanding on posture, the activity of trunk muscles, which must adjust to this burden, is increased.

7. Acknowledgment

This work was elaborated with the help of the research plan of the Ministry of Education of the Czech Republic **VZ MŠMT ČR MSM 0021620864.**
We would like to thank the Department of Swimming of the FTVS UK, and namely Mgr. Daniel Jurák for his assistance and making possible measurement in the Aquatic Sports Research Laboratory.

8. References

Clarys, J.; Robeaux, R.& Delbeke, G. (1985). Telemetrical versus conventional EMG in air and water. *Biomachnics IX: Human Kinetics,* pp.286-294, ISBN:0-931250-52-8, Champaign, France, 1985

Da Silva Carvalhoa, R.; Amorimb, C.&Perácioa L.&Coelhoa H.&Vieiraa, A.& Menzelc, H.& Szmuchrowski, A. (2010). Analysis of various conditions in order to measure electromyography of isometric contractions in water and on air. *Journal of Electromyography and Kinesiology.* Vol. 20, No. 5, (2010), pp.988-993, ISSN 1050-6411

DeLuca, C. (2002). Surface Electromyography: Detection and Recording. In: Delsys, 2.3.2006, Available from http://delsys.com/KnowledgeCenter/Tutorials.html.

Dewhurst, S.; Riches, P. & Nimmo, M. & De Vito, G. (2005). Temperature dependence of soleus H-reflex and M-wave in young and older women. *European Journal of Applied Physiology.* Vol. 94, No. 5-6, (2005), pp. 491-499, ISSN 8750-7587

Fujisawa, H,; Seunaga, N.& Minami, A. (1998). Electromyographic study during isometric exercise of the shoulder in head-out water immersion. *Journal of Shoulder and Elbow Surgery.* Vol. 7, No.5, (1998), pp. 491-494, ISSN 1058-2746

Holländerova, D. (2011). *Evaluation of EMG Activity of the Shoulder Girdle Muscles during Exercises with Thera-Band in the Aquatic Environment and on the Land.* Diploma thesis, Departmen of Physiotherapy. Faculty of Physical Education and Sport, Charles University, Prague, Czech Republic, 2011 (in Czech)

Jandová, D. (2009). *Balneologie.* Grada Publishing a.s., ISBN 978-80-247-2820-9, Prague, Czech Republic (in Czech)

Kaneda, K.; Wakabayashi, H.& Sato, D.& Uekusa, T.& Nomura, T. (2008). Lower extremity muscle activity during deep-water running on self-determined pace. *Journal of Electromyography and Kinesiology.* Vol.18, No. 6, (2008), pp. 965-972, ISSN 1050-6411

Kelly, B.; Roskin, D.& Kirkendall, D.& Speer, K. (2000). Shoulder muscle activation during aquatic and dry land exercises in nonimpaired subjects. *Journal of Orthopaedic & Sports Physical Therapy.* Vol.30. No.4, (2000), pp. 204-210, ISSN 0190-6011

Masumoto, K.; Takasugi, S. & Hotta, N. & Fujishima, K. & Iwamoto, Y. (2004). Electromyographic Analysis of Walking in Water in Healthy Humans. *Journal of Psychiological Anthropology and Applied Human Science.* Vol. 23, No. 4, (2004), pp. 119-127, ISSN 1345-3475

Masumoto, K.; Takasugi, S. & Hotta, N. & Fujishima, K. & Iwamoto, Y. (2005). Muscle activity and heart rate response during backward walking in water. *European Journal of Applied Physiology and Occupation Physiology.* Vol. 94, No. 1-2, (2005), pp. 54-61, ISSN 0301-5548

Masumoto, K. & Mercer, J. (2008). Biomechanics of Human Locomotion in Water: An Electromyographic Analysis: Methodological Considerations for Quantifying Muscle Activity During Water Locomotion. *Exercise and Sport Sciences Reviews.*, Vol. 36, No.3, (2008), pp.160-169, ISSN 0091-6331

Masumoto, K.; Delion, D. & Mercer, J. (2009). Insight into Muscle Activity during Deep Water Running. *Medicine & Science in Sports & Exercice.* Vol. 41, (2009), pp. 1958-1964, ISSN 0195-9131

Miyoshi, T.; Shirota, T. & Yamamoto, S. & Nakazawa, K. & Akai, M. (2004). Effect of the walking speed to the lower limb joint angular displasments, joint movements and ground reaction force during walking in water. *Disability & Rehabilitation.* Vol. 26, No. 12, (2004), pp. 724-732, ISSN 0963-8288

Pánek, D.; Jurák, D. & Pavlů, D. & Krajča, V. & Čemusová, J. (2010). Water Surface Electromyography –WaS-EMG. *Rehabilitation and Physical Medicine.*Vol. 17, No. 1, (2010), pp.21-25, ISSN 1211-2658 (in Czech)

Pavlů, D. & Pánek, D. (2008). EMG - Analysis of Selected Muscles of Upper Extremity Moving in Water Environment and Motion against Elastic Rezistance. *Rehabilitation and Physical Medicine.* Vol. 15, No. 4, (2008), pp. 167-173, ISSN 1211-2658 (in Czech]

Petrofsky, J. & Laymon, M. (2005). Muscle Temperature and EMG Amplitude and Frequency During Isometric Exercise. *Aviation, Space and Environment Medicine.* Vol. 76, No.11., (2005), pp. 1024- 1030, ISSN 0095-6562

Pöyhömen, T.; Kyrolainen, H. & Keskinen, K. & Hautala, A. & Savolainen, J. & Mälkiä, E. (1999). Isometric force production and electromyogram activity of knee extensor muscles in water and on dry land. *European Journal of Applied Physiology and Occupation Physiology.* Vol. 80, No. 1, (1999), pp. 52-56, 1999, ISSN 1432-1025

Pöyhönen, T.; Keskinen, K. & Kyröläinen, H. & Hautala, A. & Savolainen, J. & Mälkiä, E. (2001). Neuromuscular function during therapeutic knee exercise under water and on dry land. *Archives of Physical Medicine and Rehabilitation.* Vol. 82, No. 10, (2001), pp. 1446-1442, ISSN 0003-9993

Rainoldi, A.; Cescon, C. &, Bottin, A. & Casale, R. & Caruso, I. (2004). Surface EMG alteration induced by undewater recording. *Journal of Electromyography and Kinesiology.* Vol. 14, No.3, (2004), pp. 325-331, ISSN 1050-6411

Rouard, A. & Clarys, J. (1995). Cocontraction in the Elbow and Shoulder Muscles During Rapid Cyclic Movements in an Aquatic Environment. *Journal of Electromyography and Kinesiology. Vol.* 5, No. 3, (1995), pp. 177-183, ISSN 1050-6411

Shono, T.; Masumoto, K. & Fujishima, K. & Hotta, N. & Ogaki, T. & Adachi, T. (2007). Gait Patterns and Muscle Activity of the Lower Extremities of Elderly Women during Underwater Treadmill Walking againts Water Flow. *Journal of Physiological Anthropology.* Vol. 26, No. 6, (2007), pp. 579-586, ISSN 1880-6791

Silvers, W. & Dolny, D. (2001). Comparison and reproducibility of sEMG during manual muscle testing on land and in water. *Journal of Electromyography and Kinesiology.* Vol. 21, No.1, (2001), pp. 95-101, ISSN 1050-6411.

Sladká, H. 2011. *Compare of muscle timing during cycling on land and in water.* Diploma thesis. Departmen of Physiotherapy. Faculty of Physical Education and Sport, Charles University, Prague, Czech Republic, 2011 (in Czech)

Stejskalova, P. (2011). *Effect of water temperature on muscle contraction.* Diploma thesis. Departmen of Physiotherapy. Faculty of Physical Education and Sport, Charles University, Prague, Czech Republic, 2011 (in Czech)

Sulková, I. (2011). *Possibility of using Aquatherapy for shoulder stabilization.* Diploma thesis. Department of Physiotherapy, Faculty of Physical Education and Sport, Charles University, Prague, Czech Republic, 2011 (in Czech)

Veneziano, W.; da Rocha, A. & Goncalves, C. & Pena, A. & Carmo J. & Nascimento, F. & Rainoldi, A. (2006). Confounding factors in water EMG recordings: an approach to a definitive standard. *Medical & Biological Engineering & Computing.* Vol. 44, No. 4, (2006), pp. 348-351, ISSN 0140-0118

9

Scanning Electromyography

Javier Navallas[1], Javier Rodríguez[1] and Erik Stålberg[2]
[1]Department of Electrical and Electronic Engineering,
Public University of Navarra, Pamplona
[2]Institute of Neuroscience, Department of Clinical Neurophysiology,
Uppsala University Hospital, Uppsala
[1]Spain
[2]Sweden

1. Introduction

The study of the anatomy and physiology of the motor unit has important implications in the diagnosis and follow-up of neuromuscular pathologies. Muscle action potentials allow the use of electrophysiological techniques based on electromyography (EMG) to make inferences about muscle structure, state and behaviour. Scanning EMG is one such technique that can record the temporal and spatial distribution of electrical activity of a single motor unit, allowing for deep insight into the structure and function of motor units.

In this chapter, we describe the scanning EMG technique in detail, both from a technical and clinical point of view. A brief review of the motor unit anatomy and physiology is provided in Section 2. The technique, the apparatus setup, the recording procedure and the signal processing required are described in Section 3. Key results of studies using scanning EMG are reviewed in Section 4, including findings related to motor unit organisation in normal muscle and how changes due to pathology are reflected using this electrophysiological technique. Finally, Section 5 provides some hints regarding the use of scanning EMG in research.

2. Investigation of the motor unit structure

The motor unit is the functional building block of skeletal muscle and the target of scanning EMG. In this section, the main concepts regarding the anatomy and physiology of the motor unit are described. Several electrophysiological techniques that allow the investigation of the structure of motor units are also introduced.

2.1 Motor unit anatomy

The motor unit is the smallest functional structure in skeletal muscle, comprising a motoneuron and the set of muscle fibres innervated by its axon. An action potential propagating through the axon eventually arrives at motor end-plates at the presynaptic side of the neuromuscular junctions. The electrical stimulus is then converted into a chemical signal that subsequently induces an action potential in the muscle fibre. This single fibre action potential (SFAP) propagates in both directions toward the ends of the muscle fibre, inducing a contraction of the fibre itself. The motor unit fibres, i.e., all the muscle fibres belonging to the same motor unit, contract synchronously given upon receiving the motor control command from the same motoneuron through the arborisations of its axon.

Viewing the muscle longitudinally (Fig. 1), motor unit fibres generally run in parallel between two musculotendinous junctions, although some muscle fibres have tapered fibre-to-fibre ends (Lieber, 1992). Motor end-plates of corresponding neuromuscular junctions tend to concentrate in the central portion of the fibres, halfway between their two ends. In a muscle like the biceps brachii, motor end-plate zone occupies a thin strip about 6-10 mm in width (Aquilonius et al., 1982; Amirali et al., 2007). Action potentials generated under motor end-plates propagate through the muscle fibre at a certain conduction velocity (Stålberg, 1966); the conduction velocity of a muscle fibre is directly related to its diameter (Nandedkar & Stålberg, 1983a).

Views of muscle cross-sections (Fig. 2) reveal that fibres belonging to the same motor unit occupy only a fraction of the cross-section area (Kugelberg et al., 1970); this area is referred to as the motor unit territory, and is generally irregular, mainly rounded, although it has also been described to be oval-shaped (Bodine et al., 1988) or crescent-shaped closer to the fascia. Within this territory, fibres of the same motor unit are scattered and intermingled with fibres belonging to other motor units (Burke et al., 1974). Hence, territories of different motor units overlap. The size and shape of a single motor unit territory is considerably preserved throughout the entire length of the motor unit, as shown in three-dimensional reconstructions of complete motor units (Roy et al., 1995).

The technique employed to study motor unit cross-sections is based on glycogen depletion (Edström & Kugelberg, 1968). Briefly, a single axon is repeatedly stimulated to ensure that all the glycogen is depleted from the muscle fibres innervated by the axon. Next, the muscle is excised and stained with a glycogen reagent. In the microtome cross-section, the glycogen-depleted fibres that belong to the same motor unit can be traced. The glycogen depletion technique provides a picture of the motor unit cross-section that enables a

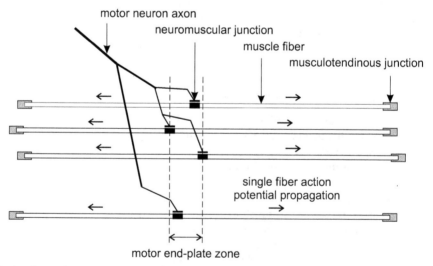

Fig. 1. A schematic representation of a motor unit with the motoneuron axon branching to innervate a set of muscle fibres.

visualisation of individual motor unit fibres. The technique also makes it possible to count individual motor unit fibres and to study their spatial distribution (Venema, 1994).

Several glycogen depletion studies have demonstrated that the number of motor unit fibres greatly varies not only among muscles (Enoka, 1995; Feinstein et al., 1955) but also within the same muscle, where the number of motor unit fibres can vary up to 10-fold (Bodine et al., 1988; Burke & Tsairis, 1973; Burke et al., 1974; Edström & Kugelberg, 1968). For example, in the medial gastrocnemius of the rat, the observed number of motor unit fibres ranges from 40 to 350 (Kanda & Hashizume, 1992). The area of the motor unit territory has also been measured in several glycogen depletion studies (Ansved et al., 1991; Bodine et al., 1988; Kanda & Hashizume, 1992; Rafuse & Gordon, 1996), which also show a broad range of variation. For example, motor unit territories of the tibialis anterior of the rat account for 10% to 24% of the muscle cross-sectional area, whereas territories of the soleus account for 25% to 75% of the cross-sectional area (Kugelberg et al., 1970).

Given the number of motor unit fibres and the area of the motor unit territory, the motor unit fibre density can be calculated (Kanda & Hashizume, 1992). Fibre density seems to be rather independent of the size of the motor unit (Weijs et al., 1993) and constant throughout the length of the motor units (Roy et al., 1995). However, fibre density can vary for different motor unit types, with smaller motor units having lower fibre densities (Kanda & Hashizume, 1992).

The spatial distribution of motor unit fibres within a motor unit territory has become a controversial issue. This spatial distribution has been described as uniform without localised collections (Burke et al., 1974), quasi-Gaussian (Miller-Larsson, 1980), evenly distributed (Willison, 1980), uniform (Gath & Stålberg, 1982), and random (Gates & Betz, 1993). A thorough statistical analysis of spatial point patterns obtained by glycogen depletion has provided more insight into this discrepancy. Short-range analysis based on adjacency tests and nearest-neighbour distributions suggest a random distribution (Bodine et al., 1988).

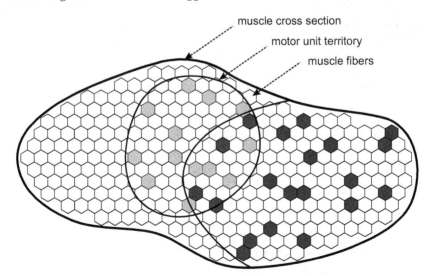

Fig. 2. A schematic representation of two motor units with overlapping territories within a muscle cross-section, and their corresponding muscle fibers.

However, long-range analysis based on quadrat analysis, point-to-nearest-neighbour distributions and inter-fibre distance distributions suggest the existence of holes within the territory and some degree of clustering in motor unit fibre distribution (Bodine-Fowler et al., 1990). The spatial clustering can be related to the axonal branching pattern established during the development of the neuromuscular system (Monti et al., 2001; Pffeifer & Friede, 1985). Other results show that, in the long-range, the randomness of the distribution may depend on the age and type of the motor unit (Ansved et al., 1991).

2.2 Electromyographic investigation of the motor unit structure

The electrical activity of the muscle can be recorded using intramuscular or surface electrodes. Intramuscular recordings are usually performed using needle electrodes. Depending on the type of needle and the recording procedure, EMG can measure the activity of muscle fibres by recording SFAPs, the activity of motor units by recording motor unit potentials (MUPs) or the activity of the entire muscle by recording the interference pattern.

2.2.1 Motor unit potentials obtained in concentric needle EMG

MUPs reveal many properties of motor unit structure because MUPs are made up of superimposed SFAPs of motor unit fibres. MUP characteristics depend on the number and relative positions of the muscle fibres generating the SFAPs and the temporal alignment of individual SFAPs (Nandedkar et al., 1988b).

The number of muscle fibres, especially within the closest uptake area of the electrode, determines the size of the resulting MUP (Nandedkar et al., 1988a). Several parameters reflect the size of MUPs, like the amplitude, the area, or the size-index (Sonoo & Stålberg, 1993). The duration of MUPs also reflects the number of fibres, but within a larger uptake area (Nandedkar et al., 1988b). A misalignment of the SFAPs contributing to an MUP increases the waveform complexity of the resulting MUP. This temporal misalignment can be caused by spatial dispersion of motor end-plates, temporal dispersion the initial depolarisation of motor end-plates, and differences in muscle fibre conduction velocities in different motor unit fibres (Navallas & Stålberg, 2009). The complexity of MUPs can be assessed with parameters like the number of phases, the number of turns (Pfeiffer & Kunze, 1992; Stålberg, 1986; Willison, 1964), or the irregularity coefficient (Zalewska & Husmanova-Petrusevich, 1995).

2.2.2 Specific techniques to estimate motor unit parameters

Quantitative analysis of MUPs is a valuable tool in diagnosis. In addition, there are other specific EMG techniques that allow us to estimate some of the physiological and anatomical parameters of the muscle and motor units. Because the glycogen depletion technique requires excising the muscle, it is unsuitable for human research, although some restricted experiments have been performed using muscle biopsies (Gollnick et al., 1973; Garnett et al., 1979). Hence, all available data pertaining to complete muscle cross-sections correspond to small mammalians. Alternative techniques based on electrophysiological recordings have been developed allowing the investigation of motor unit structures in human muscles.

The number of motor units in a certain muscle can be estimated by incrementally stimulating the nerve while simultaneously recording the compound muscle action potential (CMAP) with a surface electrode, a technique called motor unit number estimation

(MUNE) (McComas et al., 1971). This basic concept was later developed into a number of MUNE methods.

The number of motor unit fibres cannot be estimated quantitatively using electrophysiological techniques, but a relative measure can be assessed using macro EMG (Stålberg, 1980; Stålberg & Fawcett, 1982). It has been demonstrated that the amplitude of motor unit potentials recorded using the macro EMG technique is highly correlated with the number of muscle fibres involved in the generation of the signal and hence the number of motor unit fibres (Nandedkar & Stålberg, 1983b; Roeleveld et al., 1997a, 1997b). The density of motor unit fibres can also be estimated using single fibre EMG (Gath & Stålberg, 1982). This technique relies on the assumption of a homogeneous Poisson distribution of muscle fibres (Gath & Stålberg, 1981, 1982) and provides an average measure of fibre density of different motor units (Stålberg, 1986). Although this technique may average the differences in fibre densities for different motor units, recent studies in humans show no change in fibre density with a recruitment threshold up to 50% of the maximum voluntary contraction (Lukács et al., 2009).

2.2.3 Multipoint EMG techniques

The previously presented electrophysiological techniques share one thing in common: the recordings are made using electrodes with a single channel, and hence all the information is recorded from a single spatial location. Using special multilead electrodes, or multielectrodes, simultaneous recordings from different locations can be obtained, enhancing the scope of the electrophysiological technique for studying the muscle. A straightforward example is the use of a special multielectrode to assess muscle fibre conduction velocity *in situ* (Stålberg, 1966).

Using multielectrodes with recording sites lined up along the length of the needle, the main axis of the needle defines a recording corridor. It is common to position the corridor perpendicular to the muscle fibres, so that different recording sites gather information from different regions of the muscle cross-section or the motor unit territory under study.

One of the most straightforward applications of multipoint techniques is the investigation of motor unit territories. Motor unit territories have been have been studied using various EMG multielectrode configurations, one containing twelve 1.5 mm long leads distributed over 25 mm (Buchthal et al., 1957, 1959) and another containing 14 different recording sites of 25 μm diameter allowing 40 recording sites spaced 150 μm apart over 14 mm (Stålberg et al., 1976; Schwartz et al., 1976). Scanning EMG was developed as an extension of multielectrode techniques (Stålberg & Antoni, 1980), allowing higher flexibility both in the spatial interval of detection and in the type of of electrode used. In this case, any type of conventional needle electrode can be used; therefore, the technique is not restricted to a single fibre-like recording.

In addition to the investigation of motor unit topography using scanning EMG (Diószeghy, 2002; Gootzen, 1990; Gootzen et al., 1992; Stålberg & Antoni, 1980; Stålberg & Diószeghy, 1991; Stålberg & Eriksson, 1987; Tonndorf, 1994), motor end-plate topography has also been studied using this technique (Navallas & Stålberg, 2009).

3. Scanning EMG technique

In this section, the methods, procedure, and set-up required to perform scanning EMG will be reviewed. Special attention will be paid to the recording procedure and the signal processing required to condition the signal after it is recorded.

3.1 Recording setup

The main objective of scanning EMG is to record the electrical activity of a motor unit from different locations along a scanning corridor as the needle electrode passes through the motor unit territory (Fig. 3). A very important aspect is that, although a single recording is made at each location, all recordings must be synchronised in relation to the firing of the motor unit, equivalent to simultaneously recording from all the sites. To extract the firing pattern of the motor unit, a second needle electrode, called the triggering needle, is inserted into the muscle. This electrode records localised activity, ideally from a single fibre, to minimise interference from other motor units. Hence, single fibre EMG needles or facial concentric needles are used for this purpose. A given motor unit is separated from others using an amplitude trigger.

If a concentric needle is used as the scanning electrode, the signal recorded in each location corresponds to an MUP. As the scanning needle moves through the scanning corridor, the relative geometry of motor unit fibres in relation to the active region of the electrode changes; hence, the recorded MUPs will be different, reflecting these changes. However, because the triggering needle is maintained at a fixed location, all the MUPs recorded by the scanning needle will be synchronised with the firing pattern of the motor unit.

The signals from both the triggering needle and the scanning needle are amplified and digitised, and transmitted to a personal computer running specific scanning EMG software (Fig. 4). This software must provide a way to establish a voltage threshold for the signal acquired from the triggering electrode. Whenever the signal exceeds this threshold voltage, the scanning software performs three operations:

1. Records a trace of the scanning signal within the predefined bounds of a temporal window, i.e., a buffer gathering the samples some milliseconds before and after the trigger event.

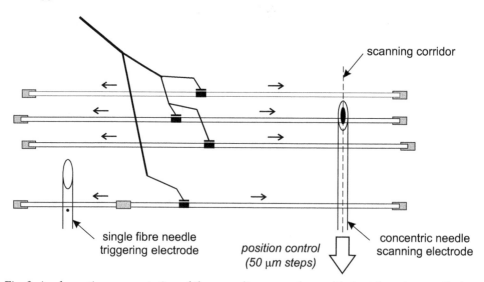

Fig. 3. A schematic representation of the recording procedure with the triggering needle in a fixed position and the scanning needle moving along the scanning corridor throughout the motor unit territory.

2. Sends a command to a micromotor controller to advance one step.

3. Waits until a new threshold event occurs. The micromotor controller is responsible for translating software commands into electrical signals that instruct the step-motor to advance a predefined distance, e.g., 50 μm.

The recorded signal is 2-dimensional in nature (Fig. 5(a)); the first dimension represents the spatial location of the recording in the scanning corridor and the second dimension represents the temporal duration of the recorded MUP. Both dimensions are discretised, the spatial dimension according to the step length controlled by the micromotor, and the temporal dimension according to the sampling time, i.e., the inverse of the sampling frequency of the acquisition system. Therefore, the signal can be thought of as a collection of MUPs from the same motor unit, where each trace is an individual MUP recorded from a different position along the scanning corridor, but also as a picture of the spatiotemporal distribution of the electric potential generated by the motor unit.

3.2 Recording procedure

In the first step, the triggering needle, a single fibre EMG electrode or facial concentric needle, is inserted to record the activity from one motor unit during slight voluntary contraction. The electromyographer should look for a stable waveform with good amplitude that is free of interference from other motor units. Next, the needle should be maintained in a fixed position to ensure a stable recording during the remainder of the process. The voltage level of the trigger must be adjusted so that a single trigger event is recorded each time the selected motor unit discharges.

The scanning needle is inserted a few centimetres away (20 mm is recommended) from the triggering electrode along the direction of the muscle fibres. The tip of the electrode must be sharp to ensure a smooth movement through the scanning corridor. The electrode must be inserted as close to perpendicular to the muscle fibres as possible (Stålberg & Antoni, 1980) to record from the actual cross-section of the muscle. Once the needle is inserted, the electromyographer should move it while looking for electrical activity synchronised with

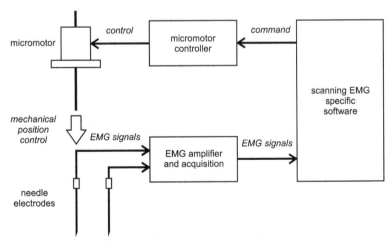

Fig. 4. A schematic representation of a scanning EMG system consisting in acquisition (needles and amplifier), processing, and control devices (micromotor and controller).

that of the triggering electrode (time-locked activity). To obtain good recordings and to ensure that the scanning needle is completely inside the motor unit territory, this time-locked activity should satisfy the same recording criteria applied to standard recordings; if a concentric needle is used for the scanning, the recorded signals should have high amplitude and a short rise-time.

Once the scanning needle is inside the motor unit territory, the electromyographer should push the needle until it reaches a position where spike activity is no longer detected. This ensures that we have completely passed through the motor unit territory. This procedure of selecting the triggering signal and finding synchronous activity with the scanning needle should take little more than one minute.

The next step is to physically connect the scanning needle to the step-motor, which should be mounted in a holder with an electrode grip and a wide-foot plate. The foot plate is held tightly against the skin over the muscle during the recording to ensure no relative movement between the step-motor and the muscle. Once the recording procedure begins, the step-motor pulls the scanning needle in small spatial increments until the recorded signal decays in amplitude or the needle exits the skin. The complete procedure should take less than five minutes.

3.3 Signal processing

The scanning EMG signal as initially recorded is a raw signal (Fig. 5(a)) that must be post-processed to obtain a cleaner version that is free of noise and interferences. There are two steps in the enhancement of the raw signal. First, a temporal filter is applied individually to each of the scanning traces (Stålberg & Antoni, 1980). A low-pass or band-pass filter can be applied to remove baseline noise produced by the needle or muscle movement and a band-pass filter will also subtract high frequency noise from the signal. The resulting signal (Fig. 5(b)) presents a smoother profile in the spatial dimension with fewer and smaller baseline jumps. Actual filter settings, like filter order and cut-off frequencies, will depend on the recording needle and should follow the recommendations for conventional recording using the needles.

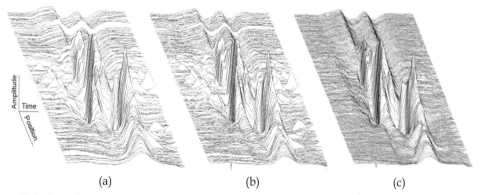

        (a)   (b)   (c)

Fig. 5. A three-dimensional representation of a scanning EMG signal: (a) a raw signal, (b) the pervious signal filtered in the temporal domain, and (c) the previous signal filtered in the spatial domain.

Significant interference due to the coactivation of other motor units may still exist in the signal, represented by superimposed MUPs scattered alongside the MUP being tracked. However, superimposed discharges are not synchronised with the firing of the tracked motor unit. Therefore, these interfering discharges are not consistently repeated and, in a trace corrupted with such an artefact, superimposed MUPs are usually found between two clean traces in the spatial domain. For this reason, a median filter is applied in the spatial dimension during the second processing step (Stålberg & Antoni, 1980). Median filters preserve smoothly changing values of synchronised activity in motor units being tracked, removing all artefacts generated by other motor units (Fig. 5(c)).

Although median filtering is a very useful technique to eliminate interfering MUPs, its influence on the signal it is not negligible. The larger the size of the median filter, the greater the reduction in the amplitude of the peaks compared to the raw data. When a 3-point median filter is used, peaks are reduced by about 10%, and when a 5- or 7-point median filter is used, peaks are reduced up to 30% (Gootzen, 1990). This should be taken into account when extracting quantitative data from the signals.

4. Scanning EMG results

Scanning EMG provides valuable information not only about the territory and arrangement of muscle fibres within a motor unit, but also about the spatiotemporal distribution of the electrical activity of a motor unit, information no other EMG technique can provide (Diószeghy, 2002). We will introduce some key aspects for qualitative interpretation of scanning EMG signals and several parameters for quantitative analysis.

4.1 Interpretation of the scanning EMG signal

In the most straightforward interpretation, a scanning EMG signal is a collection of MUPs recorded from slightly different locations through a scanning corridor. Hence, it shows the evolution of MUPs as the location of the needle electrode changes relative to the motor unit fibres of the motor unit being tracked. However, a scanning EMG signal can also be interpreted as a picture of the spatiotemporal distribution of the electric potential generated by a motor unit. Fig. 6 shows a 2-dimensional signal as a contour map that allows us to distinguish between peaks and valleys corresponding to the negative and positive phases of MUPs. In this figure, four spatial locations within the corridor are selected, and the corresponding traces representing the MUPs recorded at these sites are depicted.

Due to the recording procedure, the first part of the scanned recording corresponds to a section of the corridor outside the motor unit territory. In this case, the recording tip of the needle electrode is too far away from the generators to record their signals. However, the cannula, which is used as reference electrode in concentric needle recordings, is almost completely inside the motor unit territory. The result is that an inverted potential is recorded, similar to that of a macro EMG recording (first selected MUP in Fig. 6). This causes a trough at the beginning of the scan referred to as the cannula effect. In this way, it is possible to obtain the equivalent of an inverted macro EMG recording from the motor unit under study by averaging 50 to 100 traces that are recorded before the tip of the needle is inside the motor unit territory (Stålberg & Diószeghy, 1991). It is important to note that this method is not identical to conventional macro EMG, as the cannula used in the scanning procedure may not be partially insulated (Stålberg & Diószeghy, 1991).

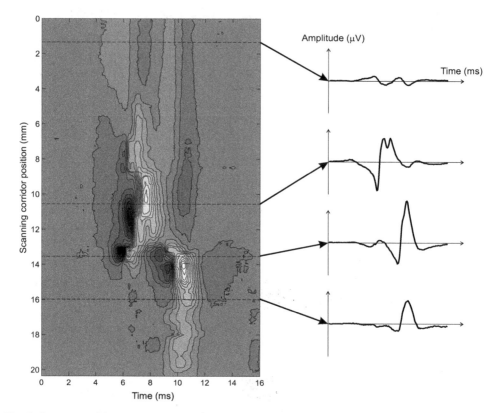

Fig. 6. A topographic representation of a scanning EMG signal in a contour plot (left) and selected MUPs at four different positions along the scanning corridor (right), with the uppermost MUP being a clear example of the cannula effect.

Once the active area of the electrode enters the motor unit territory, the recorded electric field increases and takes the shape of a conventional MUP (second to fourth MUPs in Fig. 6). Remarkably, the high variability of MUPs becomes apparent in scanning EMG recordings; as we move through the scanning corridor, the MUP waveform changes dramatically, reflecting the changes in the geometrical disposition of the set of generators, i.e., the set of motor unit fibres.

The length of the recording is characterised by regions of high activity separated by regions where the potential amplitude decays considerably. Regions of high activity are called motor unit fractions, or simply fractions, and the regions of low activity are called silent areas.

Clearly, the fractions correspond to regions close to motor unit fibres, whereas silent areas correspond to holes in the motor unit territory, or regions depleted of motor unit fibres. This arrangement of motor unit fibres, where motor unit fibres are not evenly distributed throughout the motor unit territory, is in agreement with glycogen depletion findings suggesting a certain degree of clustering of the muscle fibres within its motor unit territory (Bodine et al., 1998). Furthermore, fractions observed in scanning EMG recordings from normal muscle more commonly present distinct latencies rather than spatial separation. This observation points to the existence of different average temporal latencies of fibres belonging to different fractions (Stålberg, 1986; Navallas & Stålberg, 2009) and supports the hypothesis that each fraction represents a set of fibres innervated by a common axonal branch; therefore, the end-plates of these fibres will be in close proximity to one another compared to the overall motor end-plate zone dispersion (Stålberg, 1986; Nandedkar & Stålberg, 1986; Stålberg & Diószeghy, 1991; Navallas & Stålberg, 2009).

Sudden amplitude changes may also occur in scanning EMG profiles. These can be produced either by small uncontrolled jumps of the scanning needle or by changes in the properties of the volume conductor as the needle passes through a tendon layer or through a fascia (Stålberg & Eriksson, 1987; Diószeghy, 2002).

4.2 Analysis and parameterisation of the signal

Quantification of the EMG waveforms establishes objective criteria for comparing signals and for subsequent diagnosis. Several parameters have been proposed to quantify scanning EMG waveforms, most based on characteristics that cannot be observed in conventional EMG recordings. It is important to note that because the individual traces of scanning signals are MUPs themselves, all the conventional MUP parameters, like amplitude, area, duration, size index, etc., can be calculated in these traces. However, we will focus on specific scanning EMG parameters that exploit the two-dimensional nature of the signal and the recording through the spatial corridor.

4.2.1 Length of the motor unit cross-section

The length of the motor unit cross-section (Hilton-Brown & Stålberg, 1983a, 1983b ; Stålberg, 1986) is defined as the maximal distance between traces with amplitudes of at least 50 µV (Fig. 7). This distance represents an estimation of the length of the scanning corridor that runs inside the motor unit territory, given that as soon as the active area of the electrode enters the territory, the amplitude of the recorded MUP will exceed the 50 µV threshold. The length of the motor unit cross-section can alternatively be defined as the length between the two most distant traces with amplitudes above 15% of the maximum positive amplitude of the scan (Gootzen, 1990). However, this definition may under- or overestimate the measured length because it is relative to the amplitude of the largest MUP recorded during the scanning procedure (Stålberg & Diószeghy, 1991).

Measured length can be used as a lower bound to estimate the diameter of motor unit territories (Stålberg, 1986). It has to be noted that an actual estimation of the motor unit diameter is not feasible with this parameter, as it is not evident whether or not the recording has being done through a maximal arc of the motor unit territory bounds (Fig. 8). Statistically, the average measured length of the motor unit cross-section would be 87% of the true transverse motor unit diameter for territories with round cross-sections (Stålberg & Eriksson, 1987).

4.2.2 Number and length of silent areas

The number of silent areas (Stålberg, 1986) is defined as the number of areas within the length of a motor unit cross-section with amplitudes below 50 µV (Fig. 7). The length of the silent areas corresponds to the length measured over the cross-section of the corresponding silent areas (Stålberg and Diószeghy, 1991).

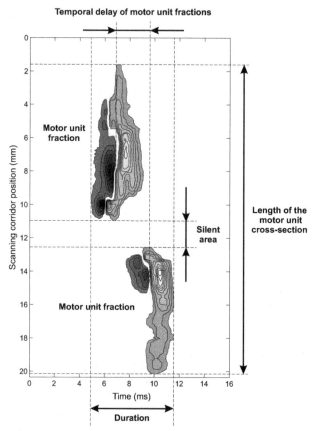

Fig. 7. Parameterisation of a scanning EMG signal after removing the signal content below the 50 μV threshold for the sake of clarity.

4.2.3 Number and length of fractions

The number of fractions (Stålberg, 1986) is defined as the number of areas within the length of a motor unit cross-section with amplitudes above 50 μV and either separated by silent areas or having clearly separated maxima along the time axis (Fig. 7). The length of the fractions corresponds to the length measured over the cross-section of the corresponding motor unit fractions (Navallas & Stålberg, 2009).

4.2.4 Number and length of polyphasic fractions

An MUP is defined a polyphasic or complex if it has more than 4 phases or more than 5 turns. Hence, the number of fractions containing polyphasic MUPs can be counted (Stålberg, 1986), and the overall length of these fractions can be measured (Stålberg & Diószeghy, 1991).

4.2.5 Temporal dispersion of fractions

The temporal dispersion of the motor unit fractions (or motor unit time dispersion) is defined as the latency difference between the earliest and latest MUP traces recorded within

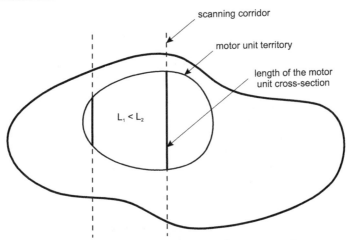

Fig. 8. An illustration of the problem regarding motor unit territory diameter estimation: how can we ensure that we are crossing a maximal arc?

a motor unit cross-section, where the latency of an MUP is measured at the steepest downward slope (Gootzen, 1990) or at the time point corresponding to 50% of the energy of the envelope signal (Navallas & Stålberg, 2009). Temporal dispersion measurements are slightly affected when the needle is not inserted orthogonally into the muscle fibres, which can produce up to 0.5 ms of error for a 20° angle deviation (Gootzen et al., 1992). It is important not to confuse this parameter with the temporal dispersion of individual SFAPs contributing to MUPs when observed from a single point (Gootzen, 1990). Rather, this parameter gives information about the average temporal dispersion of groups of SFAPs contributing to different fractions, which reside in different parts of motor unit territories and are observed essentially from different locations throughout the scanning corridor (Navallas & Stålberg, 2009).

4.2.6 Depth of the motor unit territory
Although not a parameter of a scanning EMG signal, it is important to note that the depth of the motor unit territory under study can also be estimated using the scanning procedure. A stereotactic location system can be used to assess the location of the moving EMG needle relative to the internal tendinous boundaries within the muscle under study (Tonndorf, 1994) by combining magnetic resonance imaging, scanning needle electrode optical tracking, and stereotactic reconstruction.
Furthermore, by taking into account the beginning and ending positions of the scanning electrode and the number of steps taken for each trigger, the electrode location can be estimated. Using this information, the position of the motor unit can be defined as the position in the scans corresponding to a contribution of 50% of the signal within the length of the cross-section (Roeleveld et al., 1997a, 1997b). The position of the motor unit provides an estimation of the depth of the centre of the motor unit territory.

4.3 Findings in normal conditions
A limited number of muscle types has been investigated using scanning EMG, including the biceps brachii (Hilton-Brown & Stålberg, 1983a, 1983b; Stålberg & Diószeghy, 1991; Navallas

& Stålberg, 2009), the tibialis anterior (Hilton-Brown & Stålberg, 1983a, 1983b; Stålberg & Diószeghy, 1991), the masseter (Stålberg & Eriksson, 1987), and the quadriceps (Gootzen, 1990; Gootzen et al., 1992).

The length of the motor unit cross-section has been measured in normal conditions in various muscles. In the biceps brachii, the length of the motor unit cross-section has been reported as 6.0 ± 3.9 mm (mean ± SD) (Hilton-Brown & Stålberg, 1983a, 1983b), 4.64 ± 2.14 mm with a range of 1.69 to 10.17 mm (n=59) (Stålberg & Diószeghy, 1991), and 4.39 ± 2.29 mm with a range of 1.55 to 10.70 mm (Navallas & Stålberg, 2009). In the tibial anterior, the length has been reported as 7.9 ± 1.3 mm (Hilton-Brown & Stålberg, 1983a) and 5.26 ± 2.18 mm with a range of 1.53 to 10.33 mm (n=70) (Stålberg & Diószeghy, 1991). In the masseter, the length has been reported as 3.7 ± 0.6 mm with a range of 0.6 to 12.5 mm (Stålberg & Eriksson, 1987) and 3.7 ± 2.3 mm with a range of 0.4 to 13.1 mm (Tonndorf et al, 1994b). Finally, in the quadriceps, the length has been reported with a range of 2.0 to 8.0 mm (Gootzen, 1990; Gootzen et al., 1992).

As previously stated, motor unit fractions and silent areas, which are structural properties that can only be observed using scanning EMG, suggest that adjacent motor unit fibres have adjacent motor end-plates with a lower spatial dispersion than the overall muscle motor end-plate zone width (Navallas & Stålberg, 2009). Each fibre group would correspond to a distinct axonal branch reflecting a distinct motor unit fraction in a scanning EMG recording (Stålberg, 1986; Navallas & Stålberg, 2009).

The number of fractions and silent areas gives an indication of the degree of grouping or clustering of motor unit fibres in a normal muscle. The number of fractions generally ranges from 1 to 4 fractions per scan (Stålberg, 1986), although exact counts may vary among muscles. In the biceps brachii, 3.25 ± 1.49 (mean ± SD) fractions with the range of 1 to 6 fractions (Stålberg & Diószeghy, 1991) and 1.65 ± 1.02 fractions with a range of 1 to 5 fractions (Navallas & Stålberg, 2009) have been reported. In the tibialis anterior, 3.73 ± 1.74 fractions with a range of 1 to 8 fractions have been reported (Stålberg & Diószeghy, 1991). The number of silent areas has also been measured in the biceps brachii. A mean of 0.5 silent areas (Hilton-Brown & Stålberg, 1983b) and 0.15 ± 0.36 silent areas with a range of 0 to 1 (Stålberg & Diószeghy, 1991) have been reported. In the tibialis anterior, a mean of 0.2 silent areas (Hilton-Brown & Stålberg, 1983b) and 0.19 ± 0.47 silent areas with a range of 0 to 2 (Stålberg & Diószeghy, 1991) have been reported. The length of the individual motor unit fractions in the biceps brachii has been reported as 1.56 ± 1.07 mm with a range of 0.35 to 5.10 mm (Navallas & Stålberg, 2009).

Furthermore, temporal dispersion between fractions (see section 4.2.5) has provided valuable information about innervation patterns of motor units. The temporal dispersion measured in the biceps brachii has been reported as ranging from 0.5 to 5.0 ms (Gootzen, 1990) and 0.55 ± 0.98 ms with a range of 0.01 to 4.70 ms (Navallas & Stålberg, 2009). These temporal differences can be justified by assuming 1) a variation in the depolarisation delay in different fractions due to length differences among the innervating axonal branches and/or 2) different mean motor end-plate positions along the muscle fibres (Fig. 9) (Navallas & Stålberg, 2009).

The complexity of MUPs, measured in terms of the number of phases, number of turns, or irregularity coefficient, is a key feature used to distinguish normal conditions from pathology (Zalewska et al., 2004). In scanning EMG recordings from normal muscles, the complexity parameters of individual MUP traces extracted from a scan are within the range of values of conventional multi-MUP studies. The following complexity parameters of the

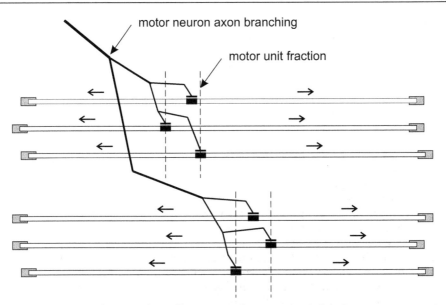

Fig. 9. The motor unit fractions hypothesis states that motor unit fractions are representing groups of motor unit fibres innervated by different axonal braches that may have a shifted motor end-plate location.

biceps brachii have been reported: a mean (± SD) of 3.26 ± 1.18 phases, a mean of 4.17 ± 1.87 turns, and an irregularity coefficient of 3.61 ± 0.82 (Navallas & Stålberg, 2009). The number of polyphasic fractions reported in the biceps brachii was 0.21 ± 0.41 with a range of 0 to 1 polyphasic sections (Stålberg & Diószeghy, 1991), and the number of polyphasic fractions reported in the tibialis anterior was 0.41 ± 0.58 with a range of 0 to 2 polyphasic sections (Stålberg & Diószeghy, 1991). Therefore, the proportion of polyphasic fractions, as the proportion of polyphasic MUPs in conventional quantitative EMG studies, is relatively low in normal conditions.

4.4 Findings in pathological conditions

In a study conducted with subjects suffering from a variety of neuropathies (including ALS, SMA, postpolio, polyneuropathy, and syringomyelia), the most relevant changes in scanning EMG recordings taken from the biceps brachii and the tibialis anterior were related to an increased complexity of motor units (Stålberg & Diószeghy, 1991). Specifically, the length of motor unit cross-sections and the number of fractions were slightly increased in both muscles, although only significant in the tibialis anterior. The number and length of silent areas were not significantly different from controls. Finally, the number and the length of polyphasic sections were significantly increased in both muscles.

These changes in scanning parameters are related to a reorganisation of motor units that occurs in neuropathies. Reorganisation is essentially due to reinnervation by collateral sprouting of surviving axons (Kugelberg et al., 1970). During reinnervation, collateral sprouts tend to be confined to the originally innervated fascicles, what derives in the observation of non increased motor unit cross-sections (Stålberg & Sanders, 1984). The increase in the number of motor unit fibres creates more compact and dense motor units;

therefore, the increase in motor unit fibres does not lead to a significant increase in silent areas or motor unit fractions (Diószeghy, 2002). However, reinnervation does cause an increase in fibre diameter variation and the dispersion of motor end-plates, which results in an increased waveform complexity throughout the region and an increased length and number of polyphasic fractions (Stålberg & Diószeghy, 1991).

Another study conducted with subjects suffering from various myopathies (including muscular dystrophies and polymyositis) found that the most relevant changes in scanning EMG recordings of the biceps brachii and the tibialis anterior were related to increased fractioning and an increased complexity of motor units (Stålberg & Diószeghy, 1991). The length of motor unit cross-sections was not significantly different from normal muscles. The number of fractions was significantly increased in both muscles. The length and number of silent areas was also significantly increased in both muscles, although more prominently in the tibialis anterior. Note that this significant change among myopathies is not identifiable using conventional EMG because, using this technique, an area with no activity cannot be ascribed to loss of muscle fibres within a given motor unit. Finally, the length and number of polyphasic sections was also significantly increased in both muscles. These results agree with previous findings in patients suffering from muscular dystrophy. The muscles of these patients showed no difference in the length of motor unit cross-sections but showed an increased number of silent areas and an increased variability in the amplitude profile and shape of scanning EMG recordings (Hilton-Brown & Stålberg, 1983a, 1983b).

Myopathic processes cause several structural changes, including fibre loss, fibre atrophy and hypertrophy, and fibre splitting (Hilton-Brown & Stålberg 1983a). Hence, an increased fibre grouping due to fibre splitting and an appearance of motor unit territories depleted of motor unit fibres explains the increased number of fractions and length and number of silent areas (Stålberg & Diószeghy, 1991; Diószeghy, 2002). The increased variability in fibre diameter due to hypertrophy and atrophy causes increased MUP complexity, which is observed as an increased length and number of the polyphasic fractions within scans (Diószeghy, 2002).

One study of juvenile myoclonic epilepsy (Gooker et al., 2009b, 2010) revealed that patients suffering from the disorder have enlarged motor unit territories compared to healthy subjects. The enlargement of motor units is not due to a reinnervation process but to a preponderance of genetically determined large lower motor units (Ertas et al., 1997).

Another study of both neuropathic and myopathic muscles (Gootzen, 1990; Gootzen et al., 1992) measured the length of motor unit cross-sections and the temporal dispersion of motor unit fractions in the biceps brachii. The results showed that scans from both patients and healthy subjects largely overlap with respect to the length of cross-sections. Both neuropathic and myopathic recordings showed an increased temporal dispersion of fractions. The temporal dispersion ranged from 0.5 ms to 6 ms in scans of healthy patients, 0.5 ms to 9 ms in scans of neuropathic patients, and 1 ms to 12.5 ms in scans of myopathic patients. Additionally, a strong positive correlation between the length of cross-sections and the temporal dispersion of the fractions was detected for the neuropathic group. Using these two parameters as a diagnostic tool, normal and pathological scans can be reliably separated, although parameters fail to distinguish between myopathy and neuropathy (Gootzen, 1990; Gootzen et al, 1992).

5. Future trends

The scanning EMG technique has evolved as a versatile and informative tool for the investigation of motor unit architecture. In combination with other EMG techniques, such as

fibre density measurements, a detailed description of motor units can be obtained using scanning EMG (Stålberg, 1986).
Further research should focus on extracting more information from the scanning signals. For example, the analysis of pathological signals suggests that parameters describing motor unit integrity, the complexity of motor end-plate zones or the variability in propagation velocities may soon be identified (Gootzen et al., 1992).
Several possible applications have been suggested in previous studies. Scanning EMG may be used to quantify the background activity of a muscle for a given degree of contraction to determine whether some regions account for many recruited motor units while others remain inactive (Stålberg, 1986). This could lead to studies relating functional compartmentalisation and recruitment strategies of muscles.
It has been also suggested that scanning EMG may be applied to verify volume conductor models by observing SFAPs (Gootzen, 1990), as scan recording profiles provide a reliable description of amplitude decay with distance. However, care must be taken to eliminate possible fibre movements to ensure there is no potential blocking.
In conclusion, scanning EMG is a valuable technique used in studies of motor unit anatomy and physiology and to study the structural and functional parameters in normal muscle and the changes that occur in pathology.

6. Acknowledgment

This work was supported by the Regional Health Ministry of the Government of Navarre under the project 1312/2010.

7. References

Amirali, A., Mu, L., Gracies, JM., & Simpson, DM. (2007) Anatomical localization of motor endplate bands in the human biceps brachii. *J Clin Neuromuscul Dis*, Vol. 9, No. 2, pp. 306-312.

Ansved, T., Wallner, P., & Larsson, L. (1991). Spatial distribution of motor unit fibres in fast- and slow-twitch rat muscles with special reference to age. *Acta Physiol Scand*, Vol. 143, No. 3, pp. 345-354.

Aquilonius, SM., Arvidsson, B., Askmark, H., & Gillberg, PG. (1982). Topographical localization of end-plates in cryosections of whole human biceps muscle. *Muscle Nerve*, Vol. 5, No. 5, pp. 418.

Bodine, SC., Garfinkel, A., Roy, RR., & Edgerton, VR. (1988). Spatial distribution of motor unit fibres in the cat soleus and tibialis anterior muscles: local interactions. *J Neurosci*, Vol. 8, No. 6, pp. 2142-2152.

Bodine-Fowler, S., Garfinkel, A., Roy, RR., & Edgerton, VR. (1990). Spatial distribution of muscle fibres within the territory of a motor unit. *Muscle Nerve*, Vol. 13, No. 12, pp. 1133-1145.

Buchthal, F., Erminio, F., & Rosenfalck, P. (1959). Motor unit territory in different human muscles. *Acta Physiol Scand*, Vol. 45, No. 1, pp. 72-87.

Buchthal, F., Guld, C., & Rosenfalck, P. (1957). Multielectrode study of the territory of a motor unit. *Acta Physiol Scand*, Vol. 39, No. 1, pp 83-104.

Burke, RE., Levine, DN., Salcman, M., Tsairis, P. (1974). Motor units in cat soleus muscle: physiological, histochemical and morphological characteristics. *J Physiol*, Vol. 238, No. 3, pp. 503-514.

Burke, RE., & Tsairis, P. (1973). Anatomy and innervation ratios in motor units of cat gastrocnemius. *J Physiol*, Vol. 234, No. 3, pp. 749-765.

Diószeghy, P. (2002). Scanning electromyography. *Muscle Nerve*, No. S11, pp. 66-71.

Edström, L., & Kugelberg, E. (1968). Histochemical composition, distribution of fibres and fatiguability of single motor units. Anterior tibial muscle of the rat. *J Neurol Neurosurg Psychiatry*, Vol. 31, No. 5, pp. 424-433.

Enoka, RM. (1995), Morphological features and activation patterns of motor units. *J Clin Neurophysiol*, Vol. 12, No. 6, pp. 538-559.

Ertas, M., Uludag, B., & Araç, N., Ertekin, C., & Stålberg E. (1997). A special kind of anterior horn cell involvement in juvenile myoclonic epilepsy demonstrated by macro electromyography. *Muscle Nerve*, Vol. 20, No. 2, pp. 148-152.

Feinstein, B., Lindegard, B., Nyman, E., & Wohlfart, G. (1955). Morphologic studies of motor units in normal human muscles. *Acta Anat (Basel)*, Vol. 23, No. 2, pp. 127-142.

Garnett, RAF., O'Donovan, MJ., Stephens, JA., & Taylor, A. (1979). Motor unit organization of human medial gastrocnemius. *J Physiol*, Vol. 287, pp. 33-43.

Gates, HJ., & Betz, WJ. (1993). Spatial distribution of muscle fibers in a lumbrical muscle of the rat. *Anat Rec*, Vol. 236, No. 2, pp. 381-389.

Gath, I., & Stålberg, E. (1979). Measurements of the uptake area of small-size electromyographic electrodes. *IEEE Trans Biomed Eng*, Vol. 26, No. 6, pp. 374-376.

Gath, I., & Stålberg, E. (1981). In situ measurement of the innervation ratio of motor units in human muscles. *Exp Brain Res*, Vol. 43, No. 3-4, pp. 377-382.

Gath, I., & Stålberg, E. (1982). On the measurement of fibre density in human muscles. *Electroencephalogr Clin Neurophysiol*, Vol. 54, No. 6, pp. 699-706.

Goker, I., Baslo, MB., Ertas, M., & Ulgen, Y. (2009a). Design of an experimental system for scanning electromyography method to investigate alterations of motor units in neurological disorders. *Digest Journal of Nanomaterials and Biostructures*, Vol. 4, No.1, pp. 133-139

Goker, I., Baslo, MB., Ertas, M., & Ulgen, Y. (2009b). Motor unit territories in juvenile myoclonic epilepsy patients. *Conf Proc IEEE Eng Med Biol Soc*, 2009, pp. 819-822.

Goker, I., Baslo, MB., Ertas, M., & Ulgen, Y. (2010). Large motor unit territories by scanning electromyography in patients with juvenile myoclonic epilepsy. *J Clin Neurophysiol*, Vol. 27, No. 3, pp. 212-215.

Gollnick, PD., Armstrong, RB., Saubert, CW., Sembrowich, WL., Shepherd, RE., & Saltin, B. (1973). Glycogen depletion patterns in human skeletal muscle fibers during prolonged work. *Pflugers Arch*, Vol. 344, No. 1, pp. 1-12.

Gootzen, TH. (1990). *Electrophysiological investigation of motor unit structure by means of scanning EMG*, University of Nijmegen, ISBN 90-9003335-1, Nijmegen.

Gootzen, TH., Vingerhoets, DJ., & Stegeman, DF. (1992). A study of motor unit structure by means of scanning EMG. *Muscle Nerve*, Vol. 15, No.3, pp. 349-357.

Hilton-Brown, P., & Stålberg, E. (1983a). The motor unit in muscular dystrophy, a single fibre EMG and scanning EMG study. *J Neurol Neurosurg Psychiatry*, Vol. 46, No. 11, pp. 981-995.

Hilton-Brown, P., & Stålberg, E. (1983b). Motor unit size in muscular dystrophy, a macro EMG and scanning EMG study. *J Neurol Neurosurg Psychiatry*, Vol. 46, No. 11, pp. 996-1005.

Kanda, K., & Hashizume, K. (1992). Factors causing difference in force output among motor units in the rat medial gastrocnemius muscle. *J Physiol,* Vol. 448, pp. 677-695.

Kugelberg, E., Edström, L., & Abbruzzese, M. (1970). Mapping of motor unit in experimentally reinnervated rat muscle. *J Neurol Neurosurg Psychiatry,* Vol. 197, No. 33, pp. 319-329.

Lieber, RL. (1992). *Skeletal Muscle Structure and Function: Implications for Rehabilitation and Sports Medicine* (1st ed.), Williams and Wilkins, ISBN 978-0683050264, London.

Lukács, M., Vécsei, L., & Beniczky, S. (2009). Fibre density of the motor units recruited at high and low force output. *Muscle Nerve,* Vol. 40, No. 1, pp. 112-114.

McComas, AJ., Fawcett, PR., Campbell, MJ., & Sica, RE. (1971). Electrophysiological estimation of the number of motor units within a human muscle. *J Neurol Neurosurg Psychiatry,* Vol. 34, No. 2, pp. 121-131.

Miller-Larsson, A. (1980). A model of spatial distribution of muscle fibres of a motor unit in normal human limb muscles. *Electromyogr Clin Neurophysiol,* Vol. 20, No. 4-5, pp. 281-298.

Monti, RJ., Roy, RR., & Edgerton, VR. (2001). Role of motor unit structure in defining function. *Muscle Nerve,* Vol. 24, No. 7, pp. 848-866.

Nandedkar, SD., Barkhaus, PE., Sanders, DB., & Stålberg, EV. (1988a). Analysis of amplitude and area of concentric needle EMG motor unit action potentials. *Electroencephalogr Clin Neurophysiol,* Vol. 69, No. 6, pp. 561-567.

Nandedkar, SD., Sanders, DB., Stålberg, EV., & Andreassen, S. (1988b). Simulation of concentric needle EMG motor unit action potentials. *Muscle Nerve,* Vol. 11, No. 2, pp. 151-159.

Nandedkar, SD., & Stålberg, E. (1983a). Simulation of single muscle fibre action potentials. *Med Biol Eng Comput,* Vol. 21, No. 2, pp. 158-165.

Nandedkar, SD., & Stålberg, E. (1983b). Simulation of macro EMG motor unit potentials. *Electroencephalogr Clin Neurophysiol,* Vol. 56, No. 1, pp. 52-62.

Navallas, J., & Stålberg, E. (2009). Studying motor end-plate topography by means of scanning electromyography. *Clin Neurophysiol,* Vol. 120, No. 7, pp. 1335-1341.

Pfeiffer, G., & Friede, RL. (1985). The localization of axon branchings in two muscle nerves of the rat. A contribution to motor unit topography. *Anat Embryol (Berl),* Vol. 172, No. 2, pp. 177-182.

Pfeiffer, G., & Kunze, K. (1992). Turn and phase counts of individual motor unit potentials: correlation and reliability. *Electroencephalogr Clin Neurophysiol.* Vol. 85, No. 3, pp. 161-165.

Rafuse, VF., & Gordon, T. (1996). Self-reinnervated cat medial gastrocnemius muscles. II. analysis of the mechanisms and significance of fiber type grouping in reinnervated muscles. *J Neurophysiol,* Vol. 75, No. 1, pp. 282-297.

Roeleveld, K., Stegeman, DF., Vingerhoets, HM., & Van Oosterom, A. (1997a). Motor unit potential contribution to surface electromyography. *Acta Physiol Scand,* Vol. 160, No. 2, pp. 175-183.

Roeleveld, K., Stegeman, DF., Vingerhoets, HM., & Van Oosterom, A. (1997b). The motor unit potential distribution over the skin surface and its use in estimating the motor unit location. *Acta Physiol Scand,* Vol. 161, No. 4, pp. 465-472.

Roy, RR., Garfinkel, A., Ounjian, M., Payne, J., Hirahara, A., Hsu, E., & Edgerton, VR. (1995). Three-dimensional structure of cat tibialis anterior motor units. *Muscle Nerve*, Vol. 18, No. 10, pp. 1187-1195.

Schwartz, MS., Stålberg, E., Schiller, HH., & Thiele, B. (1976). The reinnervated motor unit in man. A single fibre EMG multielectrode investigation. *J Neurol Sci*, Vol. 27, No. 3, pp. 303-312.

Stålberg, E. (1966). Propagation velocity in human muscle fibers in situ. *Acta Physiol Scand*, Suppl. 287, pp. 1-112.

Stålberg, E. (1980). Macro EMG, a new recording technique. *J Neurol Neurosurg Psychiatry*, Vol. 43, No. 6, pp. 475-482.

Stålberg, E. (1986). Single fibre EMG, macro EMG, and scanning EMG. New ways of looking at the motor unit. *CRC Crit Rev Clin Neurobiol*, Vol. 2, No. 2, pp. 125-167.

Stålberg, E., & Antoni, L. (1980). Electrophysiological cross section of the motor unit. *J Neurol Neurosurg Psychiatry*, Vol. 43, No. 6, pp. 469-474.

Stålberg, E., & Dioszeghy, P. (1991). Scanning EMG in normal muscle and in neuromuscular disorders. *Electroencephalogr Clin Neurophysiol*, Vol. 81, No. 6, pp. 403-416.

Stålberg, E., & Eriksson, PO. (1987). A scanning electromyographic study of the topography of human masseter single motor units. *Arch Oral Biol*, Vol. 32, No. 11, pp. 793-797.

Stålberg, E., & Fawcett, PR. (1982). Macro EMG in healthy subjects of different ages. *J Neurol Neurosurg Psychiatry*, Vol. 45, No. 10, pp. 870-878.

Stålberg, E., & Karlsson, L. (2001). Simulation of the normal concentric needle electromyogram by using a muscle model. *Clin Neurophysiol*, Vol. 112, No. 3, pp. 464-471.

Stålberg, E., & Sanders, DB. (1984). The motor unit in ALS studied with different neurophysiological techniques, In: *Research Progress in Motor Neurone Disease*, pp. 105-122, FC Rose (Ed), Pitman Books, London.

Stålberg, E., Schwartz, MS., Thiele, B., & Schiller, HH. (1976). The normal motor unit in man. A single fibre EMG multielectrode investigation. *J Neurol Sci*, Vol. 27, No. 3, pp. 291-301.

Sonoo, M., & Stålberg, E. (1993). The ability of MUP parameters to discriminate between normal and neurogenic MUPs in concentric EMG: analysis of the MUP "thickness" and the proposal of "size index". *Electroencephalogr Clin Neurophysiol*, Vol. 89, No. 5, pp. 291-303.

Tonndorf, ML., & Hannam, AG. (1994). Motor unit territory in relation to tendons in the human masseter muscle. *Muscle Nerve*, Vol. 17, No. 4, pp. 436-443.

Venema, HW. (1994). Motor unit innervation patterns and fiber type grouping. *Muscle Nerve*, Vol. 17, No. 3, pp. 360-362.

Weijs, WA., Jüch, PJ., Kwa, SH., & Korfage, JA. (1993). Motor unit territories and fiber types in rabbit masseter muscle. *J Dent Res*, Vol. 72, No. 11, pp. 1491-1498.

Willison, RG. (1964). Analysis of electrical activity in healthy and dystrophyic muscle in man. *J Neurol Neurosurg Psychiatry*, Vol. 27, No. 5, pp. 386-394.

Willison, RG. (1980). Arrangement of muscle fibers of a single motor unit in mammalian muscles. *Muscle Nerve*, Vol. 3, No. 4, pp. 360-361.

Zalewska, E., & Hausmanowa-Petrusewicz, I. (1995). Evaluation of MUAP shape irregularity--a new concept of quantification. *IEEE Trans Biomed Eng*, Vol. 42, No. 6, pp. 616-620.

Zalewska, E., Husmanova-Petrusewicz, I., & Stålberg, E. (2004). Modeling studies on irregular motor unit potentials. *Clin Neurophysiol*, Vol. 115, No. 1, pp. 543-556.

10

Man to Machine, Applications in Electromyography

Michael Wehner

Wehner Engineering, Berkeley,
USA

1. Introduction

The study of electrical signals due to muscle activation has been evolving since Francesco Redi found electrical generation in the muscles of the electric ray fish in 1666 (Fishman, Wilkins, 2011), Dubois discovered electrical activation in voluntary muscles in 1849 (Blanc, Dimanico, 2010), and Mari coined the term Electromyography in 1922 (Raz, et al., 2006). Evolving over the following decades, electromyography has found widespread use in clinical settings as well as extensive use in ergonomic assessment and biomechanics research laboratories.

As with many technologies, the discovery of electromyography occurred long before inexpensive and robust hardware was developed to utilize the vast amount of information available from myoelectric signals. Until recently, existing technology could not support efficient generation of repeatable robust signals for even highly sophisticated research laboratories, let alone the widespread availability of affordable, robust hardware required to propagate electromyography through the research communities. New high-speed computation tools make real-time analysis feasible. With the emergence of low cost hardware, high speed wireless communication technology, and low cost, high speed computing/signal processing equipment, Electromyography is becoming available to a whole new set of experimenter. With these advances making electromyography a feasible option in many situations, we see the emergence of a key period in the evolution of the technology. Surface electromyography (sEMG) provides a convenient and relatively non-invasive avenue for determining muscle activation, particularly as highly portable devices become available. Of course with the benefits of wider availability, we must consider the risks inherent in this spread, as the practitioners involved move from electromyography specialists, to technologists in other fields, using electromyography either part time, or only occasionally. Electromyography is a detailed art, and can easily lead to erroneous conclusions if not practiced carefully. With new applications, particularly where electromyography is employed as a means for humans to control electromechanical systems, care must be taken to insure that these systems are developed with robust safety systems, and improper assumptions about electromyography do not cause harm, injury, or even death.

2. Background

Recognized as a potentially powerful tool EMG was first used in measuring human movement at the turn of the 20th century (Medved, 2001). As use spread, techniques for recording, processing, and interpreting EMG signals varied widely. With a lack of standardization, various styles developed and the discipline became an art as much as it was a science (De Luca, 1997).Efforts have been underway to standardize the EMG process, with considerable efforts in the past decade to implement standards which 1) formalize scientific understanding of the concepts behind EMG (De Luca, 1997), 2) allow interpretation and repetition of previously published results (Hermens, et al., 2000) , and 3) provide standards going forward for generating as well as publishing EMG data (Hermens, et al., 2000). In the following sections, three major efforts to standardize the EMG recording, processing, interpreting, and publishing procedures are discussed

2.1 What is electromyography?

Muscle cells are surrounded by a selectively permeable membrane with a resting electrical potential of 70 to 90 millivolts. The outside of the cell is positive relative to the inside. Motoneurons carry impulses from the central nervous system to the muscle cells called the nerve action potential (NAP). All muscle cells (or fibers) innervated by one motoneuron are called a motor unit, and are stimulated simultaneously when the motoneuron fires. The muscle fibers of one motor unit are not bundled within a muscle. Rather they are spread throughout the muscle with a relatively uniform distribution. When a series of NAP's reach the cells of a muscle unit they cause a release of chemical transmitters which depolarize the cell to a threshold value, initiating an action potential as the cell wall permeability changes. This depolarization causes a brief contraction, or twitch, of the muscle cell (and all other cells in that motor unit) and comprises the basis of muscle movement. The depolarization that travels along the muscle fiber and can be detected on the surface of the muscle as a small electrical potential called the muscle action potential (MAP). Each muscle is comprised of many muscle motor units, which are comprised of many cells, and are connected to many motoneurons, thus a seemingly simple muscle contraction will correspond to a complex overall MAP waveform. An electrode properly positioned with respect to the muscle can record these MAP waveforms. The sensing and recording of these electrical waveforms is called electromyography (EMG). Though a motor unit is either on or off, based on whether or not it is being stimulated by a NAP, an increase in muscle tension beyond that caused by a single NAP can occur either from multiple NAPs stimulating the same motor unit, or from recruitment of additional motor units. Fortunately, both phenomena cause an increase in overall MAP waveform amplitude, corresponding to an increased EMG signal (Chaffin, Andersson, 1999). Properly recorded and processed EMG signal is known to correlate to muscle activation level, and in some cases can be used to determine muscle tension (De Luca, 1997). EMG recordings can be done through two basic methods; 1) Intramuscular, where needle based electrodes are inserted through the skin into the muscle of interest, or 2) Surface, where flat electrodes are adhered to the skin surface above the muscle of interest. Intramuscular EMG is the preferred method when measuring small muscles, particularly those surrounded by large muscles which may prevent accurate recording of the signal of interest or when attempting to measure only a few motor units. Surface EMG is preferred when studying large muscles, especially those near the surface and with few large muscles nearby. An added advantage of surface EMG is that the electrodes are adhered to the skin surface, thus piercing of the skin is not required.

2.2 EMG, proper signal detection and processing

In the Journal of Applied Biomechanics, De Luca details the factors affecting EMG signal and proper procedure for detecting and processing the signal (De Luca, 1997). These discussions are followed by a summary of recommendations in the use of EMG. In most biomechanics applications, EMG is used in three areas, 1) to identify the initiation of muscle activity, 2) as a surrogate for estimating muscle tension (force), and 3) as a method for estimating muscle fatigue. In this discussion we cover applications involving filtered and processed EMG signals, thus initiation and fatigue will serve only as tertiary topics of discussion, with the focus of this chapter on muscle activation level. In detecting and recording an EMG signal with maximum fidelity and minimum noise, one must consider a number of factors.

- Electrode configuration. This includes shape and area, material, and inter-electrode distance (IED) which determines the number of motor units being detected. Also to be considered are location of the electrodes on the muscle, laterally and longitudinally. This effects the amplitude and frequency of the signal detected as well as the level of cross-talk from other nearby muscle groups. An appropriate IED should be chosen which is small enough to minimize crosstalk, yet large enough to minimize risk of shunting (electrical contact between electrodes, in effect making them one larger electrode and reducing signal amplitude and signal to noise ratio).

- Intrinsic (muscle) factors. This includes the number of active motor units at any time, fiber type of the muscle, blood flow to the muscle, fiber diameter, and the depth of active muscle fibers. These considerations can affect amplitude and frequency characteristics of muscle response. Also of consideration are the amount and type of tissue between the muscle surface and the electrode. Signal may experience considerable spatial filtering due to interstitial tissue.

- Intermediate factors. These effects include electromechanical properties of the electrodes, and their ability to act as band-pass filters or integrators, and the tendency to record cross-talk from other muscles. Also of concern is the conduction velocity of action potentials and spatial filtering effects of relative electrode-muscle fiber position, as these tend to affect amplitude and frequency characteristics of an EMG signal. This is particularly important when considering anisometric EMG, as EMG signal varies as muscle fibers change in length.

- Deterministic factors. This includes the number of active and detected motor units, motor unit force twitch, fiber interaction, firing rate, characteristics of the action potentials, and recruitment characteristics.

- Other interstitial tissue properties. It can be understood that the movement of subcutaneous tissues including muscle and fat can cause signals erroneously. These signals should be considered in EMG data as a source of artifact error.

The recorded EMG signal can be used to determine muscle activation level in many situations and even to determine muscle force in some cases. These relationships are not automatic however, and care must be taken to design the experiment correctly and to draw only appropriate conclusions from the data. For the isometric case, the amplitude of the EMG signal is understood to increase with muscle force. This qualitative relationship however can not be extrapolated to a force magnitude for one subject or especially as a force comparison or magnitude measurement from subject to subject. In order to make force predictions or make comparison between subjects, EMG signals must be normalized to some applied force. This is usually done normalizing to maximum contraction of the muscle (MVC 100%) or to a reference voluntary exertion (RVE). Additionally, every time an electrode is moved (between sessions or simply due to electrode dislodging) normalization must be repeated. When electrodes are placed, no matter how carefully, they cover a slightly different set of motor units. As the muscle units under study and the spatial filtering characteristics will change with the new electrode placement, they will yield a slightly or even substantially different signal. Also, if the joint angle changes, the location of the electrodes relative to the muscle belly change. In comparing signals between subjects, the amount of subcutaneous fatty tissue can vary substantially and becomes a major concern. De Luca warns that all of these issues become magnified, and new issues arise when dynamic EMG is considered.

Several recommendations are given and are listed in an abridged form below.

- The preferred electrode configuration (general, not muscle specific) consists of two parallel bars, 1cm by 1-2 mm wide placed 1 cm apart, which record at a bandwidth 20-500 Hz.
- Locate the electrodes on the midline of the muscle belly.
- Use the RMS value of the signal for measuring amplitude of the EMG signal.
- Measure activation time of all contractions.
- Check for crosstalk
- Quantitative comparisons between EMG signals are to be performed in static cases only, and require additional precautions and procedures.
- Instantaneous EMG signals should be treated as stochastic. To obtain a force-EMG relationship, signal should be filtered over a 1 second window, among other precautions.
- In constant force isometric contractions, motor units should not be near their threshold.
- Avoid measurement of anisometric contractions. Additional considerations are required.
- Normalize EMG at values less than 80% of maximum voluntary contraction (MVC), but calibrate between electrode placements and between subjects at MVC.

2.3 EMG, and SENIAM (surface EMG for a non-invasive assessment of muscles)

European group SENIAM has a specific objective of creating collaboration, developing recommendations on sensors, sensor placement, signal processing and modeling. From 1996 – 1999, a major effort was conducted to scan the literature for existing surface-electromyography (SEMG) work, contact these researchers for details and clarifications on their SEMG work, and develop recommendations for SEMG in the future (Hermens, et al., 2000). This effort yielded results showing the breadth of hardware and procedures used, as well as those that were most common.

Based on this research as well as parallel investigation into optimum properties (as opposed to the most commonly reported ones discussed above), SENIAM generated the following recommendations for SEMG.

- There is no recommendation regarding electrode shape, but the size of the electrode should not exceed 10 mm in the direction of the muscle fiber.
- IED should be 20 mm, but this should be reduced for small muscles.
- Pre-gelled Ag/AgCl electrodes are recommended.
- Skin at the sensor location is to be shaved if covered with hair and is to be cleaned with alcohol prior to adhering the sensors.
- SENIAM refers to their CD data for proper subject posture during sensor attachment for specific muscles. This is also the case with determining proper sensor location on specific muscles.

2.4 Standards for reporting EMG data, ISEK

The International Society of Electrophysiology and Kinesiology (ISEK) has endorsed standards for reporting EMG data, and have published them in the Journal of Electromyography and Kineseology (Merletti, 1999). Standards applicable to the experiments conducted here are summarized below.

- Electrode material, shape, and size should be reported.
- Skin and electrode preparation should be given, including abrasion, shaving, cleaning, and use of gel or paste.
- Electrode orientation and location over the muscle should be given.
- Detection details, including gain range used should be given.
- Filtering details, hardware and software, should be given, and amplifier filters should be in the range of high pass 5 Hz, and low pass 500 Hz.
- If rectification and smoothing occur in hardware prior to sampling and storing data, sampling rates can be reduced to 50 – 100 Hz.
- Description of the A/D card used should be given.
- If the Mean Average Value (MAV) of the rectified signal over time T is used, then T should be given.
- EMG values should be normalized about MVC, and conditions should be described.
- When normalizing, the following information should be provided: Training, rate of rise of force, velocity of shortening or lengthening and range of angles if not isometric, load in non-isometric contractions.
- Efforts should be taken to determine that crosstalk did not contaminate the signal. And care should be taken in areas with subcutaneous adipose tissue (body fat).

In reviewing the recommendations from these sources, and especially when comparing them to published experiments, one sees some ambiguity and even some conflicting recommendations. For the most part, however, the guidelines allow the design of well organized experiments, and data can be taken with considerable confidence as to standards and repeatability. In using these agreed upon methods, EMG based devices and applications can anticipate good, robust, and recognizable result. These relatively consistent results can be used to control an array of devices.

As discussed above, EMG data is not a reliable method of predicting forces during individual events within a short task, because EMG signals do not correlate with muscle forces on a real time basis, and individual event measurement is understood as stochastic data only. De Luca expressed concern over the repeatability of tests based on calibration around maximum voluntary contraction and the consistency of subjects applying a truly maximum contraction. Depending on the application, calibration based on maximum or reference contractions are of varying importance. In many applications, truly real-time event recognition may not be necessary, so filtering over a relatively long timeframe (hundreds of milliseconds) may be perfectly acceptable. In other applications, higher speed may be necessary, but accuracy of signal magnitude may be of low concern. In such applications, different approaches to interpreting myoelectric signals should be undertaken. For yet other applications, very little lag is permissible, and high signal fidelity is also required. For such applications, EMG may not currently be the optimum sensing tool. As with most design projects, clearly understanding the parameters and scope of the endeavor is key to developing a successful device or tool. So while standards are in place for interpreting myoelectric signals, proper care and design structure is required to insure the best possible results.

3. Chapter organization

Electromyography is being used in a myriad of evolutionary and revolutionary ways, both alone and in conjunction with other technologies. Along with the widespread availability of high speed, robust computing and sensing equipment at a relatively low cost, EMG is pushing the forefront of human machine interface. We discuss several of the interesting applications of EMG, including current and emerging areas of EMG use, as well as mixed-use applications in which EMG is used in conjunction with other technologies to yield a suite of sensors providing robust signals for the application at hand. Next, we cover possible future applications of EMG, and we discuss the relative merits and cautions of using EMG in various applications.

4. Methods of utilizing EMG in engineering devices

Electromyography can be used in many ways for various applications, with various techniques and concerns corresponding to each new application. This chapter covers five of the most common methods of employing EMG. Each technique has advantages and disadvantages to be explored or avoided based on the specific application.

Methods of using EMG in engineering applications:

Method 1. Sense and emulate/amplify. Here, Electromyography is used to sense the activity of a muscle and the myoelectric signal is processed in order to determine an activation magnitude as a function of time. This magnitude is then used to determine a target force, position, or motion of a worn mechanical device emulating, or actually worn over the same limb. In this method, the myoelectric signal is interpreted in order to determine a discrete magnitude, not a target threshold value. This method is used in controlling the HAL exoskeleton discussed later (Kasaoka, Sankai, 2001)

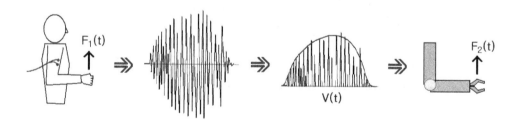

Fig. 1. Method 1 Schematic.

Method 2. Sense and interpret, proportional. Similar to method one, EMG is used to determine activation level of a muscle as a function of time. Rather than interpreting the signal in order to control a local device and directly emulate the limb being sensed, this method interprets the signal in order to provide input to another device, either locally or remotely. Signal strength is used to interpret a desired magnitude (such as speed, lift force, grip strength) For example, a prosthetic arm can not use EMG signals from the missing limb (an exception to this, using the emerging TMR techniques, will be discussed later in the chapter) but can be controlled by sensing the activity of other muscles. Likewise, myoelectric signals can be used as an input source for other devices, either locally or remotely. In this method, as in method one, signal strength is interpreted to determine a magnitude which changes over time rather than a threshold value.

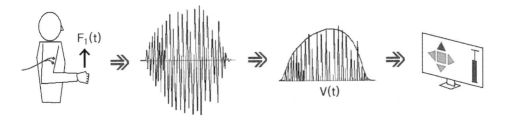

Fig. 2. Method 2 Schematic.

Method 3. Sense and interpret, threshold. A myoelectric signal is read, processed, and compared to a predetermined threshold value. When that value is reached, a condition is considered satisfied. Rather than interpreting a signal to determine a curvilinear magnitude with respect to time, this application is more similar to an on-off switch. EMG signal can be used to signal stop-go, open-close, or other two state situations. Other configurations such as three state situations or any number of two state situations are also possible. The matrix of possible states available is limited only by the number of EMG channels available, and user skill/endurance in operating the device. A simple two or three state device offers the advantage of being easier to operate and has a faster learning curve. This method is used in some prosthetic devices and is believed to cause less fatigue for users than the proportional control in method 2 when the system is designed properly with this goal in mind. This advantage is possible because with the threshold value technique, the controlling muscle is not required to maintain a consistent activation level to maintain the device state.

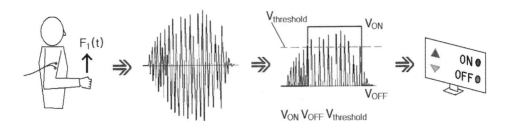

Fig. 3. Method 3 Schematic.

Method 4. Monitor to design. EMG signals are recorded and evaluated during the design and development phases of a device in order to optimize device effectiveness. After development is completed, the EMG tools are no longer used on the device. This use of EMG may be completely transparent to the end user or purchaser of the retail device. This method was used in the development of the Berkeley Lifting Exoskeleton device to evaluate the effectiveness of the device in reducing activation levels in the muscles of the lower back during lifting (Wehner, et al., 2009).

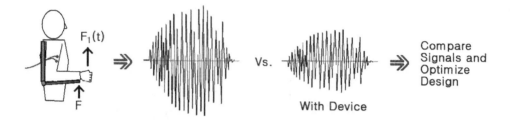

Fig. 4. Method 4 Schematic.

Method 5. Monitor to evaluate. EMG technology is used to study muscle activation levels and report on the effectiveness of a device after it has been designed, and possibly after it is already commercially available. In devices, procedures, or workplace layouts developed to reduce operator exertion or injury, this method can be used alone or with other tools such as surveys to gather data. In some of these cases, EMG was not used during the development of the device, and the developer may not even be aware of EMG technology or its use in evaluating the design. Ergonomic evaluations often fall under this method (Ulrey, Fathallah, 2011).

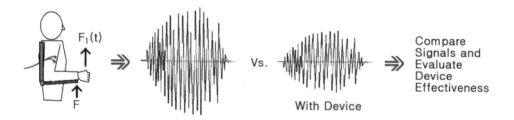

Fig. 5. Method 5 Schematic.

5. On-body devices (worn devices, human exoskeletons, and prosthetics)

Electromyography lends itself especially well to use in on-body devices, as the devices are by definition local to the user. In some applications, EMG provides a particularly intuitive and convenient interface, as the device is intended to perform an action very similar to the motion of the wearer. Because surface EMG is less invasive than some other options, it has natural advantages in non-clinical settings. EMG also has the advantage that the hardware required to record and process myoelectric signals can be relatively small and light, making it more convenient than other sensors which would be awkward or impossible to incorporate into mobile devices (MRI, fMRI). Because EMG electrodes are placed locally, it can anticipate a greater user acceptance than a full EEG sensor array, designed to cover the user's head. Social acceptance can be a considerable block to device use, so eliminating the requirement of wearing a sensor network on one's head can greatly affect a devices widespread success.

5.1 Human exoskeletons

Human exoskeletons have undergone rapid development recently, and are enjoying a surge in popularity. With the wide variety of applications for which human exoskeletons are utilized, use of EMG can fall under any of the five methods discussed earlier. For re-ambulation of patients with reduced ability due to illness or advanced age, method one can be the most suitable technology. To amplify the efforts of able bodied workers, providing additional strength, reach, or range of motion, method one may also be a valuable method and additional features can even be employed in which the wearer controls an additional device utilizing methods two or three. For paraplegic patients with no muscle signal to measure, or patients with other disorders causing spastic muscle behavior, method one would be an inappropriate and possibly dangerous choice. Many exoskeleton designs can utilize method four during the design optimization process or method five after development is complete. As with any application, the appropriate parameters must be set prior to deciding on a method.

The selection of muscle to measure and electrode placement is critical to effective use of EMG for exoskeleton and machine control, particularly if a worn device is intended to perform such complex tasks as interpreting a wearer's intent. A selection of muscles and sensor locations must maximize signal strength, and minimize noise/crosstalk. Additionally, the design must maximize sensitivity to desired signals, yet insure maximum specificity, and not read undesired signals as intended commands. In addition, the decision regarding sensor placement must consider variability in wearer physiology as well as gait variations. Body shapes and sizes vary and have a vastly varying amount of adipose tissue interfering with proper EMG sensing. Additionally, any electrode placement should not be overly invasive, cause discomfort, and can not obstruct proper use of the device. These often competing concerns make EMG sensor placement a difficult task. For example, perhaps the most readily measurable muscle contains high signal variability (false positives), and the most predictive muscle (both sensitivity and specificity) is either small, difficult to reach, or surrounded by larger muscles. Zhen, Songli, Yanan, and Jinwu discuss the relative merits of using sEMG signals of four ankle muscles for gait analysis and control (Zhen, Songli, 2007). The following is a discussion of some human exoskeleton projects, and their use of EMG.

5.1.1 Berkeley exoskeleton (BLEEX, Austin, HULC, etc)

The exoskeleton systems developed at the University of California at Berkeley are used for a variety of applications and come in both active and passive versions (application based). The Lifting Exoskeleton project employs a passive device, as it is used to reduce back forces in able bodied workers during lifting (Wehner, 2009). The Austin, medical exoskeleton, however, is active as it re-ambulates patients with no use of their lower extremities. Intended for paraplegic users, the Austin project would not be a suitable candidate for the direct use of EMG for control. Other exoskeletons, BLEEX, ExoClimber and HULC, are active exoskeleton systems, intended to amplify the movements and abilities of able-bodied users. While not using EMG for sensing or control, and not using EMG during development, method five is still a viable candidate for further experimentation, and can be incorporated with other techniques such as VO2 monitor and treadmill tests. Passive ExoHiker, shown below, uses active damping control based on stride, and swing/stance gait phase to support heavy weight, but actuation is performed by the able bodied wearer. This exoskeleton system does not use EMG for sensing or control, but could utilize method five during future experiments. The Lifting Exoskeleton project used EMG by method four to monitor and evaluate the device during design, development, and testing (Wehner, 2009). The device was developed as a research platform, intended to generate data which will serve as a knowledge base for the development of an eventual low-cost passive device to reduce back forces. It was never anticipated that the final device would include EMG capability.

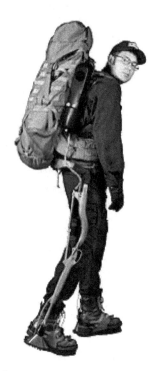

Fig. 6. Berkeley ExoHiker exoskeleton.

On the Lifting Exoskeleton project, a passive exoskeleton based device was developed to reduce back forces during lifting. During device development, a variety of techniques were used to optimize the design balancing effectiveness at reducing forces and user comfort. The device featured a spectrum of adjustable features including adjustable size of various features for wearers of varying height and body type. Additionally, the device featured adjustable overall restoring force, adjustable onset angle, and adjustable restoring moment profile, allowing wearers to vary the amount of restoring moment provided in various portions of the squat-lift cycle. Key techniques employed in optimizing the design were human subject comfort surveys, video motion tracking, force plate based lift analysis, and surface EMG, used during static squat postures and dynamic squat lifting. sEMG was used to track the activity of the lumbar erector spinae muscles during repeated lifting of objects with and without the assistance of the device. Use of these techniques facilitated tuning of the device using a variable stiffness spring profile, yielding a reduction of erector spinae muscle activity (as measured by EMG) of 27 to 52%. Tests were conducted in dynamic squat-lift scenarios as well as static squat-sustain postures. This allowed the utilization of the benefits of static EMG (well understood muscle contraction correlation, averaging over long periods, minimal electrode-to-muscle relative motion), but also generated valuable data over more realistic dynamic tasks. Issues such as crosstalk, relative muscle movement, and inability to determine momentary muscle activation were considered individually during experiment design, as should be done by any EMG practitioner.

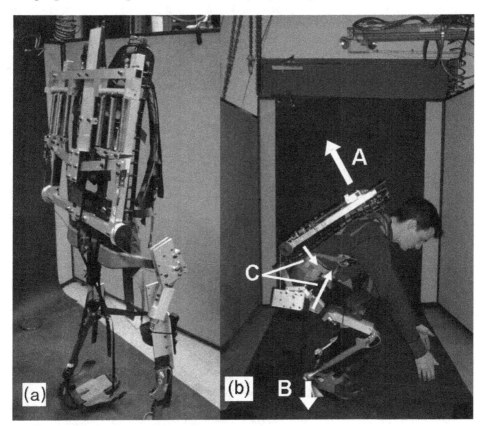

Fig. 7. Berkeley lifting exoskeleton. (a) device. (b) the device with a wearer in squat position. Forces illustrated.

5.1.2 HAL (hybrid assistive limb) exoskeleton by cyberdine
The HAL system by cyberdine (Kasaoka, Sankai, 2001) uses a number of innovative techniques in order to allow the device to function using EMG method one described above. Due to the inherent sensitivities, requirements, and considerations with EMG, specifically high noise rate, muscle movement relative to skin, and difficulty in determining momentary events (detailed in the background section), direct sensing-actuating can not be conducted with the confidence required of such a fault-intolerant application as bipedal walking. For this reason, HAL uses an assortment of techniques to anticipate user actions, adapt to each user's gait, and vary impedance in the knees of the HAL device. (Lee, Sankai, 2002). It is believed that the human limb moves most efficiently at its natural frequency, thus HAL uses

the natural frequency/pendulum model to determine initial settings for the device, modifying the dynamics based on user behavior and EMG signal based feedback (Lee, Sankai, 2003). These techniques utilize known characteristics of EMG signals, standard human gait and gait variation, using a recursive least square (RLS) technique to optimize HAL's gait and impedance realtime. These techniques allow a more natural gait, reduced energy consumption by the exoskeleton device, a robust sensing/actuation loop, and reduced energy expenditure by the user (Kawamoto, Suwoong, 2003). Further refinement, including correlation between a large amount of data from many gait studies by biomedical research groups has allowed the HAL project to develop a calibration algorithm, further developing the natural gait capabilities based solely on sensors onboard the exoskeleton system (Fleischer, Hommel, 2008), and based mainly on surface EMG signals.

5.1.3 Other exoskeletons
Though the above exoskeletons use EMG for design optimization and force amplification, several exoskeleton devices are not currently using these methods. The Sarcos/Raytheon exoskeleton (Sarcos, 2011) MIT exoskeleton (MIT, 2011) and the Berkeley BLEEX exoskeleton (BLEEX, 2011) use direct force control to sense/anticipate user intention. Use of EMG for gait control is an exceedingly difficult task, as seen by the HAL system. Despite not using EMG to directly control the motion the exoskeleton actuators, these exoskeleton systems can incorporate EMG into the development and refinement of their devices (methods 4 and 5). There is no indication if such efforts are currently underway.

5.2 Lift assist devices
Numerous knee-to-shoulder lift assist devices have been designed and are at various levels of development (We hner et al., 2009). Professor Fathallah at UC Davis has conducted extensive tests on these devices, and an additional two person device (Ulrey & Fathallah, 2011; Paskiewicz & Fathallah, 2007). Research tools include extensive use of sEMG, inclinometers, electrogoniometers, and a lumbar motion monitor were used. The worn devices evaluated are shown in figures 8, 9, and 10 below. Figure 11 shows a two-person device, GRIPSystem™. Device effectiveness varies between devices, but sEMG proves to be an effective method of evaluating relative muscle activation and is relatively easy to switch test setups between subjects. While numerous variables must be considered, sEMG provides a highly quantifiable measure of back muscle activation (magnitude and variability from lift to lift and from subject to subject) with and without the device. Other factors such as user comfort and satisfaction as well as device adaptability to various body shapes are critically important to a lift assist device. These factors are not, however, as readily quantifiable as EMG based muscle activation information. Comfort surveys can yield valuable data, but uncertainty is much greater than with EMG muscle activation data. Even if a device is ineffective or yields highly varied results, which can be shown in a quantifiable manner with EMG based experiments, making sEMG particularly useful in this suite of data options. In testing the BNDR system, investigators were able to witness and quantify the flexion relaxation (FR) phenomenon, where some subjects are able to relax the erector spinae muscles of the lower back during sustained static stoop postures, where other subjects maintain high back stresses. The device under study (BNDR) reduced erector spinae forces by 26% (p<.001) among non-FR subjects, while those experiencing FR had such low erector spinae activation that the device did not cause a significant change in activation. Without a

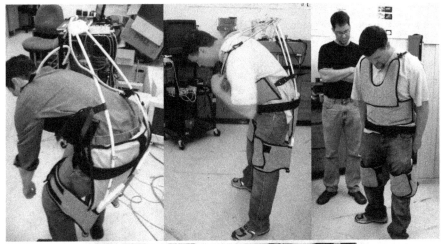

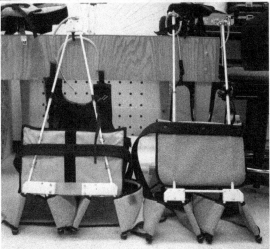

Fig. 8. Happy back, two versions. Top, in use. Bottom, both versions alone.

quantitative analysis tool such as EMG, this phenomenon would have been difficult to detect, let alone separate out the subjects experiencing FR. Device comfort and adjustability were major concerns (Ulrey, Fathallah, 2011). In a study of the GRIPSystem™, twelve subjects performed a variety of real-world lift scenarios, lifting 3 devices at various weights (weight adjusted with the addition of sandbags). EMG was used to monitor the activation levels of ten muscle groups (right and left erector spinae, latissimus dorsi, rectus abdominus, internal abdominal obliques, external abdominal obliques) with and without the use of the device. Erector spinae muscles of the low back saw reductions in low back muscle activation (erector spinae) of varying percentages, all yielding p values below 0.05. EMG allowed researchers to quantify the benefits of the device, but other concerns were evaluated through careful manual analysis. It was noted that the device couples the two workers and makes It more difficult to release an object. Thus, other safety concerns may arise from such a device.In both the GRIPSystem™ and the BNDR study, EMG was the conduit to valuable information, but the researcher was still required to make the observations and decisions which lead to the true discoveries.

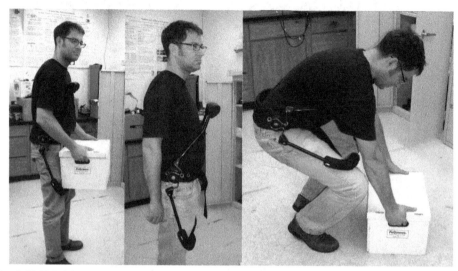

Fig. 9. BNDR lift assist system.

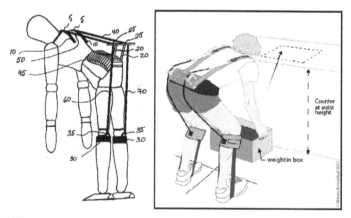

Fig. 10. PLAD lift assist system.

6. Prosthetics, upper limb

Upper limb prosthetics (hand, elbow) have been available in some form for millennia. In recent decades, these prosthetics have developed from fairly rudimentary rigid devices to single degree of freedom (DOF) devices, controlled by movment of the shoulder inside of a mechanical harness. More recently, modern upper limb prosthetics have used EMG to control much more advanced devices, incorporating more complex motion into reduced

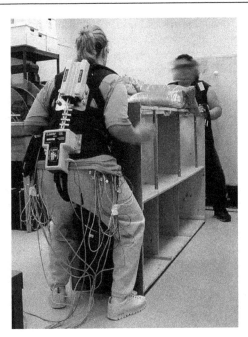

Fig. 11. GRIPSystem™.

order devices and multiple DOF devices more closely resembling actual hands and arms. EMG based prosthetic hands were first used in 1960 by Kobrinkski et al., and have been growing in popularity and capability ever since. In 1980, forty-three subjects were tested using Otto Bock EMG based as well as hook based hands. Results varied based on many factors, but overall observations included a desire for more durable fingers and finer control of the prosthetic's fingers (Northmore-Ball, et al., 1980). Since this time, of course, advances in materials science, controls, robotics, and other areas have permitted modern designs to greatly improve on the earlier models. In reviewing the five methods of using EMG in on-body devices, we can make several observations. Because prosthetics specifically deal with replacement of missing body parts, method one (amplifying existing motion) does not apply. An exception to this using emerging TMR technology is discussed below. Methods two and three (sense and interpret, proportional or threshold) are the most common use of EMG in prosthetics. Methods four and five (monitor to design or evaluate) can be used to evaluate/optimize designs, or determine metabolic cost of a design or configuration.

6.1 Proportional sensing versus threshold sensing

Upper extremity prosthetics present a considerably different set of challenges from lift assist devices and lower extremity/walking exoskeletons. Emulating a natural gait is not the goal, and precise measurement of muscle activation/muscle force is not necessarily a requirement or even a goal. One popular choice in EMG based upper limb prosthetic control is to use threshold sensing to achieve robust control of a reduced order (one or two DOF) prosthetic hand or hand/elbow system. Otto Bock has developed a full line of threshold based prosthetic hands (Ottobock, 2011a) using a myoelectric signal to activate a degree of freedom based on a threshold. Signal above a threshold initiates or ceases a command. Force is exerted based on yes/no value (breaking a threshold) rather than proportional to the signal strength. A variety of signal-logic structures are possible, the most basic of which causes a gripper to open/close based on presence of one EMG signal. More complex possible logic structures include a combination of signals all acting as 'switches' to indicate various states such as Signal 1: open, signal 2: close, signal 3: make the DOF go limp, no signal: lock DOF at present location. Of course, the matrix of possible logic states is limited only by the number of EMG sensors available, the available DOF's, and of course the ability/endurance of the patient. Another option in prosthetic control is proportional sensing. In this method, the speed or force of a DOF is controlled by the magnitude of a signal. This presents all of the traditional difficulties of EMG (crosstalk, filtering, realtime issues), and presents new challenges of safety, accuracy/repeatability, and user fatigue. While potentially much more elegant, and possibly capable of providing more realistic emulation of natural hand movement, proportional sensing includes the fundamental issue of requiring a much higher level of continuous engagement from the user. Proportional sensing, by its nature requires continuous stimulation of the controlling muscle by the user. User fatigue quickly becomes a major concern. Recent advancements in computer science and machine learning are addressing this. Current work uses EMG with downsampling techniques to reduce the exertion/fatigue issues (Castellini & Smagt, 2009) and use of a linear-nonlinear projection method to more effectively control myoelectric prosthetic hands real-time (Chu, et al., 2006).

6.2 Current research and commercial prosthetic hands

Currently, Otto Bock provides a variety of EMG based prosthetic hands to the commercial market (Ottobock, 2011b) including high speed (300mm/s) and high force (160N compression) options. i-Limb provides a hand with five independently powered digits, but is controlled by only two EMG electrodes (Touch Bionics, 2011). Antfolk et al. discuss controlling the SmartHand prosthetic using sixteen myoelectric sensors on able bodied and amputee participants (Antfolk, et al., 2010). 86% accuracy was reported on this extremely complex sixteen DOF system (three per finger plus one for thumb-opposition). Despite these considerable advances, EMG control of prosthetic hands is still far from natural hand motion, and some feel that a great deal of improvement is possible (Massa, et al., 2002).

Currently, feedback is a major concern in upper limb prosthetics. Clearly, existing prosthetics can not 'feel' in the traditional sense. While much research is underway to provide haptic touch/force feedback, for position, feedback is still obtained by visual examination of the prosthetic. Touch/force research is currently underway using vibration as a feedback mechanism to indicate contact, or even force feedback (Cipriani, et al., 2008).

6.3 Targeted Muscle Reinnervation (TMR)

Research is also underway to use targeted muscle reinnervation (TMR), in which residual nerves of an amputated limb are connected to spare muscle fibers of a target nerve. EMG signals from these newly innervated muscle fibers are then used to drive a prosthetic device (Zhou et al., 2005a) (Zhou et al., 2005b). Using this technique, a patient performs the mental action of moving the phantom extremity. The rerouted nerves stimulate the newly innervated fibers, generating a myoelectric signal. This signal can be measured similar to traditional EMG measurement of the original muscle fibers, allowing patients to generate a signal in a much more natural manner. With additional development, TMR could allow researchers to fundamentally rethink the control of prosthetics, and allow for innovative new designs. If successful, this promising technique would allow the use of EMG in prosthetics to move from Methods 2 and 3 to the highly preferable Method 1. Because TMR allows users to actuate prosthetics by "moving" their corresponding phantom muscles, prosthetics controlled by TMR based EMG signals have been shown to be much more intuitive. This new technique has been shown to yield a much shorter learning curve, and has allowed users to control far more sophisticated devices with a greatly increased number of DOF's. As this technology evolves, it will allow the development of considerably more realistic, higher order devices (Kuiken, et al., 2009). Emerging technology, targeted Sensory Reinervation (TSR) promises a complementary technique, providing a sense of touch to the missing limb. A segment of the skin over the TMR site is denervated and regenerating nerves from the TMR procedure reinnervate in this area. When this area is touched, the patient feels a touch sensation in the phantom limb Kuiken et al., 2007). These two emerging technique could allow the realistic closed loop control of multi DOF prosthetics.

7. Lower extremity prosthetics

Electromyography has been used extensively in upper limb prosthetics, and has enjoyed numerous advancements in myoelectric signal processing, as well as pattern recognition (PR) software algorithms. Rates as high as 97.4% EMG based recognition accuracy have been achieved (Chu, et al., 2007). While this is a major achievement in upper extremity control, in highly fault-intolerant tasks such as walking, a 2.6% error rate could prove disastrous. A great deal of effort has gone into EMG for lower extremity exoskeletons, and tremendous strides have been made in this extremely difficult task (see exoskeleton section for details). In EMG controlled prosthetic ankle/knee applications, where the limb is completely absent, patients would be required to control active prosthetics by enervating other muscles. This is considerably difficult in upper limb prosthetics, where real-time movement control (walking gait) is not required. For many applications, grasping can be completed at a modified pace, with position feedback being generated by observing the position of the prosthetic. This would provide overly cumbersome for EMG as a neural control system for lower limb prosthetics, and failures could be dangerous for the user. Due to the critical importance of real-time control and very fault-intolerant nature of walking, lower limb prosthetics are generally not EMG based, though recent research brings new hope about it's future viability. Even in research scenarios, there is a large variation between cycles, making PR difficult. Without the ability to sense or predict the user's intent, active control becomes difficult, because impedance and power must be varied in a feed-forward manner (Huang, et al., 2008). While several active prosthetic ankles and knees have been developed at a research level (Au, et al, 2009; Johansson, et al., 2005; Wilkenfeld, Herr, 2000). There has even been very preliminary work on the possibility of controlling an active ankle prosthetic using EMG, and it has shown promise over a neural network approach (Au, et al., 2006). For the most part, however, other techniques are largely used to control lower limb prosthetics. Despite not currently being suitable for methods one through three, methods four and five can be utilized in lower limb prosthetics development and evaluation. The Otto Bock C-Leg is a popular active lower extremity prosthetic, making it a prime candidate for EMG based gait research (Orendurff, et al., 2006).

8. Tele-operation and gesture based remote control

Just as EMG can be used to control on-body devices, it can be used to tele-operate remote devices from great distance or nearby. While tele-operation via EMG possesses the same restrictions and drawbacks of EMG control of worn devices, it can nevertheless be a powerful tool, and in certain situations the so-called drawbacks of EMG can be used as advantages. Current research in EMG teleoperation includes controlling a wheelchair through a combination of EMG and electroencephalography (EEG) (Han, et al., 2003). In this research, a novel application of EMG has been proposed. In addition to a neural control system for the wheelchair, EMG can be used as a monitoring and alarm system. Other research has used EMG and EEG to control a robot system, with the intent of future use by the handicapped (Ferreira, et al., 2008). In this application, eight subjects were able to control a computer algorithm designed to command devices, with a rightness rate of 95%. Experiments were undertaken to control a robotic arm by EMG signals in the forearm (Flexor Carpi Radialis), control a robotic wheelchair by EMG signals acquired from a neck muscle (elevator scapulae) to allow use by patients with upper and lower limb motor disabilities due to paralysis or amputation (Moon et al, 2003). Yet other research has investigated using EMG to control humanoid robots such as Honda's Asimo (Honda, 2011). Clearly, other possibilities exist, from remotely operating machinery in dangerous locations such as nuclear reactors or deep undersea, to a more intuitive control mechanism for any number of applications. Gesture based control of machinery and computer systems are well within the realm of EMG research, using methods 2 and 3 (Xu, et al., 2009). In these applications, monitoring, warning, and feedback control can be incorporated much more simply and effectively than in previously discussed applications. Each of these remotely operated applications would incorporate a method of feedback. An audio or video warning could be included indicating various states or warnings. An indicator could illuminate to indicate that the device has contacted an object. Complex haptics configurations can be eliminated or greatly reduced in these applications. In order to retain force magnitude "sensing", an array of strain gauges can record forces, and transmit this information to the controller. One is not limited to emulating human capability. Proximity sensors can also be installed to indicate when a remotely-operated device is approaching the desired object. Bar-graph style indicators could be included on a monitor to indicate magnitude based values such as force based control. In any of these applications, just as with worn devices, user comfort must be considered. To this end, a design/evaluate/optimize cycle can be included during the development process, and method four can be used to reduce user fatigue from operation.

9. Emerging applications in modern culture and technology based art

Electromyography is being used to illustrate muscle phenomena in the technology-based-art community. Experimental artists are using EMG to generate a signal from muscles to control audio or video signals, and to actuate electromechanical apparatus in performance settings. As has been the case with previous emerging technologies, artists are using EMG in creative new ways. With the availability of high-speed real-time wireless devices at ever increasingly high bandwidth and low cost, the same technology that allows convenient gathering of walking and running gate-data allows avant-garde dance troupes to collect EMG data during performances to control audio signals or video displays. Artistic applications are often more fault tolerant than traditional applications (In art, a bad myoelectric signal can hurt an artistic performance. In a prosthetic knee, a bad signal can cause injury or even death). The art community can therefore utilize technologies before the technologies are commercially viable for the mass market.

Australian performance artist Stelarc has been using technology in his art, and using the human body as an art medium since 1976 (Elsenaar & Scha, 2002). His work has explored the boundary between man and machine, using signals from his body to control machinery, and using external machinery to control parts of his body, through mechanical animation, and by electrically stimulating muscles, often using his own body as the art medium. Stelarc has used electromyography in conjunction with numerous other sensor technologies (EEG, ultrasound, electromechanical encoders, goniometers), along with other more broadly used sensors (accelerometers, thermistors, and contact microphones) to control devices in performances around the world. In one work, Stelarc developed a "Third Hand", a robotic appendage, attached to his own arm, but controlled via EMG sensors measuring activation of muscles in his abdomen and thigh. In another piece, Stelarc used a similar suite of sensors to create a variety of sounds, all generated, directly or indirectly, real-time by the human body. In this piece, he contrasted rhythmic sounds (heartbeat, breath) with more "chaotic" sounds such as those found in myoelectric signals (Elsenaar & Scha, 2002). Stelarc uses these techniques and sensors to blur the line between himself, electromechanical devices, and the audience. Many of his performances even blur the line between local and remote self, transmitting the body signals over the internet to control remote devices or manipulate audio-video displays at a performance site far from his physical body in order to question the localized self (Fleming, 2002). In another performance, Stelarc used an electromechanical device to allow audience members to manipulate his body via actuators. EMG was used to detect his muscle actuation, blurring the distinction between his voluntary movements and those caused by the audience. These myoelectric signals were then transmitted to a remote device, where a robotic actuator system was "controlled" by the signals. The audience input was done locally and remotely over the internet. In this piece, Stelarc used himself as a portion of the nonlinear control loop in which the audience indirectly controlled the robotic actuator. Additionally blurring the line between self, machine, and even location (Elsenaar & Scha, 2002).

Electronic/visual artist, Sean Clute often incorporates electronics and technology more traditionally found in other fields in his work. An upcoming piece for his performance group Double Vision (Jennings, 2011) uses EMG extensively. Professor Clute describes the piece as follows:

"Intermedia performance company Double Vision's work entitled Wishing for the Perfect Dorsiflexion depicts a solo performer controlling live-video via a wireless electromyogram interface. Conceptually, the work highlights two symptomatic conditions of Multiple Sclerosis; foot drop (dorsiflexion) and Uhthoff's phenomenon. The performer, who has MS, can be seen walking on stage with increased difficulty over time. Simultaneously, a rear video projection of a recreation trail in Stowe, Vermont can be seen. As the performer shows increased signs of weakened gait the video projection appears to both stumble and become unnaturally high in contrast. Thus, the real-time physical condition of the performer is projected visually for the audience to express the surreality of having a demyelinating disease such as MS.

Double Vision uses a wireless EMG attached to muscles in the anterior portion of the lower legs. The data is sent via the Open Sound Control (OSC) communication protocol developed at the Center for New Music and Audio Technologies at the University of California at Berkeley. The data is received by a computer using custom software created in the language Max/MSP Jitter. The software takes the incoming data, runs it through a band pass filter, and then maps to the x and y axis of prerecorded video footage. If the EMG activity is below a certain threshold then the video begins to "wiggle." This visually represents the foot drop. Additionally, the same data is used to control the contrast of the video. Artistically, this relationship is to demonstrate the unusual characteristics of Uhthoff's phenomenon including increased optic neuritis and vision abnormalities with nerve weakness.

This work is proof of the growing application of electromyography in the performing arts community. As the cost of producing works using electromechanical encoders decreases with an increase in the shared knowledge base of how to use such technologies, emerging groups such as Double Vision are experimenting with ways to map the human condition artistically" (Clute, 2011).

Such use of EMG in the art world helps expose the technology to ever growing numbers of people from more varied fields. Clute and Stelarc show that as previously arcane technologies become more robust, reliable, and affordable, the arts communities can provide a conduit to expose them to these populations. Figure 12 shows images from the work of Clute's group Double Vision (with co-director Pauline Jennings). Included are a preliminary image for the upcoming performance entitled Wishing for the Perfect Dorsiflexion, and a still image from a previous live performance.

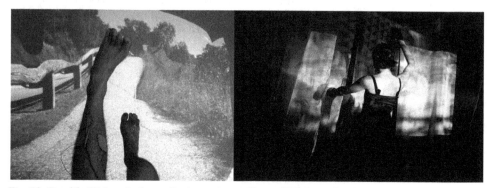

Fig. 12. Double Vision. Left, preliminary image from "Wishing for the Perfect Dorsiflexion". Right, image from a previous performance. (Jennings, 2011a, Jennings, 2011b).

10. Mixed applications - EMG in combination with other technologies

While a powerful tool on its own, some of the greatest benefits of EMG come when combined with other sensing technologies. If well planned, an application can be designed so that the weaknesses in EMG can be supplanted by strengths in other sensors, and the inherent strengths in EMG can be fully leveraged, often overcoming difficulties in other methods. Designers must also keep in mind that myoelectric signals can have a detrimental effect on other signals. Electroencephalography (EEG) practitioners have long found problems with EMG signals contaminating their data. As EEG detects brain signals of even smaller amplitudes (10 to 100 microvolts) noise from the relatively much larger EMG waves signals (10 to 100 milivolts) can completely drown out an EEG signal. As careful as EMG practitioners must be in minimizing crosstalk when studying EMG signals, EEG practitioners must deal with a much greater relative problem. Fortunately, muscles of the human body are either relatively small (cranio-ocular musculature) or relatively distant from the brain and EEG setup (shoulders, arms, back, legs) (Shackman, et al., 2009). With proper consideration, valuable data can be taken from different technologies simultaneously, valuable information can be learned, and innovative new devices can be developed, all of which would be impossible using only one type of sensor.

10.1 EMG with fMRI

Magnetic resonance imaging (MRI) and functional magnetic resonance imaging (fMRI) allow practitioners to generate detailed internal structures of the human body, often the brain. Of course, such valuable technology comes with features which can be drawbacks or even make the tool unusable in some applications. The devices are very large, not portable, and in the case of MRI, involve a very high dose of electromagnetic radiation. Additionally, the hardware and operation of the devices is very expensive. While tremendously valuable in many applications, these factors make MRI and fMRI prime candidates for mixed use applications, particularly those in which initial procedures can be completed with MRI fMRI, but can later be simplified to eliminate the large expensive machinery. It has been shown (Dai, et al., 2001) that fMRI, EMG, and joint muscle force can be correlated in some cases. Ten volunteer participants were asked to exert a hand grip force as measurements were taken. Brain images were acquired using FMRI, as participants gripped at 20, 35, 50, 65, and 80% of their maximal force. Concurrently, EMG signal data was taken on the activation levels of the flexor and extensor muscles. EMG based signals were directly proportional to brain signal amplitude. Both of these signal intensities also correlated with hand grip force. A novel technique, computed myography (CMG), uses a dense array of individual sEMG electrodes rather than traditional bipolar electrodes to determine muscle activation across several muscle groups. Multiple electrodes were attached to a human forearm to record a broad spectrum of EMG data during flexion/extension (number and locations of sensors were varied based on the experiment performed) Then, using the finite element method (on commercial analysis packages Comsol and Matlab), this array of electrode data is inverted to determine qualitatively and quantitatively the activation levels of the internal muscles. Concurrently, the arm is monitored with fMRI, yielding a well understood map of the desired muscle activation. It is believed that with further correlation, the fMRI can be eschewed completely, and an essentially fMRI level map can be generated using only EMG and this novel CMG method (Vand Den Doel et al., 2008). An EMG based prosthetic arm was used to study the mutual adaptation between the system and the human body. A 13 DOF prosthetic was used, including electrical stimulus for tactile feedback. fMRI data is recorded to clarify the plasticity of portions of the brain due to changes in the device. The experiments show adaptation in the studied areas (from fMRI data) of a phantom limb image to the prosthetic (Kato, et al., 2009).

10.2 EMG with EEG

Recently, great strides have been made in brain-machine interface using EEG. Unfortunately, because EEG signals are several orders of magnitude smaller than EMG, and because interstitial layers, particularly the skull, tends to damp out much of the frequency range of EEG signals, EEG signals are notoriously difficult to record, process, and interpret accurately (Saneei & Chambers, 2007). Just as advances have been made in interpreting EMG signals, the field of EEG has been rapidly evolving and hardware is becoming available at ever reduced cost to ever larger groups. Concurrently, much research has occurred developing a hybrid approach to human-machine interface utilizing EEG, EMG, fMRI, and recently even motion tracking systems such as the Kinect by Microsoft. EMG has been used in conjunction with EEG in a clinical setting to detect changes in sleep and shift between sleep stages in healthy patients and patients suffering from narcolepsy or other ailments, leading to increased ability to diagnose certain disorders and has lead to a greater understanding of sleep and the many musculo-physical issues associated with it (Ferri, et al., 2008; Rechtschaffen & Kales, 1968). This EMG EEG hybrid approach has also been used to control machinery and virtual conditions. Often, EEG is used as a source of multi-dimensional data, and EMG is used as a more reliable safety/backup system, utilizing the advantages of both systems. Research has been done on wheelchair control, allowing users to control the device with EEG. EMG was used to correlate desired commands with recorded EEG states. While research shows encouraging preliminary results, additional research and possible further hybridization with EMG is required (Blankertz, et al., 2006). This research was particularly encouraging, because it found that very little training was required before subjects could begin controlling the apparatus using only EMG and EEG. Robotic control using EMG and EEG has been proposed and is the subject of several experiments. A technique labeled Biopotential, using EMG and EEG to control machines was studied. Data acquisition rates in EMG and EEG realms are quite high and more work is required to process this magnitude of data real-time (McMillan, 1998). Flight control via EMG and EEG is far from a reality, as any fault could be catastrophic. However, virtual flight control research can readily be performed. EEG was used for control, with EMG as validation and backup signal (Friedman, et al., 2004). Yet another study into flight simulation via human-machine interface actually used both EMG and EEG to control the simulation. In this experiment, subjects showed the ability to control the single DOF simulation with relative accuracy (though some suffered cybersickness from immersion in the simulator). The study presented the questions of users' limits of control, suggesting future experiments including multi-DOF tasks. A program is now underway in the Netherlands to control a lower limb exoskeleton using EEG and EMG signals. Entitled MINDWALKER, the project attempts to develop a device primarily for use among those suffering from spinal cord and other injuries. An ambitious project, the use of both EEG and EEG EMG based controls will be implemented, because it is understood that those with spinal cord injuries may not be able to control such a device using EMG. The addition of EEG with EMG expands the realm of applications, and techniques used for voluntary and semi-voluntary control. Event-related potential (ERP), or the direct brain response to a perception/thought as well as P300, by which the patient can learn to control slow brain waveforms in order to control devices. These techniques along with measures of autonomic system balance (Heart Rate Variability, Skin Conductance) expand the use of EMG into entirely new realms of system control from gaming to dentistry.

11. Future directions

As technologies mature, additional applications become feasible. Just as many applications discussed above were the subject of wild fancy a short time ago, we will continue to see advancements including EMG as the primary driver, or one tool in a suite of technologies bringing us ever greater opportunities. Energy Harvesting/Scavenging is an ever growing field, in which low power and intermittently powered devices use available energy from the surroundings. Energy sources include heat and vibration, and are absorbed using pieso-electrics and thermopiles (Vullers, et al., 2009), often for applications in difficult to reach areas, where changing a battery or hard-wiring electricity is difficult or costly. In vivo devices are prime examples of such difficult to access applications. One highly plausible method for research is the study of EMG or EKG as a power source for energy harvesting. In such an application, signal clarity, timing, and interpretation are unimportant. Cross talk from other nearby muscles can actually be a benefit. The focus in this application is the magnitude of the signal. It has also been proposed that EMG and EEG can be used as a form of human/robot interaction where a robot/device would sense EMG/EEG signals to learn about nearby humans, not explicitly for control (Bien, et al., 2008). EMG techniques can also be used to monitor users for fatigue, alertness, or other variables in various situations. Work has already begun in user monitoring in wheelchair applications, in which the device will stop if EMG signals fall below a threshold or become abnormal, allowing a failsafe in wheelchair operation (Han, et al., 2003). Research has been conducted on using EMG signals to trigger a hands-free electrolarynx device (Goldstein et al., 2004), in which myoelectric signals are monitored to control initiation and termination of the device. Additional research includes EMG for voice/speech recognition even at the sub-auditory level (Jorgensen et al., 2003)

12. Discussion

The field of Electromyography is developing into new areas. As the necessary technology is developed and the devices become more reliable and less expensive, EMG can be used more reliably and at a reduced cost, making it feasible in an ever increasing range of applications. As the applications of EMG change, we must consider the benefits as well as the potential drawbacks inherent in this proliferation. The applications exploring the possible use of EMG have different priorities, and if used appropriately, many of them may use EMG as a powerful tool. If used improperly, however, erroneous data taken from a myoelectric signal can be useless, if not harmful or even fatal. In traditional applications, crosstalk is a major concern. In energy scavenging, or in spread array techniques such as CMG, crosstalk becomes less of a concern, or even an additional source of electrical energy. Some EMG applications rely on robust signal fidelity, divisible into fine resolution to obtain maximum data. Other applications, such as two state and three state conditions discussed as method three in this chapter, do not require such high signal fidelity. Table 1 below covers major applications of EMG, and addresses the relative importance of major factors for each.

When developing new devices or applications drawing EMG out of the traditional setting, one must consider the challenges, risks, drawbacks, and advantages involved in using EMG. Some challenges are being addressed through modern sensing, signal processing, and computational techniques, but other issues are inherent to the nature of the phenomenon. Advanced hardware now allows us to acquire and filter signals real-time in a ever more portable packages. Computer modeling and other software techniques are now allowing us to learn about myoelectric signal and even predict motions and muscle activity. EMG is being used in various suites of sensors to extract the best components of EMG as well as the other sensors such as fMRI, EEG, and motion tracking. As EMG becomes available to more

		Consideration				
Application		Signal Fidelity & Resolution	Realtime	Convenience	Crosstalk & Accuracy	cost
Worn Devices	Exo (lower extremities)	2	1	3	1	3
	Prosthetic hand, proportional (method 2)	2	1	3	1	3
	Prosthetic hand, gradient (method 3)	3	1	3	3	2
	Lower Limb Prosthetics	1	1	3	1	3
Device control	virtual environment control	2	2	1	3	1
	hybrid, fail-safe, signal check	3	3	3	3	2
Art/dance/culture		3	3	2	3	1
Design validation/ Optimization (methods4, 5)		2	4	2	2	2
Matrix devices/FEA/CMG		2	3	3	4	4
Energy Scavenging		4	4	4	4	3

Table 1. Relative importance, applications vs major areas of concern in EMG. 1. Critical. 2. Important. 3. Somewhat Important. 4. Not Important.

practitioners and applications, it becomes tempting to use the technology as a "black box" (simply extracting data without understanding the details), and not understand the background and limitations. As EMG becomes easier to use, it becomes easier to abuse. Untrained practitioners can draw erroneous conclusions, which can cause harm, injury, or even death. We must be mindful to maintain the integrity of EMG applications, along with the other sensing techniques used, in worn devices, devices to assist the elderly and handicapped, control machinery, and other new and emerging technologies.

13. Acknowledgment

The authors would like to thank: Professor Fadi Fathallah, Department of Biological and Agricultural Engineering, University of California at Davis for discussion of devices, models, and methodology; David Gessel of Black Rose Technology and the Massachusetts Institute of Technology for EMG concept discussion, procedures, and support; Professor Sean Clute and Pauline Jennings, department of fine and performing arts, Hohnson State College, for discussions of EMG in art and contribution of pre-release material from their upcoming performances.

14. References

Antfolk, C.; Cipriani, C.; Controzzi, M.; Carrozza, M.; Lundborg, G.; Rosen, B. & Sebelius, F. (2010) Using EMG for Real-time Prediction of Joint Angles to Control a Prosthetic

Hand Equipped with a Sensory Feedback System. *Journal of Medical and Biological Engineering*, vol 30 no 6, pp 399-406

Au,s.; Webber, J.; & Herr, H.; (2006) Initial experimental study on dynamic interaction between an amputee and a powered ankle–foot prosthesis. *Proceedings of Dyn. Walking: Mech. Control Hum. Robot Locomotion*, Ann Arbor, MI, Jul. 2006.

Au, S.; Weber, J, & and H. Herr, H (2009) Powered ankle-foot prosthesis improves walking metabolic economy. *IEEE Trans. Robotics*, vol. 25, no. 1, pp. 51–66.

Bien, Z.; Lee, H.; Do, J.; Kim, Y.; Park, K. & Yank, S. (2007) Intellignet Interaction for Human-friendly Service Robot in Smart House Environment. *International Journal of Computational Intellignece Systems*, vol. 1, no. 1, (Jan 2008), pp 77-93

Biswarup, N.; Soumyajit, M.; Soumya, G.; Sinchan, G. & Das, A. (2005) Simulation Techniques for Biologically Active Prosthetic feeet-an Overview. *International Journal of Information Technology and Knowledge Management* January-June 2011, Volume 4, No. 1, pp. 239-242

Blanc, Y.; & Dimanico, U. (2010) History of the Study of Skeletal Muscle Function with Emphasis on Kinesiological Electromyography. *The Open Rehabilitation Journal*, vol 3 pp 84-93.

Blankertz, B.; Dornhege, G.; Krauledat, M.; Müller, K.; Kunzmann, V.; Losch, F. and Curio, G. (2006) The Berlin Brain-Computer Interface: EEG-based communication without subject training. *IEEE Trans. Neural Sys. Rehab. Eng.* vol. 14 no.2. pp147-152.

BLEEX, (no date), accessed 2011, available from: <http://bleex.me.berkeley.edu/research/exoskeleton/bleex/ >

Carmena, J. M. et al. (2003) Learning to control a brain-machine interface for reaching and grasping by primates. *PLoS Biology*, Vol 1,(2003).

Castellini, C. & van der Smagt, P. (2009) Surface EMG in advanced hand prosthetics. *Biological Cybernetics*, (2009) 100, pp. 35–47.

Chaffin DB, Andersson G. Occupational Biomechanics. 3rd ed. New York: John Wiley & Sons; 1999

Chu, J-U.; Moon, I. & Mun, S. (2006) A real-time EMG pattern recognition system based on linear-nonlinear feature projection for a multifunction myoelectric hand. *IEEE Trans. Biomed. Eng.*, vol. 53, no. 11, pp. 2232-2239.

Chu, J-U.; Moon, I.; Lee, YJ.; Kim, K. & Mun, S. (2007) A supervised feature-projection-based real-time EMG pattern recognition for multifunction myoelectric hand control. *IEEE/ASME Trans. Mechatronics*, vol. 12, no. 3, pp. 282–290.

Cipriani, C.; Zaccone, F.; Micera, S. & Carrozza, MC. (2008) On the Shared Control of an EMG-Controlled Prosthetic Hand: Analysis of User Prosthesis Interaction. *IEEE Transactions on Robotics 2008*, vol 24, pp 170-184.

Clute, S. (2011) Personal conversation with Sean Clute, Assitant Professor of Fine and Performing Arts, Johnson State College. , accessed 2011, available from: < http://www.seanclute.com/bio/ >

Dai TH, Liu JZ, Sahgal V, Brown RW, Yue GH (2001) Relationship between muscle output and functional MRI-measured brain activation. *Exp Brain Res* 140:290–300

De Luca. C.J. (1997) The Use of Surface Eletromyography in Biomechanics. *Journal of Applied Biomechanics*, Volume 13, Pages 135-163, 1997

Ferreira, A.; Celeste, W.; Cheein, F.; Bastos-Filho, T.; Sarcinelli-Filho, M. and Carelli, R. (2008) Human-machine interfaces based on EMG and EEG applied to robotic systems. *Journal of NeuroEngineering and Rehabilitation*, pp. 5–10.

Elsenaar, A. and Scha, R. Electric Body Manipulation as Performance Art: A Historical Perspective. *Leonardo Music Journal, 12, 2002, 17-28.*

Ferri, R.; Franceschini, C. & Zucconi. M. (2008) *Searching for a marker of REM sleep behavior disorder: submentalis muscle EMG amplitude analysis during sleep in patients with narcolepsy/cataplexy.* Sleep. vol 31, pp 1409–17.

Fishman, L. & Wilkins, A. (2010) Functional Electromyography. (1st edition), Springer, 1607610191.

Fleischer, C. & G. Hommel, G. (2008) A Human--Exoskeleton Interface Utilizing Electromyography. *IEEE Transactions on Robotics*, vol. 24, pp. 872-882.

Friedman, D.; Leeb, R.; Antley, A.; Garau, M.; Guger, C.; Keinrath, C.;(2004). Navigating virtual reality by thought: First steps. *Proceedings of the 7th Annual International Workshop on Presence*, pp. 160–167.

Goldstein, EA.; Heaton, JT.; Kobler, JB.; Stanley, GB. & Hillman, RE. (2004) Design and implementation of a hands-free electrolarynx device controlled by neck strap muscle electromyographic activity. *IEEE Transactions on Biomedical Eng* 2004, vol 51, pp 325–332.

Han, J.; Bien, Z.; Kim, D.; Lee, H.; Kim, J.; (2003) Human–machine interface for wheelchair control with EMG and its evaluation. *Proceedings of the 25th IEEE International Conference on Engineering in Medicine and Biology Society, Cancun, Mexico, (September 2003)*, pp. 1602–1605.

Honda, (no date), accessed 2011, available from: <http://dreams.honda.com/robotics-mobility/ >

Huang, H.; Kuiken, A. & Lipschutz, R. (2008) A strategy for identifying locomotion modes using surface electromyography. *IEEE Trans. Biomed. Eng.*, vol. 56, no. 1, pp. 65–73, Jan. 2009.

Jennings, P. (2011a), accessed 2011, available from: <http://www.double-vision.biz/new/about/artistic-directors/>

Jennings, P. (2011b), Photo by Anne Peattie, Dancer: Mira Cook, accessed 2011, available from: <http://www.double-vision.biz/new/about/artistic-directors/>

Johansson, JL.; Sherrill, DM.; Riley, PO.; Bonato, P.; and Herr, H.; (2005). A clinical comparison of variable-damping and mechanically passive prosthetic knee devices. *Am. J. Phys. Med. Rehabil.* vol 84, pp 563-575.

Jorgensen, C.; Lee, D. & Agabon, S.;(2003) Sub Auditory Speech Recognition Based on EMG/EPG Signals. *Proc. of the International Joint Conference on Neural Networks*, 2003.

Kasaoka, K. & Sankai, Y. (2001)Predictive control estimating operator's intention for stepping-up motion by exo-skeleton type power assist system HAL. *Proceedings of International Conference on Intelligent Robots and Systems*, pp. 1578-1583, 2001.

Kato, R.; Yokoi, H.; Hernandez, A.; Yu, W.; and Arai, T. (2009) Mutual adaptation among man and machine by using f-MRI analysis, Robot. *Auton. Syst.* vol 57 no. 2, pp. 161–166.

Kawamoto, H.; Lee, S.; Kanbe, S. & Sankai, Y. (2003) Power assist method for HAL-3 using EMG-based feedback controller. *Proceedings of IEEE Int. Conf. Syst., Man, Cybern.*, 2003, pp. 1648–1653.

Kuiken, T. A.; Li, G.; Lock, B. A.; Lipschutz, R. D.; Miller, L. A.; Stubblefeld, K. A.; et al. (2009). Targeted muscle reinnervation for real-time myoelectric control of multifunction artifcial arms. *JAMA*, vol 301 no 6, pp 619-28.

Kuiken, T.; Miller, L.; Lipschutz, R.; Lock, B.; Stubblefield, K.; Marasco, P.; Zhou, P. & Dumanian, G. (2007) Targeted reinnervation for enhanced prosthetic arm function in a woman with a proximal amputation: a case study *The Lancet*, vol 369 pp 371-380.

Lee, S. & Sankai, Y. (2002) Power assist control for walking aid with hal-3 based on emg and impedance adjustment around knee joint. *Proceedings of IEEE/RSJ Int. Conf. Intelligent Robots and Systems*, pp. 1499–1504,2002.

Lee S. & Y. Sankai, Y. (2003) The Natural Frequency-Based Power Assist Control for Lower Body with HAL-3, *Proceedings of International Conference on Intelligent Robots and Systems*, pp. 1642-1647, 2003.

MIT, (no date), accessed 2011, available from:
    < http://biomech.media.mit.edu/research/research.htm>

Mcmillan, Grant. (1998) The technology and applications of biopotential-based control. *Proceedings of Alernative Control Technologies: Human Factors Issues*, Bretigny, France, Oct. 1998.

Massa, B.; Roccella, S.; Carrozza, M. C. & Dario, P. (2002) Design and Development of an Underactuated Prosthetic Hand. *Proceedings of the 2002 IEEE International Conference on Robotics and Automation*, pp. 3374-3379

Medved, V. (2001) *Measurement of Human Locomotion*, CRC Press, Boca Raton, Fl.

Merletti, R. (1999) Standards for Reporting EMG Data, *Journal of Electromyography and Kineseology*, vol 9, 1999.

Moon I, Lee M, Ryu J, Mun M: Intelligent Robotic Wheelchair with EMG-, Gesture-, and Voice-based Interfaces. *Proceedings of 2003 IEEE/RSJ International Conference on Intelligent Robots and Systems (IROS 2003)*, Las Vegas, Nevada 2003, 4:3453-3458

Northmore-Ball, D.; Heger, H. & Hunter, G. (1980) The below-elbow myoelectric prosthesis: a comparison of the Otto Bock myoelectric prosthesis with the hook and functional hand. *Bone Joint Surg.* vol 62B, pp 363-367.

Orendurff, M.; Segal, A.; Klute, G.; McDowell, M.; Pecoraro, J. & Czerniecki, J. (2006) Gait efficiency using the C-Leg. *J Rehabil Res Dev.* vol 43 no 2. pp239–46.

Ottobock, (2011a) accessed 2011, available from:
    <http://www.ottobock.com/cps/rde/xchg/ob_com_en/hs.xsl/384.html>

Ottobock (2011b) accessed 2011, available from:
    < http://www.ottobock.com/cps/rde/xchg/ob_com_en/hs.xsl/384.html>

Paskiewicz, J. & Fathallah, F. (2007) Effectiveness of a manual furniture handling device in reducing low back disorders risk factors. *Industrial Ergonomics.* vol 37, pp 93-102.

Raez, M.B.I.; Hussain, M.S.; & Mohd-Yasin, F. (2006). Techniques of EMG signal analysis: detection, processing, classification, and applications. *Biological Procedures Online*, vol 8, pp 11-35.

Rechtschaffen A, Kales A, eds. (1968) A manual of standardized terminology, techniques and scoring system for sleep stages of human subjects. Washington, D.C.: Government Printing Office, NIH publication no. 204. 1968.

Sanei, S. & Chambers, J. (2007) *EEG Signal Processing*. Hoboken, NJ: John Wiley & Sons, 2007.

Sarcos, (no date), accessed 2011, available from: < http://www.sarcos.com/>

Shackman, A.; McMenimin,B.; Slagter, H; Maxwell, J.; Greischar, L. & Davidson, R. (2009) Electromyogenic artifacts and Electroenecpalographic interferences. *Brian Topography*, 22(1), (June 2009), pp7-12.

Touch Bionics (2007) i-Limb system, accessed 2011, available from: <http://www.touchbionics.com>

Ulrey, B.L.; & Fathallah, F.A. (2011). Biomechanical Effects of a Personal Weight Transfer Device in the Stooped Posture. *Proceedings of the 55th Annual Meeting of the Human Factors and Ergonomics Society*. Santa Monica, CA: Human Factors and Ergonomics Society.

Van den Doel, K.; Ascher, U. & Pai, D. (2008) Computed myography: three dimensional reconstruction of motor functions from surface EMG data. *Inverse Problems*, vol 24 065010, 2008.

Vullers, R.; van Schaijk, R.; Doms, I.;van Hoof C. & Mertens, R. (2009) Micropower Energy Harvesting. *Solid-State Electronics*, vol. 53, no. 7, pp. 684 – 693.

Wehner (2009) Lower extremity exoskeleton as lift assist device. Wehner, M.; Kazerooni, H.; Ph.D. Thesis, University of California at Berkeley.

Wehner, M.; Rempel, D. & Kazerooni, H. (2009) Lower Extremity Exoskeleton Reduces Back Forces in Lifting. *Proceedings of ASME 2009 Dynamic Systems and Control Conference* October, 2009, Hollywood, California, USA,

Wilkenfeld, A.; Herr, H. (2000) "An auto-adaptive external knee prosthesis", PhD. Thesis, MIT

Zhang, X.; Chen, X.; Wang, W.; Yang, J.; Lantz, V.; & Wang, K. (2009) Hand Gesture Recognition and Virtual Game Control Based on 3D Accelerometer and EMG Sensors. *Proc ACM IUI* 2009, pp 401-406.

Zhen, Z.; Songli, Y.; Yanan, Z. & Jinwu, Q. (2007) On the surface electromyography sensor network of human ankle movement. Proceedings *of IEEE International Conference on Robotics and Biomimetics*, pp. 1688-1692, 2007.

Zhou, P.; Lowery, M.A.; Dewald, J. & Kuiken, T. (2005a) Towards Improved Myoelectric Prosthesis Control: High Density Surface EMG Recording After Targeted Muscle Reinnervation. *Conf Proc IEEE Eng Med Biol Soc*. 2005, 4:4064-7

Zhou, P.; Lowery, M.A. & Kuiken, T. (2005b) Elimination of ECG Artifacts from Myoelectric Prosthesis Control Signals Developed by Targeted Muscle Reinnervation. *Conf Proc IEEE Eng Med Biol Soc*. 2005;5:5276-9

11

EMG PSD Measures in Orthodontic Appliances

Şükrü Okkesim[1], Tancan Uysal[2], Aslı Baysal[3] and Sadık Kara[1]
[1]Fatih University, Institute of Biomedical Engineering, İstanbul
[2]İzmir Katip Çelebi University, Faculty of Dentistry, İzmir
[3]Kocaeli University, Faculty of Dentistry, Kocaeli
Turkey

1. Introduction

The human body consists of different systems which include the nervous system, the cardiovascular system, the musculoskeletal system, etc. Each system performs some kind of vital task and carries on many physiological processes. For example, the primary functions of the musculoskeletal system can be summarized as generating forces, producing motion, moving substance within the body, providing stabilization, and generating heat. Physiological processes are multifaceted fact and most of them manifest themselves as signals that reflect their nature and activities. These types of signals may be hormonal, physical or electrical. The general name of the electrical signals taken from the related organ or physiologic process with invasive or non-invasive methods is called Biomedical Signals. This signal is normally a function of time and is definable in terms of its amplitude, frequency and phase (Rangayyan, 2002).

The electromyography (EMG) signal is a biomedical signal that detects the electrical potential generated by muscle cells when these cells contract, and also when the cells are at rest. Three types of muscle tissue can be identified. One of them is the skeletal muscle, and the others are the smooth muscle and the cardiac muscle. The EMG is applied to the study of skeletal muscle (Reaz et al., 2006).

Skeletal muscles are comprised by nearly parallel cells and the muscle fibers which constitute the contractile structural units. Muscle fibers are activated by the central nervous system through electrical signals transmitted by motoneurons. A single motoneuron together with the muscle fibers that it contacts is called a motor unit which is the smallest functional subdivision of the neuromuscular system (Moritani, et al. 2004) The central nervous system controls the activation of motor units to optimize the interaction between our body and the surrounding environment. When the motor units are activated by the central nervous system, they produce an action potential trains of the active motor units add together to generate the interference EMG signal.

Surface and needle electrodes have been used to detect EMG of muscles. Surface electrodes have been widely used to investigate neuromuscular functions because of their several advantages, for example, it is noninvasive, easy to adhere to the skin and to detect the total activities of the muscle and it was called Surface EMG (SEMG). Bu the real advantage of this technique is that it is more beneficial in studies, in which simultaneous movement of many muscles is examined in vast muscle groups. On the other hand, surface electrodes have disadvantages as well. Due to the broad area for receiving signals on respective muscle bundle, signals received by surface electrodes may stem from proximal muscle groups. This situation leaves questions about the accuracy of records. Although a great deal of effort is spent to determine and characterize the effect of such artefacts, a technique of analysis that completely allays questions has not been developed yet (Cobbold, 1974).

SEMG has advantages and disadvantages; they are used widely for several issues. SEMG signals are used widely for diagnosis and to assess the treatment of some neuropathic, myopathic and neuromuscular junction diseases in the hospital and in research about biomechanics, sport medicine and rehabilitation ...etc.

Orthodontics is the branch of science dealing with teeth, jaw and face structure in terms of treatment of abnormalities/irregularities.

In orthodontics treatment performed with two different 'point of views'. One of them is the jaw orthopaedics in which the malposition of the jaws related to face or related to each other is corrected with special appliances. The other is called orthodontics and related with the correction of teeth. Generally patients are treated simultaneously with orthodontic and orthopaedic approaches.

Malocclusion is the general name of the orthodontic abnormalities arising from misalignment of teeth and incorrect relation between the upper and lower jaw and divided into Class I, II and III. Class II malocclusion is one of the most common orthodontic problems, and it is reported to constitute nearly one-third of all orthodontic disorders (Kraus, 1956 ; and Kleissen et al., 1998).

Class II malocclusions can be skeletal or dental. In skeletal Class II malocclusions the maxilla and the maxillary arch may be positioned anteriorly related to cranial base, the mandibula and the mandibular arch may be positioned posteriorly related to cranial base or the combination of these two factors. Treatment of Class II malocclusions achieved with orthopaedic and orthodontic approaches (Riedel, 1952; McNamara, 1981; Renfroe, 1948; Blair, 1954). Dental Class II malocclusions are arising from the increase in the inclination of upper incisor, crowding etc. As dental Class II malocclusion does not include skeletal problems, orthodontic corrections are sufficient for this type of malocclusions. The variability of Class II malocclusions cause to arise a lot of treatment options. Treatment options include non-oral or oral appliances, arch expansion mechanics and treatment with dental extractions (Proffit et al., 1998).

Non-oral appliances are one of the oldest treatment methods that are used widespread. The most common widespread non-oral appliance is headgear. As headgear can be used for steering or curbing the growth of upper jaw to the forward and downward (overbite), it can also be used for activating teeth in distal direction. Therefore, it can be said for this appliance that it has both orthopaedic and orthodontic effects. In addition to such advantages, the use of this appliance being difficult and the length of its service life diminish its chance for success. Additionally, the sight formed because of the appliance being placed upon the face and skull causes aesthetic considerations and for this reason, adaptation problems with patients come into existence. Non-oral appliances entail cooperation of patients given that they both pay attention to service life of apparatus and ignore the abovementioned disadvantages. Oral appliances were designed that do not entail cooperation with patients, increase his/her quality of life to be able to prevent this situation called patient cooperation (McNamara & Brudon, 2001; Hunter, 1967; Rogers, 1984).

The aim of treatment using oral appliances is to change the bone structure of the face and direction of development. Although oral appliances are designed to treat each type of malocclusion, they are most successful in the Class II malocclusion. Oral appliances can be divided three groups, called active, passive and functional (Basciftci et al., 2003).

Limiting maxillary growth, the possible development in mandibular position and its growth and the change in teeth position and muscle structure are the expected effects of functional appliances (Clark, 2002). In addition to that the use of functional appliance leads to alterations in tissues around teeth and mouth of patients, it was observed in conducted studies that it can restrict the growth of mid-face to forward, bring about a change in the location of the glenoid fossa and also changes that increase bone construction and destruction in the neuromuscular anatomy and function (Jena et al., 2006 ; Harvold, 1985 ; Pancherz, 1982 ; Birkeback et al., 1984)

Functional appliances are designed for the available pace of adaptive skeletal growth in people keeping the mandible forward (McNamara, 1981). Additionally, it produces a reciprocal effect between the maxillary and mandibular structures and the appliance itself by stimulating muscular and circulatory systems.

It is stated in the Orthodontic literature that Herbst and Twin-Block appliances are the most frequently used functional appliances. Both appliances are effective in correction of class II malocclusions (Lund & Sandler, 1998). In particular, the studies conducted in the last 10 years proved the effectiveness of Twin-Block appliance (Mills C & McCulloch, 1998).

Albeit the Twin-Block appliance is placed within the mouth, it is an appliance having unrestraint in fulfilling normal functions of mouth, at the same time providing higher level freedom in anterior and lateral movements in comparison with other appliances and that is used the whole day (Clark, 1982; Clark, 1988).

The Twin-Block appliance consisting of bite blocks and acrylic artificial palate pertaining to mandibular and maxillary bones was presented by Clark in 1970's. This appliance consists of sub and upper parts arriving to the contact point (junction) at a 70-degree angle. These parts provide stability in closing the jaw (Clark, 1982; Clark, 1988) (Figure 1.)

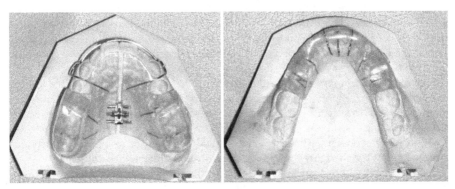

Fig. 1. Sub and Upper Parts of the Twin-block Appliance.

This appliance was preferred in our study owing to these advantages provided by the Twin-Block appliance and they being used incrementally by dentists in the last 10 years. Orthodontists are obliged to inform their patients about the different appliances, duration of treatment and about the possible changes in this period. For this aim, image of the skull is obtained; using X-ray or ultrasound techniques, thereafter jaw and teeth abnormalities are diagnosed. The name of this method is cephalometry (Figure 2). However, advantages of the appliances compared to one another and which one is more useful for one kind of abnormalities is determined by only experiences of Orthodontists.

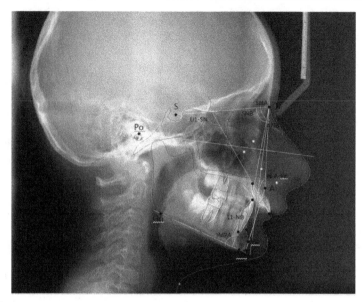

Fig. 2. Cephalometry image and some points of measurement.

Results taken from cephalometric records proved that functional appliances used in the treatment of malocclusion allay the abnormality in the mouth by affecting the alignment of teeth and bone tissue (Graber, 1985). Having said that, many different approaches/hypotheses are proposed regarding how neuromuscular periphery of teeth and bone tissue adapt to the change developed after treatment and the interaction between functional appliance and neuromuscular structure. Protraction in sizes of muscle fibers after the start of use of appliances (Woodside, 1983), the change in muscle dimensions caused by rotation of bone structure and hypertrophy of muscle structure can be given as examples to these hypotheses (McNamara, 1973).

One of the most important reasons for this difference between hypotheses is that there is no reliable and precise reference line in cephalometric image analysis used in evaluating treatment results. This situation complicates the assessment of significant changes occurring in skeletal and tooth structure (Pancherz, 1984). Additionally, it is impossible to obtain information about cephalometric image analysis and neuromuscular adaptation process and be informed about the changing muscle and bone structure during treatment process.

The principle objective of this study is to be able to put forth the interaction between functional appliances and neuromuscular structure with more scientific findings. If treatment can be assessed by quantitative data, as orthodontists can inform their patients about the issues such as treatment process, possible success ratio and etc. and also they can clearly decide which appliance is more suitable for patient as well. The electrophysiological signal that allows non-invasive assessment for changes in muscle structure is EMG. For these reasons, EMG studies continue with an increasing interest to find quantitative solutions such as problems and to measure of muscular activity changes because of the appliances.

In order to achieve this aim, we use EMG signals and their appropriate features to measure and evaluate Twin-Blok related muscular activity changes in Anterior Temporal and Masseter muscles in children with Class II malocclusion.

For this aim power spectral density (PSD) graphics were obtained using EMG and maximum power spectral density value (Max PSD) and area of the PSD graphics (Area PSD) were calculated and changes between before treatment and at the end of the six months were analyzed statistically. Furthermore, Cephalometric images were taken before treatment and at the end of six months and changes in the position with respect to base of the skull were measured to make a comparison.

1.1 Advancement of functional appliances

Albeit first trials were worthy of note, treatment with functional appliances progressed by Roux's studies pertaining to natural forces and functional stimulation. Subsequently, Rogers advocated functional treatment and associated facial muscles with the development and form of the masticatory system (Woodside, 1983).

In 1920's, Andreasen set out to use the appliance that he developed in Class II malocclusions. Emil Herbst introduced the Herbst appliance in 1905 and published findings in 1935. In 1970's, Pancerz's studies on the Herbst appliance and findings that he attained led to this appliance used by dentists more frequently. The advantages of the Herbst appliance are that it is fixed on teeth and treatment period is short. Many studies have been conducted on short and long term effects of the appliance (Pancherz, 1991;. Mcnamara & Fränkel, 2002; Pancherz & Fackel, 1990). Following the introduction of the Herbst appliance, different disadvantages caused the development of various appliances to be used in treatment of Class II malocclusion (Vogt, 2003; Awbrey, 1999). disadvantages experienced in treatment by the Herbst appliance can be summarized as that it is not hygienic, it is rigid and therefore, it restricts lateral movements of the mandible quite a lot (Pancherz, 1985). Another functional appliance similar to this appliance is the Jasper Jumper appliance. This appliance brings about food accumulation inside as well due to its structure. The Bite Fixer appliance was developed to be able to overcome such disadvantages. The Bite Fixer appliance is more flexible and does not allow food accumulation thanks to polyurethane tube situating inside but it was observed to cause open bite in the posterior area in some cases (open bite: occlusion not being able to materialize between the mandible and maxilla in the respective region) (Awbrey, 1999).

Inspired by a case in which the left gonial area disappeared, Bimler saw that mandible movements deliver force to the maxilla and the maxillary arch broadened. The Bimler appliance appeared in the literature in 1949 after many modifications since the day this study was conducted to the present day (Rogers, 1984).

Kesling presented the positioner appliance in 1944. In 1950, Balters began to modify the appliance that Andreasen developed and ensured via modifications he made that talking with this appliance is achieved in a more comfortable fashion (Pancherz et.al, 1989). In 1957, taking into account the structure of skeletal-muscular system that leads to structural and functional changes, Frankel designed his appliance (Proffit & Fields, 2000). Different than other functional appliances, the appliance he named as Kinetor and defined by Stockfish incorporates elastic tubes between two plaques and is considered to optimize oral muscle pressures.

2. Materials and methods

2.1 Measurement of surface EMG signals

EMG recordings were extracted from patients fitting Class II malocclusion criteria below, from the right anterior temporal and right masseter muscles of 15 patients whose ages varied 8 and 13. Treatments of patients, who fit the criteria, were launched via the Twin-Block appliance in the Department of Orthodontics of the Faculty of Dentistry in Erciyes University [Figure 3]. None of the participants underwent orthodontic treatment before. Before each recording session, the procedure was explained in detail to the patient and their parents to allay anxiety.

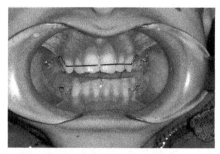

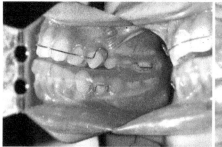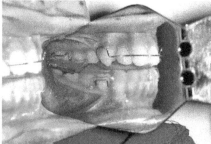

Fig. 3. Twin-block placement in situ.

Class II malocclusion criteria applied in our study:
Inclusion criteria
- Skeletal Class II relationship (ANB > 4°)
- Mandibular retrognathy (SNB < 78°)
- Overjet ≥ 5 mm
- Minimal crowding in dental arches (≤4 mm)
- Bilateral Class II molar and canine relation (at least 3.5 mm)
Exclusion criteria
- Previous history of orthodontic treatment
- Congenitally missing or extracted permanent tooth (except third molars)
- Posterior crossbites or severe maxillary transverse deficiency
- Severe facial asymmetry determined by clinical or radiographical examination
- Systemic diseases that may affect the orthodontic treatment results

Patients were asked to wash their faces with soap for face grease not to affect recordings and then recorded regions were wiped with alcohol and dried. Patients were suggested to sit up straight and look across while recordings were being kept. Electrodes were attached on the muscle bundles, which were found by palpating, by surgical plastic strips (adhesive washers) that do not irritate the skin. Filling silver-surfaced, bipolar electrodes with 4 mm. radius with electrode gel, they were sticked in a way that inter-electrode distance will be 2 cm. The common ground electrodes were adhered onto the forehead of the subject and the active electrodes were placed on the right anterior temporal and right masseter muscles as shown in Figure 4.

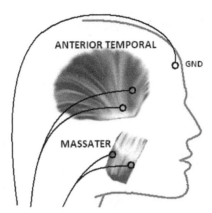

Fig. 4. Placement of surface electrodes on the anterior temporal and masseter muscles.

An important factor that affects recording quality is whether the spot where electrodes adhered and the region where muscle bundle is situated is the same. When the muscle, whose EMG recordings are sought to be taken, possesses a small area, electrodes also perceive signals coming from adjacent muscles and appear as noisy within EMG signals pertaining to the interested muscle bundle (Duchêne & Gouble 1993). Such noises can be avoided by selecting the electrode surface proportional with inter-electrode distance. The selection of appropriate electrode surface size and inter-electrode distance to be kept small diminishes the affect that will stem from the distance between electrode and source and shifts EMG bandwidth to high frequency region. Electrode diameter for bipolar recording should be as big as that can perceive muscle activity in acceptable amounts and at the same time as small as that does not pick activities of other muscles. Inter-electrode distance is described as the distance between the centres of conductive surfaces of electrodes. Inter-electrode distance recommended for bipolar recording is 20 mm (Pozzo, 2004).

Temporal and masseter muscles are muscles taking a part in the mandibular protrusion and EMG recording was extracted from these muscles considering that they may be effective in re-positioning of the mandible during treatment, ensure the mandibular growth and their adaptations may have an impact on treatment results. Mouth activity, in which these muscles play the most active role, is the jaw clenching. Therefore, recordings were taken during clenching activity. The movement was previously practiced by copying the observer.

The signals were recorded in two periods: before the treatment (0 month) and at the end of 6 months [Figure 5]. At each session, EMG recordings were made during the appliances is not in situ.

The MP150 biomedical data acquisition unit (Biopac Systems, Goleta, CA, USA) was used for recording signals. All of the signals were sampled at 5000 Hz and digitized (A/D converted) at a resolution of 12 bits per sample by the MP150 unit.

The EMG100C amplifier module of the MP150 unit was used to amplify and filter with the following settings: 500 Hz Low-Pass (LP) filter, 1.0 Hz High-Pass (HP) filter, and 2000 gain.

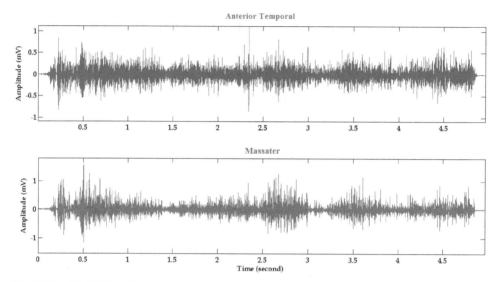

Fig. 5. Raw EMG Signals.

2.2 Analysis of surface EMG signals

There are two usual methods that have been used for the processing of EMG signals: frequency and time domain signal processing method. Some of the time domain signals processing methods are integration, linear envelope, and root mean square (RMS). However, these are are commonly not suitable, since obtained results depend on the selection of threshold [9].

The most powerful and generally used method for signal analysis in frequency domain had been the Fourier Transform (FT). FT is a method that assumes any signal is stationary. However, EMG signals are non-stationary (Panagiotacopulos, 1998)

Hence, the Fourier Transform cannot present satisfactory frequency resolution. In some respects, the Short Time Fourier Transform (STFT) is not perfectly suitable for processing of EMG signals. The main weakness inherent in the STFT is that trade off is inevitable between temporal and spectral resolution (Kim, 1989; Farina, 2004). If one uses a longer sliding time window to obtain higher spectral resolution, the underlying non-stationary will be smeared out, resulting in lower temporal resolution. Conversely, using a shorter window to achieve better temporal resolution will give lower spectral resolution. Because of these signal processing of the EMG signals were achieved using autoregressive (AR) model which is appropriate for non stationary signals and not having windowing problem (Kay, 1981). AR method is a parametric signal analysis method and first, model parameters of the available signal are estimated for such spectrum projection and then, the power spectral density value is calculated from these projection values (Kay, 1988). AR method is one of the most commonly used parametric methods owing to the fact that projection of AR parameters can be carried out easily with the resolution of linear equations. Signal that is modelled in AR method is causal.

The analysis conducted to demonstrate the distribution of power, which any physical signal that is carried to the frequency axis comprises, over frequency field is called as spectral analysis. In this way, graphs exhibiting the power density in frequency axis are denominated as the power spectral density (PSD) graph (Figure 6.).

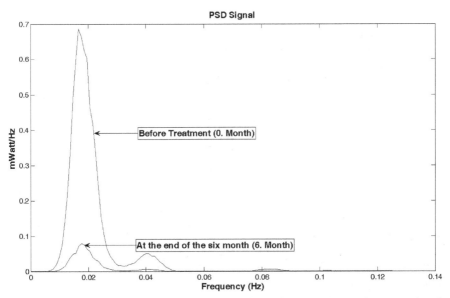

Fig. 6. The comparative display of PSD graphs calculated from EMG signals received at the end of the first and 6. Months.

EMG signal analysis that will be performed by addressing the power spectral density displaying the distribution of signal's energy capability in the frequency spectrum provides information about the neuromuscular conditions of motor units taking part during the activity (Okeson, 1998). The PSD values of EMG signals form as a result of the sum of spectral characteristics of action potentials of motor units. Consequently, it can be said that there is a characteristic power spectrum pertaining to every muscle (Blinowska, 1979). For these reasons, the PSD was used as a criterion in assessing the effect of appliance.

The maximum power spectral density value, which is a value of the PSD graph at its maximum point, varies by contraction density of motor units becoming active within that signal. The area below the PSD graph provides information about strain productivities of motor units carrying out contraction activity (Kwatny, 1970). Therefore maximum power spectral density value and area of the PSD graphics were calculated as a feature.

The AR model is a model revealing important informations in signal by using signal information in the past. It is employed widespread in biomedical signal processing because it responds well against noise. The dependence of past values to the future values is defined as autocorrelation function.

$$\Gamma_{xx}(k) = \frac{1}{N} \sum_{n=1}^{N-k} x[n]x[n+k] \tag{1}$$

where $\Gamma_{xx}[k]$ displays the signal's sample, which is shifted as much as k, and its autocorrelation. The AR model;

$$x[n] = \sum_{i=1}^{p} a_i x[n-i] + \varepsilon[n] \tag{2}$$

$x[n]$ shows the current value of time series, $a_1, \ldots, a_p$ displays the AR model parameters, which are weighting coefficients, and p is the model degree showing the number of past values that will be used to estimate the current value and $\varepsilon[n]$ displays the approximate error with 1 scale.

By using the AR method, the power spectrum is attained as;

$$P_{xx}^{AR}(f) = \frac{q_e^2}{\left| 1 - \sum_{i=1}^{p} a_i e^{-j2\pi fi} \right|} \tag{3}$$

Where q_e^2, is the variance of $\varepsilon[n]$ error.

To calculate the AR parameters, whether numerical signal samples, whose spectral analysis will be directly conducted, are employed or autocorrelation function pertaining to these signal parameters is used. The Burg method was used for estimating the AR parameters (Marple, 1987).

One of the significant issues for employing the AR method is the selection of model degree. Many researchers studied on this problem and the Akaike Information Criteria (AIC) introduced by Akaike is used most commonly in the literature (Kaluzynski, 1989). The selection of AIC model degree is in the form of making the below statement minimum.

$$AIC(p) = \ln \sigma_{wp}^2 + 2p/N \tag{4}$$

Here, σ_{wp}^2 is the estimated variance of linear prediction error and N is the data length. σ_{wp}^2 decreases with the increase of the AR model degree and therefore, $\ln\sigma_{wp}^2$ decreases as well. That being said, $2p/N$ increases too with the increase of p. In this case, a minimum value should be designated for p (Kay, 1988; Kaluzynski, 1989). The p value calculated via the AIC criteria was obtained as 12.

In order to take the fact that measurements were obtained from the same subjects into account, we used paired sample t-test for statistical comparison between 0 month and 6 months. A p-value of less than 0.05 was considered as statistically significant.

All of the data processing was carried out using in-house programs developed under MATLAB R2009b Software (MathWorks Inc., Natick MA, USA).

3. Results and discussion

The aim of present study is to use EMG signals and their appropriate features to measure and evaluate Twin-Blok related muscular activity changes in Anterior Temporal and Masseter muscles in children with Class II malocclusion.

For this aim power spectral density (PSD) graphics were obtained using EMG and Max PSD and Area PSD were calculated and changes between before treatment and at the end of the six months were analyzed statistically. Furthermore, Cephalometric images were taken before treatment and at the end of six months and changes in the position with respect to base of the skull were measured to make a comparison.

Subject	Anterior Temporal			
	Before the Treatment		**At the end of 6 months**	
	Max PSD	Area PSD	Max PSD	Area PSD
1	0,00015	0,01137	0,00001	0,00109
2	0,00009	0,00638	0,00001	0,00101
3	0,00028	0,02380	0,00001	0,00076
4	0,00031	0,02548	0,00002	0,00128
5	0,00008	0,00492	0,00001	0,00072
6	0,00033	0,02871	0,00001	0,00049
7	0,00011	0,00956	0,00011	0,00811
8	0,00015	0,01323	0,00009	0,00549
9	0,00023	0,01278	0,00012	0,00668
10	0,00048	0,02936	0,00005	0,00217
11	0,00054	0,03590	0,00000	0,00006
12	0,00026	0,02064	0,00001	0,00106
13	0,00003	0,00250	0,00001	0,00047
14	0,00032	0,01215	0,00004	0,00259
15	0,00027	0,01883	0,00001	0,00062
Mean±SEM	0,00024±0,00004	0,01704±0,00258	0,00003±0,00001	0,00217±0,00065

Table 1. Max PSD and Area PSD values calculated from EMG signals received right before placing the Twin Block appliance in the mouth over anterior temporal muscle and after 6 months treatment.

The mean values of Max PSD and Area PSD values, calculated from EMG signals for each patient, appear in the last lines of tables. The abbreviation SEM in the tables refers to "standard error of the mean."

Subject	Massater			
	Before the Treatment		**At the end of 6 months**	
	Max PSD	Area PSD	Max PSD	Area PSD
1	0,00012	0,01055	0,00017	0,01362
2	0,00014	0,00997	0,00001	0,00018
3	0,00011	0,01032	0,00001	0,00018
4	0,00006	0,00593	0,00004	0,00327
5	0,00007	0,00565	0,00015	0,01131
6	0,00035	0,02834	0,00031	0,02579
7	0,00011	0,01028	0,00073	0,06498
8	0,00002	0,00148	0,00007	0,00557
9	0,00083	0,05027	0,00037	0,02382

Subject	Massater			
	Before the Treatment		At the end of 6 months	
	Max PSD	Area PSD	Max PSD	Area PSD
10	0,00012	0,00925	0,00001	0,00088
11	0,00015	0,01340	0,00001	0,00035
12	0,00016	0,01464	0,00012	0,00843
13	0,00012	0,00945	0,00018	0,01456
14	0,00032	0,02377	0,00003	0,00270
15	0,00006	0,00497	0,00002	0,00046
Mean±SEM	0,00018±0,00005	0,01388±0,00315	0,00015±0,00005	0,01174±0,00438

Table 2. Max PSD and Area PSD values calculated from EMG signals received right before placing the Twin Block appliance in the mouth over masseter muscle and after 6 months treatment.

Before the treatment values (0. month) are greater for both the anterior temporal and masseter muscles, as seen in Table 1 and 2. However, the difference between 0. month and 6 months values more pronounced for anterior temporal. This difference is statistically significant for both features for anterior temporal but there was no significant difference for the masseter muscle (Table 3).

In addition, changes in the position with respect to base of the skull are significant (p: 0.001).

	Max PSD	Area PSD
Anterior Temporal	**0.00014**	**0.00012**
Masseter	0.5689	0.65591

Table 3. p-values for "across treatment time" comparisons.

These observations are in-line with the results in the literature that "as a consequence of the use of functional appliances the length of the muscles around the jaw gets longer" (Du & Hägg, 2003).

The PSD values of the EMG signals are depending on the power of the motor unit action potentials which makes up these EMG signals (Blinowska, 1979). Six-month-long treatment leads to a decrease in the amplitude and narrowing in the frequency range of motor unit action potentials and so PSD.

Looking at results obtained for anterior temporal muscle, it is seen that there is a significant difference between the onset of treatment and its values after 6 months for both attributes. This result is not valid for the masseter muscle. Albeit both muscles lie among jaw-closing muscles, the Twin-Block Appliance had a different impact.

It is known that the lower jaws of the people who have Class II malocclusion is placed behind their upper jaws. Twin Block appliances tries to keep lower jaw and upper jaw in the same position due to the fact that lower palate and upper palate have a contiguous structure. This can only be accomplished by forcing the lower jaw through forward. In this case, length of the jaw closing muscles must be changed so that the new position of the jaw becomes permanent. For that reason, it is a natural result for jaw closing muscles to clench with lower power density after 6 months. This result is matching the when the functional appliances is placed in the mouth, the jaw closing muscles become elongated ((Du & Hägg, 2003; Miles et al., 1986; Woodside et al., 1983). Hence, the brawn of the jaw closing muscles reduces and the PSD values tend to decrease to lower amplitude.

However, this outcome was not realized for the masseter muscle. Therefore, it can be inferred that the effect of the Twin-Block Appliance on the masseter muscle did not come into existence in the first 6 months.

The critical objective of treatment by the Twin –Block appliance is to trigger the formation of an additional extension on jawbone. This objective can be achieved by increasing the development of cartilage belonging to condyle and also restricting the maxillary growth. The change also seen in the sizes of proximal muscles as a result of elongation of jawbone particularly reflected to EMG signals extracted for anterior temporal muscle. The reason why a similar difference did not form on the masseter muscle can be explained by that a position shift materialized on jawbone rather than an actual growth. Likewise, in studies carried out on Twin-Block treatment, it is seen that the question whether the observed change is an actual growth or a position shift has been debated. (Baccetti et. al. 2000; Trenouth, 2000). Additionally, it is observed that posterior teeth do not still contact one another when the appliance is removed at the end of 6 months in patients treated by the Twin-Block. This case brings about more intensive occlusion of anterior teeth of patients and further contraction on front fibers of the masseter muscle. This impact hinders the occurrence of adaptation coming into being in masseter muscles in EMG recordings received during jaw closing/ constriction.

The patient must be observed in a longer period in order to follow the consequences which will be resulted from this condition.

4. Conclusion

The use of EMG signals in studies related to face muscles continues with an increasing interest. Muscle structure responsible for masticatory function and soft tissue belonging to face does not only affect bone development but also affects the period of orthodontic treatments and permanency of success achieved after treatment. EMG is a primary instrument to record this functional process and for the effect of skull traction. For these reasons, analysis of non-invasive EMG by appropriate methods can provide further information regarding the effect of treatment and service lives of appliances (Eckardt et al. 1997).

In the literature, there are some EMG studies that they are based one removable appliances. However, these kinds of appliances are worn only during night time (Tallgren et al. 1998; Ahlgren , 1960). Hence, the appliances act as a splint rather than an activator. On the other hand, the functional appliances that are worn full-time like the Twin-Block stimulate greater than those worn only part-time. For that reason, this study which is about the EMG and the Twin-Block, is important in order to investigate the muscle response.

The PSD is the feature regularly used for frequency domain analysis of EMG. An integration of the PSD over all frequencies yields the entire power. PSD value was chosen as a feature in order to evaluate the effects of the appliances. That's because PSD value is a parameter which is frequently used in the evaluation of the EMG signals and it gives information on power of total action potential formed by the muscles during tightening.

EMG and PSD are quite successful in showing the change occurred in the muscles. However, criteria must be determined for different age groups in using different trainers.

Moreover, if an expert system, which evaluates the functionality of the orthodontic appliances for the orthodontists; which estimates the treatment period; and which enables a follow-up for the effect of the applied orthodontic appliances on the person, is desired to be developed with artificial intelligence applications, PSD attribution will be insufficient for the input value. For that reason, orthodontists and engineers must enable different parameters to become evaluable by continuing their interdisciplinary studies.

5. Acknowledgment

The authors are grateful for the grant support provided by The Scientific & Technological Research Council of Turkey – TÜBİTAK, contract number 106E144.

6. References

Rangayyan R. M., (2002). Introduction to Biomedical Signals, In: *Biomedical Signal Analysis: A Case-Study Approach*, Akay, M., (Ed),. pp. 1-14, Wiley-IEEE Press, ISBN 0-471-20811-6, New York

Reaz, M. B. I., Hussain M. S., Mohd-Yasin F., (2006). Techniques of EMG signal analysis: detection, processing, classification and applications. *Biological Procedures Online* Vol.8, No. 1, pp. 11 – 35.

Moritani, T., Stegeman, D., Merletti R., (2004). Basic physiology and biophysics of EMG signal generation . In: *Electromyography: Physiology, Engineering, and Non-Invasive Applications*, Merletti, R., Parker, P. (Eds), pp. 1 – 26, Wiley-IEEE Pres,

Cobbold, R. S. C., Transducers for Biomedical Measurements: Principles and Applications, John Wiley & Sons, Inc., New York, (1974).

Kraus F., (1956) Vestibular and oral screens. Trans Eur Orthod Soc.; 32: 217–224

Kleissen R.F., Buurke J.H., Harlaar J., Zilvold G., Electromyography in the biomechanical analysis of human movement and it clinical application, Gait Posture, 8, 143–158, (1998).

Riedel R. A., The relation of maxillary structures to cranium in malocclusion and normal occlusion. Angle Orthod;22:142-145, (1952).

McNamara J. A. Components of Class II malocclusion in children 8-10 years of age. Angle Orthod.; 51:177-202 (1981).

Renfroe EW. A study of the facial patterns associated with Class I, Class II division 1 and Class II, division 2 malocclusions Angle Orthod;19:12-15, (1948).

Blair E.S. A cephalometric roentgenographic appraisal of the skeletal morphology of Class I, Class II, division 1 and Class II, division 2 malocclusion. Angle Orthod.;24:106-119, (1954).

Proffit W. R., Fields H. W., Moray L. J., Prevelance of malocclusion and orthodontic treatment need in the United States: estimates from the N-HANES III survey Int. J. Adult Orthod. Orthog. Surg.;13:97-106 (1998).

McNamara JA Jr. Brudon WL. Orthodontics and dentofacial orthopedics. Ann Arbor: Needham Pres;:67-80 (2001).

Hunter W. S., The vertical dimensions of the face and skeletodental retrognatizm. Am J Orthod; 53:586-595, (1967).

Rogers A. Concepts of functional jaw orthopedics. In: Graber TM, Neumann B, editors. Removable orthodontic appliances. 2nd ed. Philadelphia: Saunders;. p. 87. (1984).

Basciftci F. A., Uysal T, Büyükerkmen A, Sarı Z. (2003) "The effects of activator treatment on the craniofacial structure of Class II division 1 patients". Eur J Orthod.;25:87–93.

Clark WJ. Twin block functional theraphy applications in dentofacial orthopedics. 2nd ed. Mosby-Wolfe Press, St Louis (2002).

Jena AK, Duggal R, Parkashc H. Skeletal and dentoalveolar effects of Twinblock and bionator appliances in the treatment of Class II malocclusion: A comparative study. Am. J. Orthod. Dentofacial Orthop. 130:594-602, (2006).

Harvold EP. Bone remodelling and orthodontics. Eur J Orthod;7:217-230, (1985).

Pancherz H. The mechanism of Class II correction in Herbst appliance treatment. A cephalometric investigation. Am J Orthod;82:104-113, (1982).

Birkeback L, Melsen B, Terp S. A laminographic study of the alterations in the temporomandibular joint following activator treatment Eur J Orthod;6:267-276, (1984).

Lund D. L., Sandler P.J., The effects of Twin Blocks: a prospective controlled study. Am J Orthod Dentofacial Orthop;113: 104-10, (1998).

Mills C, McCulloch K. Treatment effects of the Twin-block appliance: a cephalometric study. Am J Orthod 1998;114:15-24.

Toth LR, McNamara JA, Jr. Skeletal and dentoalveolar adaptations produced by Twin-block appliance treatment. AmJ Orthod Dentofacial Orthop 1999;116:597-609.

Clark WJ. The Twin-block traction technique. Eur J Orthod 1982;4:129-38.

Clark WJ. The Twin-block technique. Am J Orthod Dentofacial Orthop 1988;93:1-18.

Graber TM, Rakosi T, Petrovic AG. "Dentofacial orthopedics with functional appliances". St Louis: CV Mosby; 1985.

Graber TM. Physiologic principles of functional appliances. St Louis: CV Mosby; 1985

Woodside DG, Altuna G, Harvold E, Herbert M, Metaxas A. Primate experiments in malocclusion and bone induction. Am J Orthod 1983;83:460-8.

McNamara Jr JA. Neuromuscular and skeletal adaptations to altered function in the orofacial region. Am J Orthod 1973;64:578-606.

Pancherz H. A Cephalometric analysis of skeletal and dental changes contributing to Class II correction in activator treatment. Am J Orthod 1984;85:125-34.

Pancherz H., The nature of Class II relapse after Herbst appliance treatment: a cephalometric long-term investigation. Am J Orthod Dentofacial Orthop;100:220-33, (1991).

Mcnamara JA Jr. Rolf Fränkel, 1908-2001 (in memoriam). Am. J. Orthod. Dentofacial Orthop.;121:238-9 (2002).

Pancherz H, Fackel U. The skeletofacial growth pattern pre- and post-dentofacial orthopaedics. A long-term study of Class II malocclusions treated with the Herbst appliance. Eur J Orthod;12:209-18, (1990).

Vogt W. A new fixed interarch device for Class II correction, J. Clin. Orthod. 2003;37:36-41

Awbrey J.J. The Bite-Fixer, Clinical Impressions, Ormco/A Company. 1999;8:10-16.

Pancherz H. The Herbst appliance. Its biologic effects and clinical use, Am. J. Orthod. 1985;87:1-20

Pancherz H., Malmgren O, Ha¨gg U, Omblus J, Hansen K. Class II correction in Herbst and Bass therapy. Eur J Orthod;11:17-30, (1989).

Proffit WR, Fields HW, editors. Contemporary orthodontics. 3rd ed. St Louis: Mosby; (2000).

Duchêne J. and Gouble F. Surface electromyogram during voluntary contraction: Processing tools and relation to physiological events. Critical Reviews in Biomedical Engineering 21(4): 313–397, (1993).

Pozzo M., Farina D., Merletti R., Electromyography:Detection, Processing and Applications Biomedical Technology and Devices Handbook, CRC press, 2004.

Panagiotacopulos N. D., J. S. Lee, M. H. Pope, K. Friesen, (1998) Evaluation of EMG signals from rehabilitated patients with low back pain using wavelets. J. of Electromyog. and Kinesiology, vol. 8, pp. 269 – 278,.

Kim, R. B. Hanson, T. L. Abell, and J. R. Malagelada. (1989) Effect of inhibition of prostaglandin synthesis on epinephrine-induced gastroduodenal electromechanical changes in humans. Mayo Clinic Proc. 64:149–157,.

Farina D., R. Merletti, D. F. Stegeman, (2004) Biophysics of the generation of EMG signals. In: Electromyography: Physiology, Engineering, and Non-Invasive Applications, New York, Wiley-IEEE Pres. , pp. 81 – 107.

Kay, S.M. , and Marple, S.L., (1981) Spectrum Analysis – A Modern Perspective, Proceedings of IEEE Transactions 69(11):1380–1419.

Kay S.M., Modern Spectral Estimation: Theory and Application. Prentice Hall-Englewood Cliffs, NJ, (1988).

Okeson J. P.,: "Management of Temporomandibular disorders and occlusion", Mosby, St. Louis Fourth edition (1998), pp:160-162.

Blinowska, A., Verroust, J., Cannet, G., "The Determination of motor unit characteristics from the low frequency electromyographic power spectra". Electromyography and Clinical Neurophysiology, 19, 281 – 290, (1979).

Kwatny, E., Thomas, D., Kwatng, H., (1970). An application of signal processing techniques to the study of myoelectric signals. IEEE Transactions on Biomedical Engineering 17, 303 – 312.

Marple S.L., Digital Spectral Analysis with Applications. Prentice Hall-Englewood Cliffs, NJ, 1987.

Kaluzynski K., Order Selection in Doppler Blood Flow Signal Spectral Analysis Using Autoregressive Modelling, Medical & Biological Engineering & Computing, 27, 89-92, (1989).

Du X., Hägg U. "Muscular adaptation to gradual advancement of the mandible". Angle Orthod., vol. 73, pp. 525 – 531, (2003).

Miles T. S., Nordstrom M. A., Turker K. S., "Length – related changes in activation threshold and waveform of motor units in human massater muscle", Journal of Physiology (London) vol. 370, pp. 457 – 465, (1986).

Baccetti T. et al. Treatment timing for Twin-block therapy. Am J Orthod dentofacial Orhop 2000;118:159-70.

Trenouth M. Cephalometric evaluation of the Twin block appliance in the treatment of Class II Division 1 malocclusion with matched normative growth data. Am J Orthod Dentofacial Orthop 2000;117:54-59.

Eckardt, L., Harzer, W., Schneevoigt, R., 1997. Comparative study of excitation patterns in the masseter muscle before and after orthognathic surgery. Journal of Cranio-Maxillojacial Surgery 25, 344-352

Tallgren, A., Christiansen, R., Ash, M. M., Miller, R. L., (1998) Effects of a myofunctional appliance on orofacial muscle activity and structures. Angle Orthodontists. 3, 249–258.

Ahlgren J., (1960) An Electromyographic analysis of the response to activator therapy. Odontol Revy 11, 125.

12

New Measurement Techniques of Surface Electromyographic Signals in Rest Position for Application in the Ophthalmological Field

Edoardo Fiorucci, Fabrizio Ciancetta and Annalisa Monaco
Università dell'Aquila,
Italy

1. Introduction

The Stomatognatic apparatus is a component of the craniomandibular system, and it represents an entryway to external stimuli: relationship among occlusion, masticatory muscle system (Murch, 1974; Oddsson, 1989) and head posture (Barber & Sharpe, 1988) have been recently confirmed.

Proprioception messages from the neck muscles are integrated in the central nervous system and contribute to control balance and body orientation. Centripetal impulses from neck proprioceptors cooperate with the labyrinth impulses to promote oculomotor muscular activity through the cervical–vestibular–ocular reflex (Ito, 1995). Some important encephalic nuclei (trigeminal nuclei, oculomotor nuclei, vestibular nuclei, accessorial nerve nuclei) are integrated in the medial longitudinal fasciculus.

Ocular proprioceptive receptors send afferent signals to trigeminal and cuneate nuclei. The anatomic and physiologic links of these anatomical structures imply a co-ordinated integration of proprioceptive ocular and stomatognathic afferences.

The ocular system and the stomatognathic one are anatomically and physiologically connected. Vision plays an important role in the multi-sensorial process of postural stabilisation: among visual inputs, the postural one allows to draw a moving object ocular nuclei control the eye position in the orbit; the ocular nuclei send fibers to nuclei which control neck and head movements and receive afferences from vestibular nuclei.

It has been observed that a modification of ocular proprioception modifies head and body posture (Donaldson & Knox, 1991; Buisseret-Delmas & Buisseret, 1990; Schmid et al., 1981).

Ocular proprioception is linked with stomatognathic muscular system: neuromuscular spindles and myotendinous receptors (Rose et al., 1991; Lukas et al., 1994; Rose & Abrahams, 1975) of extraocular muscles send afferences to trigeminal and cuneate nuclei (Porter, 1986). Moreover oculomotor, vestibular, trigeminal and accessorial nerve nuclei are connected through the medial longitudinal fasciculus. The role of trigeminal afferences on tonic-postural regulation has been underlined too (Meyer & Baron, 1976)

Several studies supported anatomical linkage between stomatognathic and ocular systems. Patients with Temporomandibular disorders (TMD) and this prevalence increase in those patients with head, neck, and shoulder pain. A similar association has been found in children with a mandibular functional lateral-deviation respect to healthy subjects in pediatric age. It is also stated that in TMD subjects, head rotation (as a compensatory adjustment for the eye dominance) is significantly associated to a mandibular shifting toward the contralateral side. These relationships, recorded by measuring transverse head postural change by means of temporary eye dominance change, have been confirmed (Lin SY & White, 1996). Passive soft-tissue viscoelasticity and stretch reflexes in the jaw-closing muscles are involved in mandibular postural stability during locomotion as a consequence of the influence of head support and body posture on the mandibular rest position. Relationship between oculomotors and neck cephalogyric muscles have been reported by Meyer & Baron, 1976. These authors showed that desmodontal receptors and temporo-mandibular joint, like sternocleidomatoid, trapezius and cervical muscles are connected with oculomotor muscles. A study confirmed that the alteration of dental occlusion can induce some fluctuations in visual focusing (Sharifi et al., 1998)

Electromyography has been widely applied to estimate oro-facial muscle function or dysfunction.

Association between EMG activity of jaw and neck muscles with TMD signs/symptoms as well as malocclusion, parafunctions and posture has been investigated

Some works shows the effects of body position on the EMG activity of sternocleidomastoid and masseter muscles in healthy subjects. Many sEMG studies are concerned with functional activity, such as clenching, and few of them have studied the rest position and the difference between the anterior temporalis sEMG in open and closed eye conditions.

Patients with myogenous facial pain show that the open eyes condition, compared with the closed eyes one, is associated with a change in the head and neck sEMG activity in the mandibular rest position (Monaco et al., 2010). This behaviour is not present in the healthy control subjects. A recent study (Spadaro et al., 2010) involving young healthy subjects with normal occlusion and without visual defects, compared the EMG values of the the anterior temporalis area at mandible rest position, in the closed eyes and open eyes conditions: the results showed no significant difference in the EMG values, suggesting that subjects with class I without myogenous facial pain signs or symptoms and with clinically verified correct vision, accept the exteroceptive visual input without an adaptive mechanism on the sEMG pattern of the stomatognathic system.

These observations suggest that the visual input effect could be a good provocation test for assessing a neuromuscular reply that will be more significant in neurogenic facilitation areas (Schmid & Mongini , 1985) .

The alteration of dental occlusion can induce some fluctuations in visual focusing, and the visual input effect on the EMG activity of Sternocleidomastoid and Masseter muscles at rest has been proved too. The different pattern of EMG activity of anterior temporalis with respect to masseter, sternocleidomastoid, and anterior digastric observed at rest, upon variation in the visual input, suggests a differential innervation of stomatognathic muscles. In fact the innervations of the sternocleidomastoid and anterior digastric muscles is provided by spinal and hypoglossal (XI and XII) nerves, while that of masseter and anterior temporalis muscles is provided by the trigeminal (V) nerve.

Interactions between neck and the extraocular muscles in the myopic eye have been reported (Valentino & Fabozzo, 1993). Monaco et al., 2006 confirmed that myopic defects can induce some alterations on EMG activity of masticatory muscles.

Nevertheless, there is a low interest about the influence of visual inputs on EMG values, as well about the relationship between visual defects and EMG values.

New Measurement Techniques of Surface Electromyographic Signals in Rest Position for Application in
the Ophthalmological Field

231

Among the neuromuscular factors that are able to affect the EMG values of the jaw elevators, the activity of the extraocular muscles, that is explicated by the activity of anterior temporalis, could be of interest.

2. Electrical characteristics of SEMG signals in rest position

In the intramuscular EMG, the contribution of each different motor units (UM) is distinguished according to the morphology of the electrical potentials. On the contrary, in the surface EMG (SEMG), the filtering effect of human tissues drastically reduces the morphological difference between the voltages that cannot be used as a classification element.

The human body is a good electrical conductor, but unfortunately the conductivity varies with tissue thickness. Because the of amplitude EMG signals is inversely proportional to the square of the distance from the source, the Ums, whose activity is possible to detect, are those located at a maximum distance of 15 mm from the electrodes. The interposed tissues can attenuate the high-frequency of component signals, and generally this mitigation is proportionally to the UM depth.

Moreover, in case of size-recuded muscles, neighbouring muscles may produce a significant amount of EMG noise (crosstalk); this issue is omnipresent when dealing with SEMG signals. However, all possible efforts must be made to eliminate or reduce the presence of the crosstalk. Despite this disadvantage, the use of surface electrodes simplifies the signal pick-up, making possible to record the signals in static and dynamic conditions, such as during the execution of functional movements or exercises.

The isometric activities generate electrical voltages whose root mean square (rms) values range from less than 50 μV to 20-30 mV, depending on the investigated muscle. The typical amplitude of noise amount at 5 μV rms, so the S/N is enough for the correct evaluation of the muscle activity with an acceptable accuracy (Fig. 1). The signal is generally amplified by a factor from 500 to 2000.

The frequency range of a SEMG amplifier is from 10 Hz to 500 Hz. The typical repetition rate of UM firing is about 7 to 20 Hz, depending on the size of the muscle. The high frequency cut-off corresponds to the maximum frequency of the SEMG signals. Moreover, because of the movement of electrodes and cables, the low frequency components of the collected signal should be removed. The SEMG signal is filtered, to eliminate the disturbances and highlight the relevant components (e.g. a low-pass filtering to analyze low-frequency components, or a high-pass filtering to analyze high frequency components, or a notch-filtering to eliminate components at a specific band). Therefore, the signal is processed to extract the desired quantity concerning the muscular fibres.

The Study of the activities of superficial muscles in rest position has been considered with scant regard, for two main reasons: i) the activity of signals is not measured with needle electrodes during rest time, with a consequently worsening in the transmission of the signal; ii) the amplitudes of the acquired electromyographic signals in rest conditions are in the same range of the noise (1 to 5 μV rms), and are difficult to evaluate.

Nevertheless, some interesting phenomena were observed during the application of surface electromyography in rest position (Ferrario et al., 1993; Rilo et al., 1997). For example, the records of electrical signal from the anterior temporal muscle showed different results in rest condition of the mandible, according to the open or closed eyes condition. Those signals varied by subject, but were constant for the same person, during the same recording session and without changing the recording apparatus or the electrodes themselves; furthermore, this variation was independent from the state of the eyes. In the electromyographic measurement practice, keeping open or closed the eyes is usually required for about 15 s at a time (Miralles et al., 1998; Kawamura, 1967).

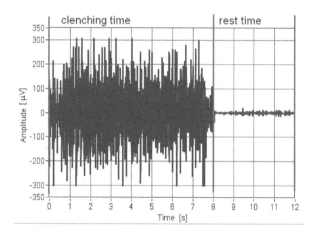

Fig. 1. The amplitude of electromyographic signal during the clenching and rest time.

From the preliminary measurements, the voltage amplitude of the investigated signals seems to be related to the sequence of the open-eyes and closed-eyes conditions. The signals appeared to be in the range of 1 to 6 μV rms, comparable with the noise level, and with a frequency lower than 20 Hz. This effect of movement could not be recorded because of the band pass (20 to 500 Hz filter), usually integrated in surface electromyographic equipment. Due to the limitation of these instruments, the clinical analysis of subjects could not unequivocally highlight the real cause of the obtained results (Bucci et al., 2009; Monaco et al., 2006; Shahani, 1977; Sharifi et al., 1998).

Considering that several clinical report questionated this issue, we decided to investigate the phenomenon with an ad hoc measurement station, that is capable to fully capture and analyze these signals. Briefly, the main goal of our research was the implementation and characterization of suitable measurement techniques for the identification of the biological signals, by reducing the effect of the superimposed noise without removing the signals related to non isometric muscle activities.

3. First preliminary study: evaluation of the influence of ocular defects on of the activity of stomatognatic muscles

The aim of this first preliminary study was to determine how the activity of the stomatognatic muscles is influenced by ocular defects. We expect a significant modification of SEMG values by changing visual input and visual defects.

A total of 20 children aged between 7 and 13 years (mean age 9±8 months), was evaluated.

In the study group 10 children with myopic defects were enlisted, selected among the patients afferent to the Pediatric Dentistry Department of the University of L'Aquila.

Ten subjects with normal vision, the control group, were chosen through the Pair Matching procedures, so that each myopic child had a matching age case control. All subjects were investigated by SEMG. Each subject underwent to two recordings of SEMG at rest: during the first SEMG each child was asked to keep his/her eyes closed, while during the second SEMG recordings each child was asked to keep his/her eyes open while looking straight ahead and to keep the lips in normal soft contact. The group of myopic children performed the recordings without lenses.Time for each recording was 15 seconds. Each individual was seated in a wooden chair with headrest in a comfortable stance. SEMG activity was recorded by K7 (Myotronic Inc.; Seattle,Washington, USA), using bipolar surface electrodes at single differential with interelectrode distance of 1 cm. The surface electrodes were placed with adhesive tape to the skin over the superficial masseter (LMM, RMM), anterior temporal (LTA, RTA), anterior digastric (RDA, LDA) and sternocleidomastoid (LSC, RSC) bilaterally and parallel to the muscle fibres. Eight channel surface electromyographic equipment was used (Myotronic Inc.; Seattle,Washington, USA). The obtained signals were amplified, recorded and computed using a clinical aimed software (K7- Myotronic Inc.; Seattle,Washington, USA); the Root Mean Square (RMS), expressed in µvolt, was used as amplitude indicator of the signal. SEMG of the subjects was examined by the same operator without knowledge of the recording purpose. A paired t-test for independent samples was performed to obtain a comparison between mean and variance values of electromyographic data. The p value < .05 was assumed as the level of significance. To facilitate the introduction of the data in the statistic software program, all the absolute values expressed in µvolt RMS were multiplied by 10.

Comparison according to the age of the individuals showed no significant differences between the groups (p > .05). Tables 1 and 2 illustrate the mean values, in µvolt, and standard deviations (parenthesis) of SEMG activity at rest with closed and open eyes for the anterior temporal, masseter, sternocleidomastoid and anterior digastric muscles of the children with normal vision (control group).

	LTA	LMM	RMM	RTA	LSC	LDA	RDA	RSC
Observations	10	10	10	10	10	10	10	10
Mean	17.2	13.6	14.5	17.7	23.6	24.5	32.0	24.7
SD	7.4	3.6	4.6	6.2	6.8	11.2	19.5	10.3

Table 1. Mean Value and Standard Deviation of Electromyographic Activity at Rest with closed eyes in the Stomatognatic Muscles of Control subjects.

	LTA	LMM	RMM	RTA	LSC	LDA	RDA	RSC
Observations	10	10	10	10	10	10	10	10
Mean	18.7	13.0	12.8	17.8	23.1	24.4	26.8	22.9
SD	8.6	3.8	2.5	10.2	10.2	10.7	8.5	8.5

Table 2. Mean Value and Standard Deviation of Electromyographic Activity with opened eyes in the Stomatognatic Muscles of Control Patients.

Tables 3 and 4 show the mean values and standard deviation of EMG activity at rest with closed eyes and open eyes for the anterior temporal, masseter, sternocleidomastoid and anterior digastric muscles of the children with myopic vision (study group). In myopic patients (study group) a significant difference was observed in LTA muscles.

	LTA	LMM	RMM	RTA	LSC	LDA	RDA	RSC
Observations	10	10	10	10	10	10	10	10
Mean	22.5	16.2	15.3	19.5	24.6	24.3	22.4	22.3
SD	11.5	8.1	10.4	7.2	8.3	11.2	8.05	10.9

Table 3. Mean Value and Standard Deviation of Electromyographic Activity with closed eyes in the Stomatognatic Muscles of Control Patients.

	LTA	LMM	RMM	RTA	LSC	LDA	RDA	RSC
Observations	10	10	10	10	10	10	10	10
Mean	32.6	17.3	14.6	24.2	20.8	27	25.9	18.4
SD	13.3	7.9	9.7	9.8	6.5	10.7	10.2	6.3

Table 4. Mean Value and Standard Deviation of Electromyographic Activity with opened eyes in the Stomatognatic Muscles of Control Patients.

In the closed eyes condition it is possible to observe an identical pattern of SEMG activity in both control and study group. SEMG values of left and right anterior temporal muscles were significantly different. These results underline that: i) a change in the visual input does not induce a modification in the basic tone of the stomatognatic system in children with normal vision; ii) the myopic children showed an increase of anterior temporal activity at rest. the activity of masticatory muscles, controlled by the trigeminal nerve, is regulated by several inputs coming from the proprioception of neuromuscular spindles. These inputs have an important role in the maintenance and in the modifications of muscular basal tone. Proprioception messages coming from the muscles of the neck are integrated in the central nervous system and contribute to control the balance and the body orientation in the space-time. Centripetal impulses from the muscles of the neck proprioceptors cooperate with the labyrinth impulses to promote the oculomotor muscular activity through the cervical-vestibular-ocular reflex.

Some important encephalic nuclei (trigeminal nuclei, oculomotor nuclei, vestibular nuclei, accessorial nerve nuclei) are integrated in the medial longitudinal fasciculus. Moreover, ocular proprioceptive receptors send afferences to the trigeminal and cuneate nuclei.

This study confirms the physiologic link of these anatomical structures: a modification of the proprioceptive ocular afferences can be reflected on the stomatognatic one. The EMG evaluations comported different RMS values as a consequence of the proprioceptive input change.

The results suggest that the relation between stomatognatic and oculomotor system is underestimated and the use of EMG could permit the integrate study of the two systems.

4. Second preliminary study: evaluation of the electromyographic activity of stomatognathic muscles at rest with eyes closed and with eyes open

The aim of the second preliminary study was to evaluate the electromyographic activity of stomatognathic muscles at rest with eyes closed and with eyes open and the effects of ocular correction on electromyographic activity and muscular balance. This knowledge could be clinically relevant in order to evaluate if, in subjects with functional lateral deviation, the ocular correction could contribute to variations of muscular tone and its symmetry.

New Measurement Techniques of Surface Electromyographic Signals in Rest Position for Application in
the Ophthalmological Field

235

The study was performed at the Dental Clinic of the University of L'Aquila. This study included 32 subjects with functional lateral-deviated mandible selected among children with tooth midline deviation, listed to paediatric dentistry clinic for dental care. All the patients presented natural dentition, an observable deviation of mandibular and anterior tooth midlines on functional base diagnosed by clinical examination, frontal and basal tele-radiographs. The subjects were chosen according to the following parameters: deviated chin from mid-sagittal plane (recognized by perpendicular line to horizontal bipupillary and bicommisural lines); the lack of alignment of the upper and lower labial frena; asymmetry of interincisive lines and molars/canine classes; deviation of incisor midline in maximal intercuspidation both in centric relation and at rest position; mandibular deviation during opening; noise and tenderness referred to temporomandibular joint (TMJ). The frontal teleradiograph, taken at open mouth, confirmed the symmetry of maxillary and mandibular structures. In order to be considered for the study, the following characteristics had to be present: i) negative history of orthodontic treatment; ii) observable deviation of anterior tooth midlines >1,5 mm with alignment at mouth open; iii) absence of skeletal asymmetry; iv) absence of any anterior or posterior/lateral crossbite; v) muscular ocular-extrinsic tone alteration. In the first visit all subjects underwent complete ophthalmological and orthoptical evaluation by the same ophthalmologist.

The oculo-extrinsic muscular tone disorders were classified as eso (convergence latent strabismus) and exophories (divergence latent strabismus) and measured by using cover test and Berens prisms. The values expressed as angle of deviation were measured in prismathic diottries (DP). Thirthy-two children with functional mandibular lateral deviation and muscular extrinsic ocular tone disorders, 19 girls and 13 boys, ranging from 8 to 12 years of age, with mean age of 10.1 (sd 1.1) in study group and 9.6 (sd 1.6) in control group (Table 1), were selected. No statistical differences were observed in the mean age for the two groups. Therefore, all subjects received a prescription for their ocular alterations. The subjects were randomly divided into two groups: study and control. The study group received ocular correction that needed to be balanced upon EMG control at the next visit, while the control group received a conventional ocular correction through lenses.

At second visit, all subjects were investigated by SEMG. Recordings were performed by placing bipolar surface electrodes (Instruments Co. Seattle) on the left and right anterior temporal, masseter, sternocleidomastoid and digastric muscles. During the recordings, EMG was monitored using a system K7 (Myotronic Inc., Seattle, Washington, USA). Each subject underwent three recordings of the integrated SEMG activity at rest, with eyes open and closed and after ocular correction. During the first SEMG recording each child was asked to keep his/her eyes closed. During the second SEMG recording, each child was asked to keep his/her eyes open while looking straight ahead and to keep the lips in normal soft contact. During the third SEMG recording children in the control group wore glasses for ocular correction through orthoptic examination only, while children in the the study group wore lenses centred and balanced through orthoptic evaluation integrated by means electromyography control. Recordings were performed with previous instruction to the children. SEMG recording time for each trial was 15 seconds. Two-samples paired comparison test (t-test) was performed on SEMG at rest, with and without visual input and with ocular correction, for each investigated muscle. The SEMG values are based on RMS measured in µvolt and using Symmetry Index (rightleft / right+left) (SI). SI values range from 0 to 1 (0 = perfect symmetry).

Each patient was seated in a wood chair with headrest in a comfortable stance, and patients were asked to closed the eyes, to avoid enviromental input. SEMG activity was recorded by

K7 software (K7 Myotronic Inc.-Seattle, Washington, USA) using bipolar surface electrodes at single differential with interelectrode distance of 1 cm. The surface electrodes were affixed with adhesive tape to the skin over the superficial masseter (LMM,RMM), anterior temporal (LTA,RTA), anterior digastric (RDA, LDA) and sternocleidomastoid (LSC, RSC), bilaterally and parallel to the muscle fibers. Eight channel surface electromyographic equipment was used (Myotronics). The signal obtained were amplified, recorded and computed using a clinical aimed software (K7-Myotronics); the Root Mean Square (RMS), expresses in μvolt, was used as amplitude indicator of the signal. SEMG of the subjects were examined by the same operator without knowledge of recording purpose.

The subjects of both groups were analysed with respect to the rate of lateral deviation from tooth midline and electromyographycally examined. Therefore the subjects of the study gruop wore lenses centred and balanced by means SEMG, the control group wore lenses fabricated according to conventional orthoptic evaluation.

The SEMG values were compared and statistically analysed. A paired t-test for independent samples was performed to obtain a comparison between mean and variance values of electromyographic data. The level of significance was set at the p value of $<.05$. A correlation analysis was performed between the rate of lateral deviation and the DP rate. A correlation coefficient (r) equal or greater than 0.600 was considered significant. A linear regression statistics coefficient was performed between the rate of lateral deviation and the DP rate.

To facilitate the introduction of the data in the statistic software, all absolute values expressed in μvolt rms were multiplied by 10. Tables 5 and 6 illustrate the mean values, in μvolt, of SEMG activity at rest with closed eyes for the anterior temporal, masseter, sternocleidomastoid and anterior digastric muscles respectively of the study and control group. Tables 7 and 8 show the mean values of SEMG activity at rest for the anterior temporal, masseter, sternocleidomastoid and anterior digastric muscles with eyes open in the study and the control groups, respectively.

Tables 9 and 10 report the mean values of SEMG activity at rest for the anterior temporal, masseter, sternocleidomastoid and anterior digastric muscles with ocular correction in the study and the control group, respectively. The comparison between the results in Tables 5 and 7 shows that EMG activity of the anterior temporal increases significantly in children with conventional ocular correction (control group) (p<0.05). In the study group children the ocular correction obtained by means SEMG did not show an increase of muscular values of TA.

	LTA	LMM	RMM	RTA	LSC	LDA	RDA	RSC
Observations	16	16	16	16	16	16	16	16
Mean	20.3	19.5	19.9	17.5	22.9	29.0	36.5	22.4
SD	10.5	13.0	13.7	6.7	6.4	18.1	22.7	10.5

Table 5. Mean Value and Standard Deviation of Electromyographic Activity at Rest with closed eyes in the Stomatognatic Muscles of study subjects.

	LTA	LMM	RMM	RTA	LSC	LDA	RDA	RSC
Observations	16	16	16	16	16	16	16	16
Mean	20.5	13.6	11.6	18.9	18.0	17.9	19.4	18.0
SD	9.4	7.0	5.1	8.0	10.9	8.6	8.2	8.7

Table 6. Mean Value and Standard Deviation of Electromyographic Activity at Rest with closed eyes in the Stomatognatic Muscles of control subjects.

	LTA	LMM	RMM	RTA	LSC	LDA	RDA	RSC
Observations	16	16	16	16	16	16	16	16
Mean	24.5	19.5	18.1	27.9	22.5	30.7	30.6	22.0
SD	12.4	12.3	13.2	15.1	8.5	21.5	18.5	9.7

Table 7. Mean Value and Standard Deviation of Electromyographic Activity at Rest with opened eyes in the Stomatognatic Muscles of study subjects.

	LTA	LMM	RMM	RTA	LSC	LDA	RDA	RSC
Observations	16	16	16	16	16	16	16	16
Mean	25.3	13.6	12.0	27.9	19.4	19.4	19.9	18.2
SD	12.7	6.3	5.2	15.1	10.0	8.9	8.1	9.2

Table 8. Mean Value and Standard Deviation of Electromyographic Activity at Rest with opened eyes in the Stomatognatic Muscles of control subjects.

	LTA	LMM	RMM	RTA	LSC	LDA	RDA	RSC
Observations	16	16	16	16	16	16	16	16
Mean	22.2	19.4	16.3	20.8	20.5	30.7	25.8	25.0
SD	10.4	8.0	5.7	9.0	6.7	21.5	10.8	17.3

Table 9. Mean Value and Standard Deviation of Electromyographic Activity at with ocular correction by means EMG in the Stomatognatic Muscles of study subjects.

	LTA	LMM	RMM	RTA	LSC	LDA	RDA	RSC
Observations	16	16	16	16	16	16	16	16
Mean	22.2	19.4	16.3	20.8	20.5	30.7	25.8	25.0
SD	10.4	8.0	5.7	9.0	6.7	21.5	10.8	17.3

Table 10. Mean Value and Standard Deviation of Electromyographic Activity at with conventional ocular correction in the Stomatognatic Muscles of control subjects.

5. The new measurement equipment

To extract useful information about the effect of incorrect lenses, the electromyographic signal in rest conditions should be suitably acquired and processed, in order to reduce the effect of the noise and to supply the oculist with a reliable quantitative indication.

To this aim, we developed an ad hoc measurement system, whose block diagram is reported in Fig. 2; the proposed system can operate in parallel with the conventional instrument to compare the supplied results.

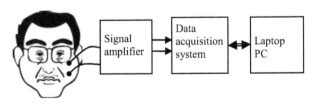

Fig. 2. The block diagram of the measurement setup.

The bio-electrical signal can be detected using two single electrodes (one active electrode located in correspondence of the muscle under analysis and another reference electrode located on a neutral point), or a bipolar electrode (two active electrodes located on the muscle). This last differential configuration has a better noise immunity, even if it presents some difficulties with muscles of reduced dimensions.

Because the SEMG signal is low in amplitude, with respect to other ambient signals on the surface of the skin, we decided to detect it with a differential configuration. The electrodes are placed in the midline of the belly of the muscle, where the signal has the maximum amplitude. The electrode signal is amplified, acquired and processed. The amplifier is the EG&G PARC 113 Low-Noise Preamp, with a bandwidth from DC to 300 kHz. Its main features are: i) adjustable high and low frequency rolloffs; ii) two input channels, AC or DC coupled, with single-ended or differential input section; iii) maximum input voltage of 1 Vrms; iv) gain ranging from x10 to x10000, in the 1-2-5 sequence; v) input impedance of 1 GΩ, shunted by 15 pF; vi) common mode rejection of 100 dB in the range from DC to 1 kHz; input DC drift < 10 μV/°C, output DC drift < 1 mV/°C.

The amplified signal has been acquired by a USB data acquisition module, the Keithley KUSB-3108 High Gain Multifunction, whose main features are: i) resolution of 16 bits, effective number of bits of 14.1; ii) sampling rate of 50 kSamples/s; iii) accuracy of +/- 0.04 %; iv) nonlinearity of +/- 4 LSB; v) input impedance of 100 MΩ, 100 pF; vi) common mode rejection > 74 dB; vii) A/D converter noise of 0.4 LSB rms. A Laptop PC supplied by a battery has been used; data acquisition and processing have been programmed using the NI LabVIEW tool (Bucci et al, 2009; Fiorucci et al., 2011).

In order to analyze the behaviour of the proposed system, a plot of the signal acquired during the sequence closed-open-closed eyes, is shown in Fig. 3, while Fig. 4 reports the same signal acquired with a traditional instrument.

The effects produced by the internal blocks of a standard SEMG that, practically, processes this signal as a noise, are evident.

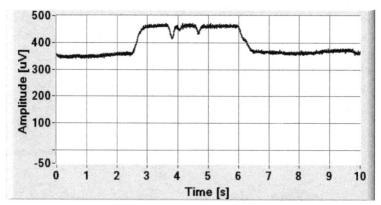

Fig. 3. Signal v(i) corresponding to the sequence closed-open-closed eyes, acquired with gain 10000.

Fig. 3 also shows that suitable signal processing techniques should be implemented in order to: i) detect the signal transitions that indicate the beginning (closed-open in the figure) and the ending (open-closed) of the time interval of interest; ii) process the signal during this time interval (up time) in order to extract the useful information.

New Measurement Techniques of Surface Electromyographic Signals in Rest Position for Application in
the Ophthalmological Field

239

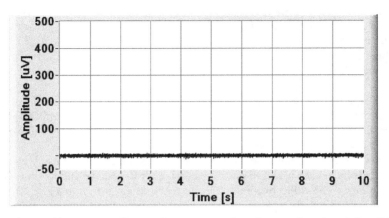

Fig. 4. Signal vemg(i) corresponding to the sequence closed-open-closed eyes (traditional
SEMG) acquired with gain 10000.

6. The measurement technique and the signals analysis

The goal of the present research is the analysis of the surface electromyographic signals on
patients wearing eyeglasses (Miralles et al., 1998; Kawamura, 1967; Shahani, 1977;). In detail,
our experimental activity has been focused on the acquisition and analysis of the SEMG
signals of anterior temporalis muscles at mandible rest conditions, in occurrence with some
particular voluntary and involuntary movements of the patient, such as closed-open eyes
condition; those signals can not be acquired with a traditional SEMG measurement
apparatus, because of the presence of pass-band filters and of the electronic noise, which
could mask the closed-open eyes effect (Airi Oksanen et al., 2007; Sharifi et al., 1998).

The acquisitions are performed in both dark and illuminated rooms, and each patient has
been asked to open the eyes after 1 s and, after 3 s, to close them; the voluntary movement of
opening and closing the eyes produces a rectangular shape in the digitized input voltage
v(i).

With the aim to emphasize the low frequency voltage variations, we adopted the rms sliding
window technique. In SEMG techniques, the rms of the signal can be considered as an index
of the power of the signal itself, and it can be correlated to the muscular stress. We are
interested in evaluating the variation of that stress during the time, to identify the
conditions in which it is higher or lower; the adoption of the rms sliding window technique
allows the observation of that variation. Moreover, the rms signal is filtered by the DEMG
high frequency components, so it can be adopted to implement a threshold technique for the
automatic identification of the time interval corresponding to the opened-eyes, in which the
muscular stress must be measured.

Specifically, the input voltage v has been digitized and processed to calculate the rms
voltage waveform v_{rms}. At any instant of time i, a new rms voltage value has been calculated
from n samples of the acquired voltage v (j), using the formula:

$$v_{rms}(i) = \sqrt{\frac{1}{n} \sum_{j=i}^{i+n-1} v(j)^2} \tag{1}$$

where n is the number of samples contained in each summation interval (variable from 20 ms to 100 ms). The new value $v_{rms}(i+1)$ has been calculated by sliding forward a sample of the input voltage.

This technique improves the transitory response and guarantees a better temporal resolution: the $v_{rms}(i)$ is updated at each sampling point, so it is possible to directly compare $v(i)$ and $v_{rms}(i)$.

During the experimental activity, by analyzing the features of the acquired SEMG signals and comparing them with the movements of the patients, we identified two stress symptoms, that can be directly related with the incorrect prescription of eyeglasses; they can be described comparing Figs. 5 and 6.

Fig 5 shows the SEMG signal acquired, in an illuminated room, on a patient without eyeglasses, that have been asked to open the eyes, to try to focalize and to close the eyes. In those conditions there is the maximum stress, whose main symptoms are: A) the partial closing and opening of the eyes due to the winking movement as a consequence of the difficulty in focusing the image; B) the amplitude increasing of the SEMG high frequency components, that is related to the increased activity of the masticatory muscles. The signal in Fig. 6 shows the minimum stress conditions, as it has been acquired in an illuminated room, on a patient wearing the correct eyeglasses: the A and B phenomena are absent.

To quantify the patient stress, we introduced a new signal, $v^*(i)$, calculated as the point-by-point difference between $v(i)$ and $v_{rms}(i)$:

$$v^*(i) = v(i) - v_{rms}(i) \tag{2}$$

It represents the dynamic component of the muscle activity, that takes into account the winking movement (high frequency components). We observed that two quantitative parameters of the $v^*(i)$ signal can be adopted as indexes of the stress of a patient wearing incorrect eyeglasses: the average power and the voltage range in open-eyes condition. We verified that these parameters are smallest when the muscle stress is minimum, that is when the prescription of eyeglasses is correct. The measurement of the average power and voltage range was performed only in the time interval in which the rms signal $v_{rms}(i)$ is higher than a suitable threshold.

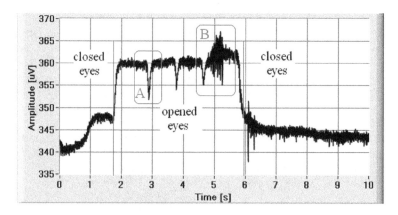

Fig. 5. Results in case of no lenses (maximum stress).

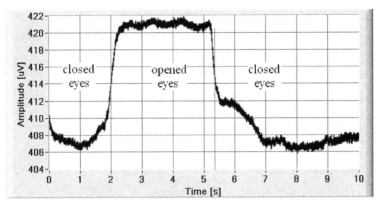

Fig. 6. Results in case of correct lenses (minimum stress).

We also performed the amplitude spectrum measurement, in order to investigate about the possible presence of frequency components whose amplitude could be related to the muscular stress.

In Fig.7 a flowchart of the signal processing algorithm implemented on the proposed measurement system is synthesized. Figs. 8 to 11 show $v_{rms}(i)$ and $v^*(i)$ signals obtained with the proposed technique starting, respectively, in dark and illuminated rooms. The acquisitions in an illuminated room have been performed asking the patient, without sight defects, to open the eyes, to try to focalize a sign and then to close the eyes. Fig. 10 shows the voltage level variations due to the voluntary movement of opening and closing the eyes, superimposed to the high-frequency signal due to the muscle stress; the voltage drop at 2.2 s is due to the focalizing movement involving a partial closing of the eyes.

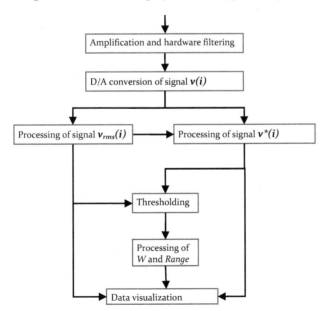

Fig. 7. Data analysis procedure.

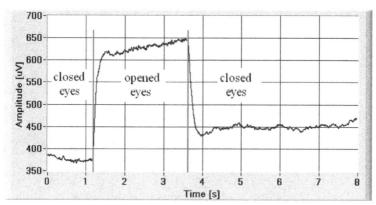

Fig. 8. Rms signal $v_{rms}(i)$ corresponding to the sequence closed-opened-closed eyes in a dark room.

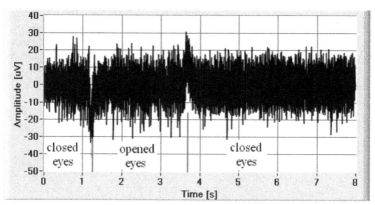

Fig. 9. Dynamic component $v^*(i)$ of the signal, corresponding to the sequence closed-opened-closed eyes in a dark room.

As part of the development phase, the measurement system has been tested to investigate its performance. The first test was the measurement of the frequency response, with different gain values: 500, 1000, 2000, 5000 and 10000. The reference signal has been generated using the Stanford Research DS360 Ultra Low Distortion Function Generator, whose main specifications are: i) output range from 20 µVpp to 40 Vpp; ii) THD 0.001%; iii) frequency accuracy of 25 ppm; iv) 20 bit D/A converter. The tests have been carried out by varying the amplitude and the frequency of a sinusoidal waveform in the ranges (50 to 500) µVrms, (5 to 5000) Hz. Successively we measured the total RMS noise voltage and the noise figure for the selected gains. The measurement of the total RMS noise, the noise figure and the system noise spectrum have been performed according to (Van Putten, 1988). In detail, the total RMS noise voltage eN, measured in the frequency range DC-1 kHz, adopted for all our experimental activity can be expressed as:

$$e_N = \sqrt{e_n^2 + i_n^2 R_{gen}^2 + e_R^2} \cdot \sqrt{1000} \qquad (3)$$

where e_n is the equivalent short-circuit input RMS noise voltage, in is the equivalent open
circuit RMS noise current, R_{gen} is the internal resistance of the voltage source, and e_R is the
thermal noise voltage developed across R_{gen}.
As suggested in (Gerleman & Cook, 1992) a typical value of surface electrode impedance is
R_{gen} = 20 kΩ, en has been measured by shunting a 20 kΩ resistor across the input terminals
of the EG&G PARC 113, at 290 K, measuring the preamp output rms voltage and dividing it
by the amplifier gains reported in Tab III. The Noise Figure has been calculated as:

$$NF = 10\log\left[\frac{e_N^2}{e_R^2}\right]$$ (4)

where:

$$e_R^2 = 4kTRB$$ (5)

K is the Boltzmann's constant, T the temperature, B the bandwidth and R the considered
resistance. The obtained results, tabulated in Table 11, show a good response of the
instrument, because the noise amplitude is quite irrelevant for the bio-electrical signal
detection.
We also calculated the system dynamic range, considering that the CMRR of the EG&G
PARC 113 in the range from DC to 1 kHz is greater than 100 dB; and that the 16 bits data
acquisition board presents a theoretical dynamic range of 96 dB; from the tests we carried
out that the overall system dynamic range can be assumed as 86 dB.

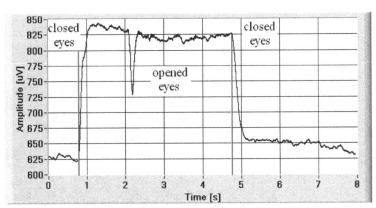

Fig. 10. Rms signal $v_{rms}(i)$ corresponding to the sequence closed-opened-closed eyes in an
illuminated room with no eyeglasses.

Gain	Noise Figure [dB]	Total RMS noise voltage [nV rms]
500	2.56	952
1000	2.04	897
2000	7.60	1702
5000	3.10	1014
10000	2.15	908

Table 11. Noise figures and total RMS noise voltages for different gain settings.

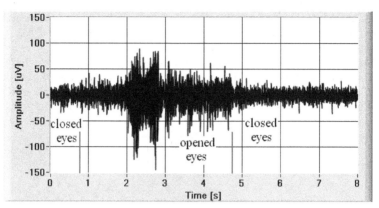

Fig. 11. Dynamic component v*(i) of the signal, corresponding to the sequence closed-opened-closed eyes in an illuminated room, without eyeglasses.

7. Experimental results

We conducted some test to investigate about the effectiveness of the processed parameters to provide useful information concerning the eyeglass prescription. To evaluate the stress of wearing eyeglasses, an experimental activity has been carried out in the Dental Clinic of the University of L'Aquila on a group of 30 patients with different visual defects.

As a first step, the correct eye glasses prescription is detected by the ophthalmologist of our team, by using a set of optical test lenses and a trial frame (Fig.12).

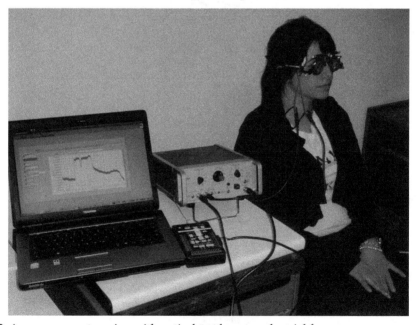

Fig. 12. A measurement session with optical test lenses and a trial frame.

After that, the closed-open-closed EMG signals are acquired while the patient is wearing
correct and wrong (obtained by adding +/-0.25, +/-2 and +/5 cylindrical correction degrees)
lenses. In all the tests, both the increasing and decreasing of the corrective lenses graduation
have been characterized by an increase of the average power and by the presence of focalizing
movements, involving an increase of the SEMG signal range. In other words, the minimum
values of both the parameters are reached when the correct prescription is applied. To
underline the relation between muscular stress and incorrect eyeglasses, the SEMG signals v(i)
acquired on the same patient are presented in Figs. 13-17, with the previously described
correction degrees; they have been obtained by adding respectively the following cylindrical
correction degrees: +0.25, -0.25, + 2, -2, +5, -5. The measured values of voltage range and
average power are reported in Table 12; it is possible, by using the proposed measurement and
analysis approach, to determine the eyeglasses prescription minimizing the muscular stress. In
Figs. 19-24 we propose the comparison between the amplitude spectrum of signal in Fig. 6,
adopted as a reference for the minimum stress conditions, and the amplitude spectra of the
signals in Figs. 13-18. It is possible to identify two frequency bands, in which the effect of the
muscular stress seems to be more evident: 10-400 Hz, and 720-740 Hz.
In all the figures, the correct eyeglasses reduce the amplitude of the frequency components.

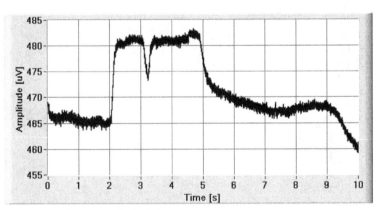

Fig. 13. Signal acquired in case of +0.25 degrees.

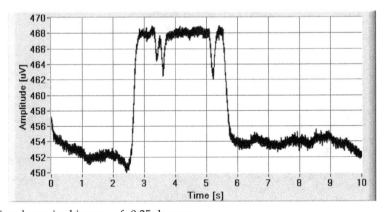

Fig. 14. Signal acquired in case of -0.25 degrees.

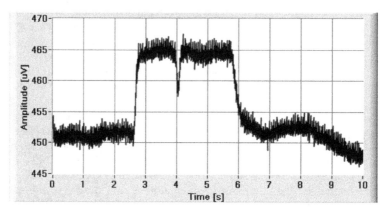

Fig. 15. Signal acquired in case of +2 degrees.

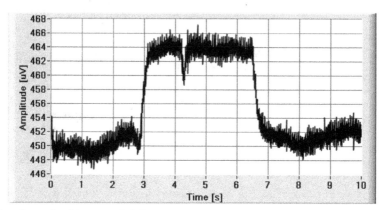

Fig. 16. Signal acquired in case of -2 degrees.

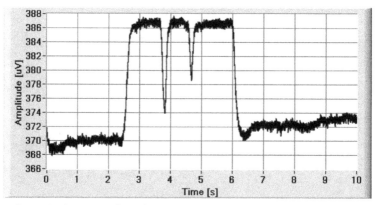

Fig. 17. Signal acquired in case of + 5 degrees.

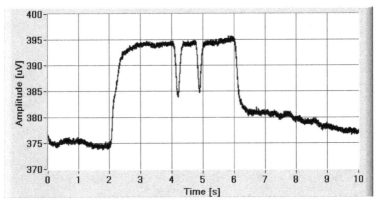

Fig. 18. Signal acquired in case of - 5 degrees.

Deviation from correct prescription [cylindrical correction degrees]	Range [uV]	Average power [pW]
-5	6.8	0.61
-2	6.7	0.35
-0,25	5.0	0.28
0	1.5	0.04
0,25	4.3	0.31
2	6.3	0.40
5	8.5	0.72

Table 12. Measured voltage range and average power values.

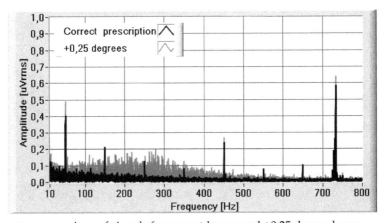

Fig. 19. Spectra comparison of signals for correct lenses and +0,25 degree lenses.

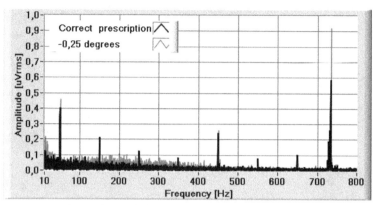

Fig. 20. Spectra comparison of signals for correct lenses and -0,25 degree lenses.

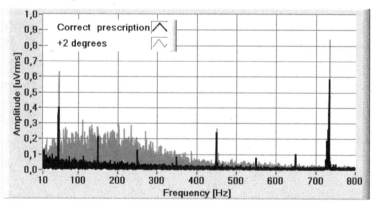

Fig. 21. Spectra comparison of signals for correct lenses and +2 degree lenses.

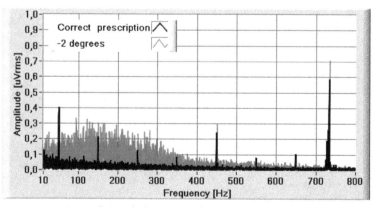

Fig. 22. Spectra comparison of signals for correct lenses and -2 degree lenses.

New Measurement Techniques of Surface Electromyographic Signals in Rest Position for Application in
the Ophthalmological Field

249

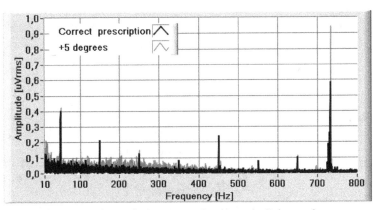

Fig. 23. Spectra comparison of signals for correct lenses and +5 degree lenses.

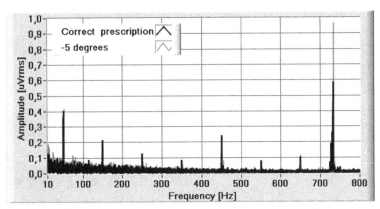

Fig. 24. Spectra comparison of signals for correct lenses and -5 degree lenses.

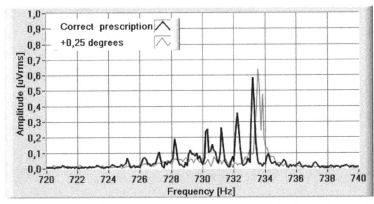

Fig. 25. Spectra comparison of signals for correct lenses and +0,25 degree lenses, in the range
720-740 Hz.

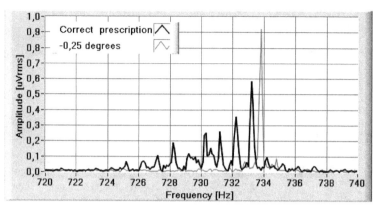

Fig. 26. Spectra comparison of signals for correct lenses and -0,25 degree lenses, in the range 720-740 Hz.

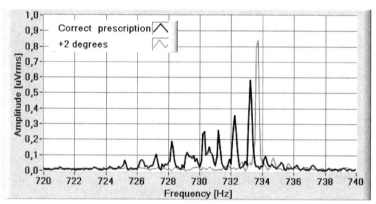

Fig. 27. Spectra comparison of signals for correct lenses and +2 degree lenses, in the range 720-740 Hz.

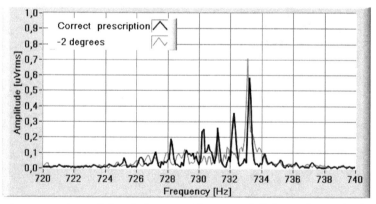

Fig. 28. Spectra comparison of signals for correct lenses and -2 degree lenses, in the range 720-740 Hz.

New Measurement Techniques of Surface Electromyographic Signals in Rest Position for Application in
the Ophthalmological Field

251

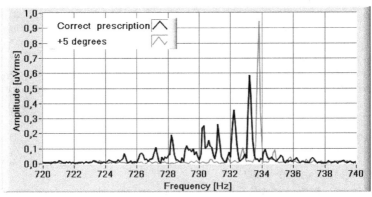

Fig. 29. Spectra comparison of signals for correct lenses and +5 degree lenses, in the range
720-740 Hz.

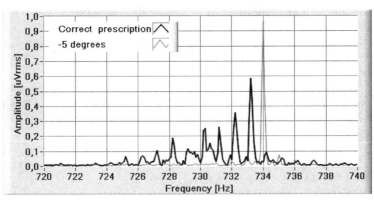

Fig. 30. Spectra comparison of signals for correct lenses and -5 degree lenses, in the range
720-740 Hz.

8. Conclusion

The main aim of this chapter was the implementation of new measurement techniques of
surface electromyographic signals, that are of great importance for the analysis of
neuromuscular functions. Traditional SEMG apparatuses can not be adopted for this
application, mainly because of the presence of built-in filtering sections that eliminate the
related signal components (Ferdjallah et al., 2000), but also because it is required a special
signal processing. By adopting the proposed technique, it is possible to acquire the raw
signals, to identify the presence of voluntary movements during the acquisition period with
the proposed rms sliding window technique, and to calculate some indexes of the signal
$v^*(i)$, such as average power and the voltage range in open-eyes conditions. The proposed
approach has been applied to evaluate the effects of the graduation of eyeglasses and
contact lens on the muscle stress in rest conditions. By processing the SEMG, it is possible to
define the right choice for the grade of glasses or contact lenses, with a direct and objective

evaluation of the generated muscular stress. Currently, we are working to elaborate a protocol by analysing a greater number of patients. Further improvement of the present paper will investigate the relation between the eyeglasses and contact lens and the amplitude spectrum of the SEMG signal in the frequency range 720 – 740 Hz, in which the amplitudes of the frequency components can supply information about the stress of the patients as suggested by Figs. 23-28. Finally, the adoption of an image acquisition device will be possible to directly compare the EMG signals to the filmed movement of the patient's face.

9. References

Barber HO. & Sharpe JA. (1988) *Vestibular disorder*. Year Book Medical Publisher Inc. Chicago, ISBN 0815104197.

Buisseret-Delmas C & Buisseret P. (1990) Central projections of extraocular muscle afferents in cat. C. *Neuroscience Letters*. Vol. 109, No. 1-2, pp.48-53, ISSN 0304-3940

Bucci G., Fiorucci E., Monaco A. & Cattaneo R. (2009), Development of an ad hoc measurement station for the human surface electromyography in rest position" *Proceedings of IEEE MEMEA 2009*, ISBN: 978-1-4244-3599-9, Cetraro Italy, May 2009

Donaldson IM & Knox PC. (1991) Afferent signals from pigeon extraocular muscles modify the vestibular responses of units in the abducens nucleus. *Proceedings Biological Sciences*. Vol. 244, No. 1311, pp.233-239, ISSN 09628452

Ferrario VF, Sforza c, Miani JR, D'Addona & Barbini E. (1993) Electromyographic activity of human masticatory muscles in normal young people. Statistical evaluation of reference values for clinical applications. *Journal of Oral Rehabilitation*. Vol. 20, No. 3, pp. 271-280, ISSN 1365-2842

Ferdjallah M.; Myers K., Starsky A. & Harris G.F. (2000) Dynamic electromyography. *Pediatric Gait, 2000. A new Millennium in Clinical Care and Motion Analysis Technology*, ISBN 0-7803-6469-4, Chicago USA , July 2000.

Fiorucci E., Bucci G., Ciancetta F. & Monaco A. (2011) Measurement and analysis of surface electromyographic signals on patients wearing eyeglasses *Proceedings of IEEE MEMEA 2011*, BARI Italy, May 2011

Gerleman D. G. & Cook T. M., (1992) *Selected Topics in Surface Electromyography for Use in the Occupational Setting: Expert Perspectives- Chapter 4: Instrumentation* U.S. Department of Health and Human Services.

Ito S., Taketomi M. &Hirano M. (1995) Effects on tonic neck reflex on optokinetic nystagmus in rabbits. *Acta Otolaryngologica* , Vol. 115, No. 2, pp 134–136.

Kawamura Y. (1967), Neurophysiologic background of occlusion. *Periodontics*. 1967; Vol.5:, pp. 175-183.

Lin SY. & White GE. (1996) Mandibular position and head posture as a function of eye dominance. *Journal of Clinical Pediatric Dentistry*, Vol. 20, No. 2, pp. 133-140, ISSN 1053-4628

Lukas JR. & Aigner M, Heinzl H, & Mayr R. (1994) Number and distribution of neuromuscular spindles in human extraocular muscles. *Investigative Ophtalmology & Visual Science*, Vol. 35, No. 13 , pp. 4317-4327, ISSN 1552-5783

Meyer J. & Baron JB. (1976) Participation of trigeminal afferences in tonic postural regulation. Static and dynamic aspects. *Aggressiologie* , Vol. 17, pp:33-40, ISSN 00021148

Miralles R., Gutierrez C., Zucchino G., Cavada G., Carvajal R., Valenzuela S. & Palazzi C. (1998) Visual input effect on EMG activity of sternocleidomastoid and masseter muscles in healthy subjects and in patients with myogenic cranio-cervical-mandibular dysfunction. *Cranio*, Vol. 16, No. 3, pp. 168-184, ISSN 0886-9634

Monaco A., Cattaneo R., Spadaro A., Giannoni M., Di Martino S. & Gatto R. (2006) Visual input effect on EMG activity of masticatory and postural muscles in healthy and myopic children. *European Journal of Paediatric Dentistry*, Vol. 7, No.1, pp. 18-22, ISSN 2035-648X .

Monaco A, Spadaro A, Cattaneo R. & Giannoni M. (2010) Effects of myogenous facial pain on muscle activity of head and neck. *International Journal of Oral & Maxillofacial Surgery* ; Vol. 39, No. 8, pp. 767-773, ISSN 0901-5027

Murch GM. (1973) *Visual and Auditory Perception*. New York: Bobbs-Merril Company Inc.;

Oddsson L. (1989) Motor patterns of a fast voluntary postural task in man: trunk extension in standing. *Acta physiologica Scandinavica*, Vol. 136, No. 1, pp. 47-58, ISSN 0302-2994

Oksanen A., Ylinen J., Pöyhönen T., Anttila P., Laimi K., Hiekkanen H. & Salminen J. (2007) Repeatability of electromyography and force measurements of the neck muscles in adolescents with and without headache. *Journal of Electromyography and Kinesiology*, Vol.17, No. 4, pp.493-503, ISSN 1050-6411

Porter JD. (1986) Branstem terminations of extraocular muscle primary afferent neuron in the monkey. *Journal of Comparative Neurology*, Vol. 247, No.2, pp. 133-143, ISSN 1096-9861

Rilo B., Santana U., Mora MJ. & Cadarso CM., (1997) Myoelectrical activity of clinical rest position and jaw muscle activity in young adults. *Journal of Oral Rehabilitation*. Vol. 24, No. 10, pp. 735-740, ISSN 1365-2842.

Rose PK. & Abrahams VC. (1975) The effect of passive eye movement on unit discharge in the superior colliculus of the cat. *Brain Research*, Vol 97, No. 1, pp 95-106, ISSN 00068993

Rose PK., Mac Donald J. & Abrahams VC, (1991) Projections of the tectospinal tract to the upper cervical spinal cord of the cat: a study with the anterograde tracer PHA-L. *Journal of Comparative Neurololgy* ; Vol. 314, No. 1, pp. 91-105, ISSN 0021-9967

Schmid W & Mongini F. (1985) Orthodontic treatment and mandibular modelling in growth. *Fortschr Kieferorthop* , Vol. 46, No. 5, pp. 352-357, ISSN 0015-816X

Schmid R., Zambarbieri D. & Magenes G. (1981) Modifications of vestibular nystagmus produced by fixation of visual and nonvisual targets. *Annals of the New York Academy of Sciences*, Vol. 374, pp. 689-705, ISSN 1749-6632

Shahani M, (1977) Influence of visual input on monosynaptic reflex. *Electromyography and Clinical. Neurophysiology*, Vol. 17, No. 1, pp. 3-11 ISSN

Sharifi Milani R, Deville de Periere D. & Micallef JP, (1988) Relationship between dental occlusion and visual focusing. *Cranio*. Vol. 16, No. 2, pp. 109-118, ISSN 0886-9634

Spadaro A, Monaco A, Cattaneo R., Masci C. & Gatto R. (2010) Effect on anterior temporalis surface EMG of eyes open-closed condition. *European Journal of Paediatric Dentistry* Vol. 11, No. 4, pp. 210-212, ISSN 2035-648X

Valentino B. & Fabozzo A. (1993) Interaction between the muscles of the neck and the extraocular muscles of the myopic eye. An electromyographic study. *Surgical and Radiologic Anatomy* , Vol. 15, No. 4, pp. 321-323, ISSN 0930-1038

Van Putten A. F. P. (1988) *Electronic Measurement Systems*, Prentice Hall, ISBN 9780132518857

Permissions

The contributors of this book come from diverse backgrounds, making this book a truly international effort. This book will bring forth new frontiers with its revolutionizing research information and detailed analysis of the nascent developments around the world.

We would like to thank Mark Schwartz, for lending his expertise to make the book truly unique. He has played a crucial role in the development of this book. Without his invaluable contribution this book wouldn't have been possible. He has made vital efforts to compile up to date information on the varied aspects of this subject to make this book a valuable addition to the collection of many professionals and students.

This book was conceptualized with the vision of imparting up-to-date information and advanced data in this field. To ensure the same, a matchless editorial board was set up. Every individual on the board went through rigorous rounds of assessment to prove their worth. After which they invested a large part of their time researching and compiling the most relevant data for our readers. Conferences and sessions were held from time to time between the editorial board and the contributing authors to present the data in the most comprehensible form. The editorial team has worked tirelessly to provide valuable and valid information to help people across the globe.

Every chapter published in this book has been scrutinized by our experts. Their significance has been extensively debated. The topics covered herein carry significant findings which will fuel the growth of the discipline. They may even be implemented as practical applications or may be referred to as a beginning point for another development. Chapters in this book were first published by InTech; hereby published with permission under the Creative Commons Attribution License or equivalent.

The editorial board has been involved in producing this book since its inception. They have spent rigorous hours researching and exploring the diverse topics which have resulted in the successful publishing of this book. They have passed on their knowledge of decades through this book. To expedite this challenging task, the publisher supported the team at every step. A small team of assistant editors was also appointed to further simplify the editing procedure and attain best results for the readers.

Our editorial team has been hand-picked from every corner of the world. Their multi-ethnicity adds dynamic inputs to the discussions which result in innovative outcomes. These outcomes are then further discussed with the researchers and contributors who give their valuable feedback and opinion regarding the same. The feedback is then collaborated with the researches and they are edited in a comprehensive manner to aid the understanding of the subject.

Apart from the editorial board, the designing team has also invested a significant amount of their time in understanding the subject and creating the most relevant covers. They scrutinized every image to scout for the most suitable representation of the subject and create an appropriate cover for the book.

The publishing team has been involved in this book since its early stages. They were actively engaged in every process, be it collecting the data, connecting with the contributors or procuring relevant information. The team has been an ardent support to the editorial, designing and production team. Their endless efforts to recruit the best for this project, has resulted in the accomplishment of this book. They are a veteran in the field of academics and their pool of knowledge is as vast as their experience in printing. Their expertise and guidance has proved useful at every step. Their uncompromising quality standards have made this book an exceptional effort. Their encouragement from time to time has been an inspiration for everyone.

The publisher and the editorial board hope that this book will prove to be a valuable piece of knowledge for researchers, students, practitioners and scholars across the globe.

List of Contributors

Ashraf Zaher
Department of Neurology, Faculty of Medicine, University of Mansoura, Mansoura, Egypt

Induk Chung and Arthur A. Grigorian
Georgia Neurosurgical Institute and Mercer University School of Medicine, Macon, GA, USA

Masafumi Yamada and Kentaro Nagata
Kanagawa Rehabilitation Institute, Kanagawa Rehabilitation Center, Japan

Faranak Farzan, Mera S. Barr and Zafiris J. Daskalakis
Centre for Addiction and Mental Health, University of Toronto, Toronto, Canada

Paul B. Fitzgerald
Monash Alfred Psychiatry Research Centre, The Alfred and Monash University School of Psychology and Psychiatry, Melbourne, Australia

Enguo Cao, Yoshio Inoue, Tao Liu and Kyoko Shibata
Kochi University of Technology, Japan

N. Terzi
INSERM, ERI27, Caen; Univ Caen, Caen; CHRU Caen, Service de Réanimation Médicale, Caen, France

N. Terzi, D. Orlikowski, H. Prigent and F. Lofaso
Centre d'Investigation Clinique - Innovations Technologiques, Hôpital Raymond, Poincaré, AP-HP, Université de Versailles-Saint Quentin en Yvelines, Garches, France

D. Orlikowski
Centre d'Investigation Clinique - Innovations Technologiques 805, Service de, Réanimation et Unité de Ventilation à Domicile, Hôpital Raymond Poincaré, AP-HP, France

H. Prigent and F. Lofaso
Services de Physiologie - Explorations Fonctionnelles, Hôpital Raymond Poincaré, AP-HP, France

F. Lofaso
INSERM, U 955, Créteil, France

Pierre Denise and H. Normand
INSERM, ERI27, Caen, Univ Caen, CHRU Caen, Service d'Explorations Fonctionnelles, Caen, France

Pedro Guerra, Alicia Sánchez-Adam, Lourdes Anllo-Vento and Jaime Vila
University of Granada, Spain

David Pánek, Dagmar Pavlů and Jitka Čemusová
Department of Physiotherapy, Faculty of Physical Education and Sport, Charles University, Czech Republic

Javier Navallas and Javier Rodríguez
Department of Electrical and Electronic Engineering, Public University of Navarra, Pamplona, Spain

Erik Stålberg
Institute of Neuroscience, Department of Clinical Neurophysiology, Uppsala University Hospital, Uppsala, Sweden

Michael Wehner
Wehner Engineering, Berkeley, USA

Şükrü Okkesim and Sadık Kara
Fatih University, Institute of Biomedical Engineering, İstanbul, Turkey

Tancan Uysal
İzmir Katip Çelebi University, Faculty of Dentistry, İzmir, Turkey

Aslı Baysal
Kocaeli University, Faculty of Dentistry, Kocaeli, Turkey

Edoardo Fiorucci, Fabrizio Ciancetta and Annalisa Monaco
Università dell'Aquila, Italy

Printed in the USA
CPSIA information can be obtained
at www.ICGtesting.com
JSHW011442221024
72173JS00004B/901